Pregnancy
and Birth
Your Questions
Answered

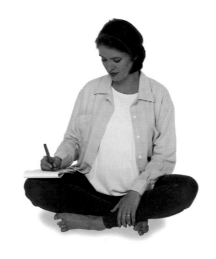

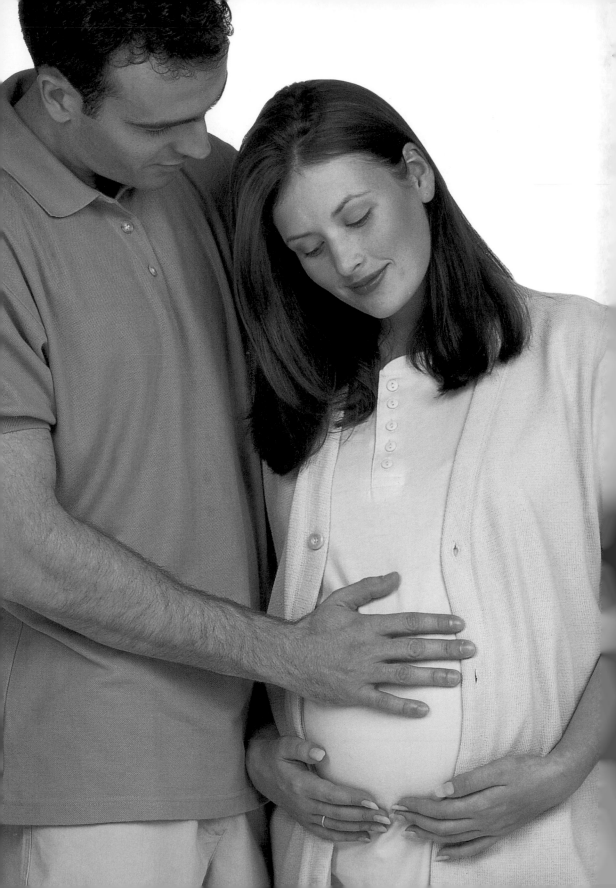

Pregnancy *and* Birth

Your Questions Answered

Dr. Christoph Lees

Dr. Karina Reynolds

Grainne McCartan

FIREFLY BOOKS

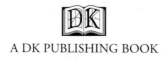

A DK PUBLISHING BOOK

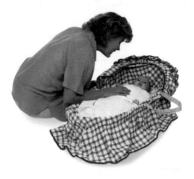

First Canadian Edition, 1999
2 4 6 8 10 9 7 5 3 1

Published in Canada by
Firefly Books Ltd
3680 Victoria Park Avenue, Willowdale, Ontario M2H 3K1

Canadian Cataloguing in Publication Data
Lees, Christoph
    Pregnancy and birth: your questions answered

    Includes index
    ISBN 1-55209-295-X

    1. Pregnancy-Miscellanea.
    2. Childbirth-Miscellanea.
    3. Infants (Newborn)-Care-Miscellanea. I. Reynolds, Karina.
    II. McCartan, Grainne. III. Title

RG525.L436 1998   618.2   C98-931643-2

MANAGING EDITOR Jemima Dunne
PROJECT EDITOR Jacqueline Jackson
EDITOR Claire Cross

MANAGING ART EDITOR Philip Gilderdale
SENIOR ART EDITOR Karen Ward
ART EDITOR Glenda Fisher
DESIGNER Chloë Steers

PHOTOGRAPHY Steve Gorton and Andy Crawford
PRODUCTION Antony Heller

Dr. Romero wrote this foreword as a private citizen and not as an agent of the United
States Federal Government or the universities in which he holds appointment. The content
of this foreword does not necessarily reflect the views or policies of the Department of
Health and Human Services of the US Government, nor does it mention trade names,
commercial organizations or imply an endorsement by the Federal Government.

Reproduced by Bright Arts, Hong Kong. Printed and bound in Italy by New Interlitho, Milan

FOREWORD

No period in a person's life is as important in determining his or her future health as the months spent developing in the womb. Exposure in early pregnancy to chemicals found in something as innocent as liver pâté may cause malformations, while the timely intake of a vitamin – folic acid – can prevent defects. There is also an emerging realization that many problems acquired later in life, such as high blood pressure, diabetes, and some cases of infertility, may have their origins in intrauterine life. The events of pregnancy may therefore reverberate throughout our lives.

Being pregnant today is far different than being pregnant 25 years ago. Technological innovations in assisted reproduction and prenatal diagnosis have made parenthood more complex but not less rewarding. For example, a question such as whether the fetal chromosome number is normal can be approached by amniocentesis, chorionic villus sampling, maternal blood tests, and ultrasound. Each test has different diagnostic precision and risks; how do you decide? Couples can choose what is best for their family; a responsible parent today needs to be informed.

Written by a team of highly respected experts in obstetrics and midwifery, *Pregnancy and Birth: Your Questions Answered* uses a concise and friendly question-and-answer format to provide the information required to make intelligent choices and to address the medical and emotional questions of parenthood. This book is both comprehensive and authoritative and I believe that it will be of great practical value to parents and will serve to enhance the experience of pregnancy.

Roberto Romero, MD
Chief
Perinatology Research Branch
National Institutes of Child Health
and Human Development

CONTENTS

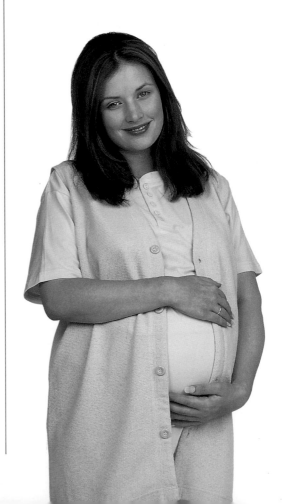

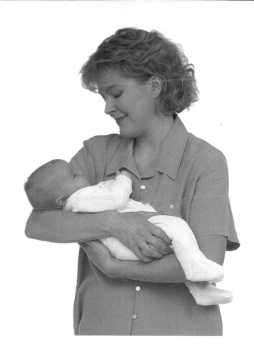

STAYING FIT AND HEALTHY

ISSUES IN PREGNANCY

LABOR AND BIRTH

THE FIRST SIX WEEKS

INTRODUCTION

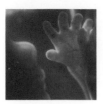

Without a doubt, having a baby is one of the most exciting, challenging, and life-changing experiences that life offers women. For most women, to produce a healthy, happy baby is all-important, and so you therefore want the best advice and care for yourselves and your babies. However, pregnancy and childbirth can be uncharted territory for new mothers-to-be and their partners; you suddenly find that you need to understand and decide on vital issues such as who provides your prenatal care, what type of pain relief you use in labor, and where and how to have your baby.

Traditional methods

Childbirth has changed dramatically during the past few decades, particularly in the developed world. Traditionally, until the 1950s, most births took place in the home, but with the introduction of structured prenatal care available for all women, by the 1960s most deliveries were taking place in the hospital. As we approach the end of the twentieth century, we are now seeing a small swing away from the largely medical management of childbirth toward more "natural" or alternative birthing methods, and prenatal care is, to some degree, moving away from complete (and often impersonal) medical supervision toward total care by a midwife and birth partner. With such major alternatives in approach, prospective parents today may be understandably uncertain about what method best meets their needs during pregnancy and childbirth.

What this book offers

No matter what kind of labor and birth you want, one thing is certain: women nowadays play a much more active part in their pregnancies and labors than their mothers and grandmothers did before them, which means that doctors and midwives are increasingly giving you the chance to decide what you want. But if you want to make an informed decision, you need all the facts.

This book aims to provide, in a simple question-and-answer format, detailed, balanced, and up-to-date information for pregnant women and their partners, so that – armed with knowledge and confidence – you can assess, decide, and take an active part in your pregnancy and labor, working with (not against) your medical advisors.

Why we wrote this book

As practicing medical professionals – two obstetricians and a midwife – we have written this book from our collective knowledge. We have learned that each pregnancy is unique and special. We also recognize that there are many ways of doing things – even in medical procedures – and instead of approaching the subject from one particular professional bias, we have combined our diverse interests and expertise to give authorative and objective information. The questions and answers within this book reflect some of the many queries, from the highly technical (*How does an epidural work?*) to the emotional (*Why do I get upset so easily?*), that we are frequently asked by pregnant women and women in labor.

Easily accessible information

Information in *Pregnancy and Birth: Your Questions Answered* is organized into eight color-coded thematic sections: Preparing for Pregnancy, Prenatal Care, Your Developing Baby, Your Changing Body, Issues in Pregnancy, Staying Fit and Healthy, Labor and Birth, and The First Six Weeks. Each section is then further subdivided into topics, such as physical changes, diet, and pain relief. Instead of having to read through lengthy narrative text, you can simply turn to the relevant section to find the information you need.

Useful features

Not only does *Pregnancy and Birth: Your Questions Answered* address many major concerns and issues, but it also focuses on more minor anxieties, which you might be reluctant to discuss with your doctor. Discussion-point boxes provide space to explore controversial ideas or approaches. The advice is explanatory rather than dictatorial, with additional sources of information in the Reference section at the back of the book. There are also checklists of questions that you can ask the professionals whom you meet during your prenatal care and labor.

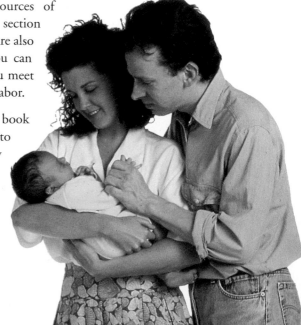

We hope that you will find this book offers the guidance you need to help you have a happy, healthy pregnancy and labor.

Dr. Christoph Lees
Dr. Karina Reynolds
Grainne McCartan

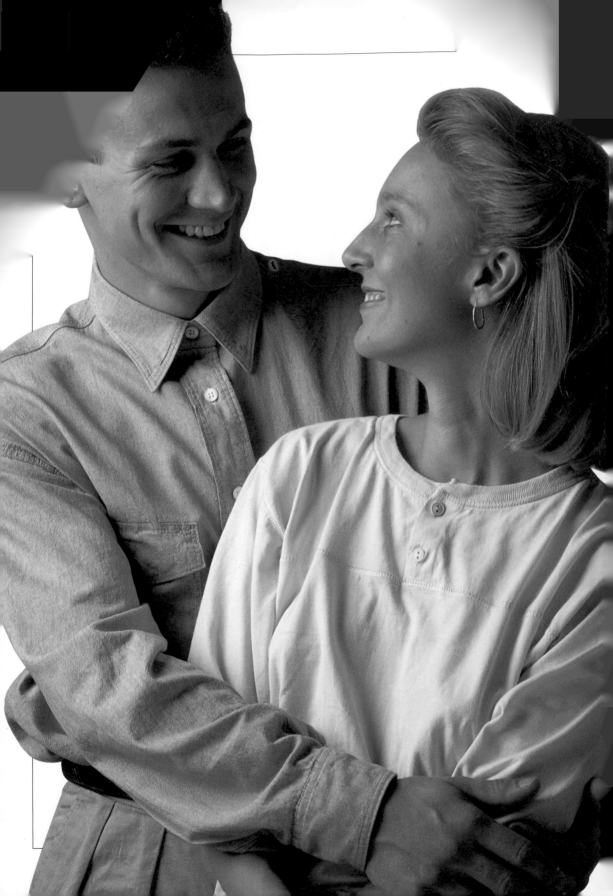

PREPARING
FOR
PREGNANCY

Deciding to have a baby is one of the most momentous decisions you can ever make. The impact that it will have on your body and daily life will be huge and possibly unsettling, but for most people the prospect of having a son or a daughter far outweighs any physical problems or lifestyle changes. Being fully prepared for pregnancy in both mind and body is extremely important; this chapter explains why you and your partner should attempt to improve your general health before trying to conceive, as well as discussing fertility problems. As you begin your preparations, your questions and concerns as prospective parents are answered.

PREPARING YOURSELF

Q DO I NEED A MEDICAL CHECKUP BEFORE TRYING TO CONCEIVE?

A It's generally a good idea to check with your doctor, gynecologist, or midwife to make sure that your Pap smear, to screen for cervical dysplasia, is up-to-date and normal. Any treatment for abnormal smears should be carried out before pregnancy. A checkup will also establish whether you are immune to rubella (German measles). If not, you can be protected by an injection before conception (see opposite). More thorough medical investigations are usually not necessary unless you have had problems with previous pregnancies or have a long-standing or serious medical condition.

Q WHAT CAN I DO TO IMPROVE MY CHANCES OF CONCEIVING?

A The best strategy is to be sure that you and your partner are in good health by improving your diet and your lifestyle. Ideally, you should stop using cigarettes, alcohol, and street drugs six months before conception and try to reduce your stress levels both at home and at work. You should also try to make love around the time that you ovulate (see below) because this is when you are most fertile. Taking folic acid supplements for three months before conceiving and during your pregnancy can reduce the risk of neural tube defects such as spina bifida.

WHEN IS CONCEPTION MOST LIKELY?

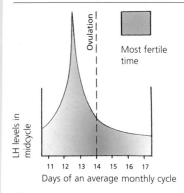

Most fertile time

HORMONAL SURGE
The diagram (above) shows the LH surge, indicating that an egg is about to be released.

The two or three days around ovulation (the time that an egg is produced from your ovary) is when you are most likely to become pregnant. This normally occurs about 14 days before your next period is due. You can work out your most fertile period by one of two methods: by using an ovulation predictor kit or by the Basal Body Temperature method (BBT) described below.

Using an ovulation kit
The kit tests urine for an LH (luteinizing hormone) surge. This hormone, produced by the brain, causes the release of eggs from the ovaries each month. Begin testing a few days before the middle of your cycle.

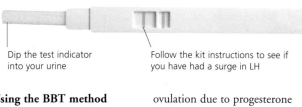

Dip the test indicator into your urine

Follow the kit instructions to see if you have had a surge in LH

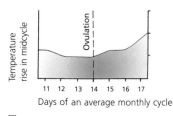

TEMPERATURE RISE
The diagram (above) shows the small rise in temperature that occurs around the time of ovulation.

Using the BBT method
Take your temperature at the same time each day; it rises at ovulation due to progesterone release from the ovary and stays constant until menstruation.

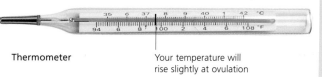

Thermometer

Your temperature will rise slightly at ovulation

Q WHY SHOULD WE GIVE UP SMOKING, STREET DRUGS, AND ALCOHOL?

A Healthy parents have healthier babies, so if you smoke (even as few as five to ten cigarettes daily), regularly drink alcohol, or take street drugs, you may reduce your chances of conception. Once pregnant, you also risk having a smaller and possibly a less healthy baby who will need expert care at birth and perhaps throughout life (see p. 214).

Q I TAKE DRUGS FOR A MEDICAL CONDITION. SHOULD I STOP?

A No, do not stop taking your medication unless advised by your doctor. If you have epilepsy, high blood pressure, diabetes, or other conditions that need long-term medication, your medication may need to be adapted once you are pregnant. Do not take any over-the-counter drugs unless you have consulted your doctor (see p. 103).

Q WILL TAKING VITAMINS MEAN A HEALTHIER BABY?

A Most caregivers routinely recommend prenatal vitamins containing 500 to 1,000 mg of folic acid (to prevent neural tube defects); some also recommend iron-enriched vitamins for potentially anemic women. Women on restricted diets, such as vegetarians and especially vegans, may need to take iron and vitamin B12 supplements if their diet provides insufficient amounts. Ask your doctor or midwife about this.

Q WHAT IF I DON'T WANT TO TAKE FOLIC ACID SUPPLEMENTS?

A Certain foods, such as dark green, leafy vegetables, are high in folic acid (see p. 100), but you must be certain to include them in your diet. Folic acid is sometimes added to grain products, but you must eat enough of the right products. Discuss this with your doctor or midwife, who will best be able to advise you about specific nutrition requirements. Folic acid supplements are advisable.

Q HOW SOON AFTER STOPPING CONTRACEPTION CAN I CONCEIVE?

A Ideally, you should stop taking birth control pills a few months before you consider pregnancy. This allows time for your normal period cycle to become reestablished. If you have an IUD (intrauterine contraceptive device), it is quite safe to conceive as soon as it is removed. If you have contraceptive implants, have them removed before you try to conceive.

WHEN IS THE BEST TIME TO GET PREGNANT?

The ideal age
There is no ideal time to get pregnant; the advantages and disadvantages at any age will depend on your state of health, work situation, and relationship. Young women may not be as psychologically and emotionally prepared for pregnancy and the demands of childcare, while more mature women – that is, mothers over 35 – are at greater risk of developing complications such as high blood pressure and diabetes; and there is a higher risk of their children having fetal chromosomal abnormalities such as Down syndrome (see p. 132).

After a miscarriage
Although it is possible for you to conceive as soon as your next period, most practitioners recommend waiting for three months until the next conception. If you have had several miscarriages, specific tests might determine the cause; it is probably best to wait for the results of such evaluations before trying again.

After a rubella (German measles) injection
The injection contains a small amount of inactivated live virus that your body recognizes as foreign, which allows it to build up immunity. It takes three months to establish this immunity; it is unwise to risk exposing a developing fetus to the rubella virus. (If you are already pregnant and do not have rubella immunity, get immunized after the baby's birth.)

Spacing between pregnancies
This depends on various issues, such as personal relationships and work commitments, but from a medical viewpoint, at least a year between pregnancies is recommended to ensure your recovery. If you get pregnant while you have a young, possibly breastfeeding, infant, you may exert a costly toll on your physical and mental reserves. Your health and infant could suffer as your body tries to cope with these demands.

After a cesarean
A cesarean delivery involves abdominal surgery that can take some time to heal. You might need much longer to recover than if you had had a vaginal delivery.

FERTILITY AND CONCEPTION

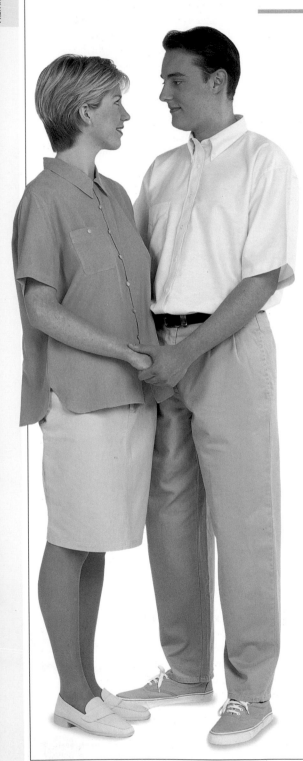

COMMON QUESTIONS ABOUT FERTILITY

QUESTIONS	ANSWERS
Will conception be difficult	
because I have painful or heavy periods?	Probably not. If your symptoms are severe see your doctor to rule out an underlying cause such as fibroids, endometriosis, or a pelvic infection.
because my periods are infrequent or irregular?	Irregularity makes planning a pregnancy harder. You may need medical advice to work out when you are most likely to conceive (see p. 12).
because both my partner and I are over 30?	Male fertility is not greatly affected by age, but the fertility of women over 35 does gradually decline.
because we both lead very busy, stressful lives, and hardly ever feel like making love?	Too much stress tends to undermine your appetite for sex, and can make your periods irregular. Exercise and relaxation can help to relieve stress. If regular sex is unlikely, figure out when you ovulate (see p. 12) and try to make love then.
because my partner had a sperm test and was told he had a low sperm count?	A low sperm count, which reduces a man's fertility, may be caused by the testicles being too warm. Looser underwear or pants may help, as may cutting down on smoking and alcohol. Your partner may need special tests or treatment.
because I recently had a pelvic infection?	Severe or recurrent pelvic infections may lead to blocked or damaged fallopian tubes (see opposite).

Q WHAT CAN REDUCE MY CHANCES OF CONCEPTION?

A Even if you are having sexual intercourse regularly, three main factors can reduce your chances of becoming pregnant: irregular or infrequent ovulation; damage to the fallopian tubes; and abnormal or poor quality sperm. (See left, for other factors.)

Q WHEN SHOULD WE CONSULT A DOCTOR?

A If you don't conceive right away, don't worry. You have a 90 percent chance of becoming pregnant within one year and a 95 percent chance within two. However, you should probably consult your doctor after a year of trying. If either of you suffers from a medical condition or if you are older than 35 years, ask for medical advice earlier.

Q MY PARTNER IS GOING TO HAVE A SPERM TEST – WHAT IS THIS?

A If you have had problems conceiving, a sperm test will determine your partner's fertility. Your partner's sperm will be examined to see how well they move and how many abnormal sperm there are. The lower the proportion of healthy sperm, the more difficult it will be for you to become pregnant, and the longer it may take.

Q MY FALLOPIAN TUBES ARE BLOCKED – AM I INFERTILE?

A The egg travels from the ovary to the womb through a fallopian tube. This can be blocked or damaged by pelvic or abdominal infections or by an ectopic pregnancy (see p. 134), which reduces, but does not rule out, your chances of pregnancy.

Q WHEN ARE FERTILITY DRUGS USED?

A Hormonal problems can prevent normal ovulation (the release of eggs) occurring. Fertility drugs boost ovulation, and improve the uterine environment.

Q IF I TAKE FERTILITY DRUGS, WILL I HAVE TWINS OR MORE?

A Not necessarily, but the odds increase; your chance of twins is one in ten, compared with one in 90 for women who don't take fertility drugs.

Q WHAT OTHER OPTIONS ARE THERE TO HELP ME CONCEIVE?

A If simple treatments fail, options include surgery to unblock your fallopian tubes, stronger fertility drugs, or your partner having treatment to improve his sperm count. If these fail, you may be offered assisted conception (see below).

WHAT IS ASSISTED CONCEPTION?

How is conception assisted?
Conception can be assisted by GIFT or IVF methods. GIFT (Gamete Intra-Fallopian Transfer) is a method by which sperm and eggs are mixed externally, then injected back into your fallopian tube. IVF, for In Vitro (in glass) Fertilization, is more complicated. It involves eggs being removed and then fertilized by sperm. As many as ten or as few as three resultant embryos (fertilized eggs) are replaced in the womb.

When is assisted conception an option?
Assisted conception can be considered after a couple has been trying to conceive, without success, for several years, or when tests suggest that you are unlikely to become pregnant naturally. Reasons include blocked fallopian tubes, problems with sperm, or even when all tests are normal but pregnancy simply does not occur.

What is the success rate?
The success rate varies widely depending on the cause of infertility and the treatment you ultimately receive. One treatment cycle for IVF results in approximately a 25 percent chance of pregnancy; with GIFT, there is a 20 percent chance. Becoming pregnant, unfortunately, does not guarantee "success" in the form of a healthy, full-term baby. Be sure to ask about both pregnancy and birth rates.

Will my pregnancy be any different from one that happens normally?
Medically, the pregnancy should be no different from a normal pregnancy. You may feel somewhat more concerned about the chance of miscarriage, and inevitably, your emotional investment will be higher, especially if you regard this as your last chance to have a child.

NOW THAT YOU'RE PREGNANT

Q I THINK I'M PREGNANT. HOW CAN I CONFIRM IT?

A There are three ways of confirming your pregnancy: urine test, blood test, and ultrasound. A urine test is the most popular method by far and can be done at home, with a pregnancy test kit, or by taking a urine sample to your doctor, midwife, or family-planning clinic and asking them to test it. It takes a few days to get the results from an office urine test. Your doctor can also do a blood test, which detects pregnancy two weeks after conception. Although not a routine procedure, ultrasound can be used to confirm a pregnancy (particularly if you are not sure about your dates) but not for at least three weeks after a missed period.

Q ARE HOME TEST KITS RELIABLE?

A If you follow the instructions carefully (see below), a home test kit is as accurate as a urine test done in the office by your doctor or midwife. Its advantage is that it gives you an immediate answer; a sensitive testing kit can tell you that you are pregnant the day after your period is due.

Q WHAT ARE THE FIRST SIGNS OF PREGNANCY?

A A missed period is the most common sign of pregnancy, but sometimes a period may not happen for other reasons, such as illness, shock, or even jet lag. However, if you are experiencing other symptoms (see below), you should consider having a pregnancy test. Although not every woman feels the full range of symptoms as soon as she becomes pregnant, you may experience some of the following, which are most characteristic:

Signs of pregnancy

- You have missed one or more periods.
- You need to urinate frequently.
- You may find that certain tastes and smells become unpleasant suddenly; or you may crave odd foods. There may be a strange metallic taste in the mouth.
- You feel nauseated and may vomit in the mornings (or at other times of the day).
- Your breasts are tingling, tender, or more swollen than usual.
- You feel particularly tired.
- You feel emotional or tearful.
- You suddenly become constipated.

HOW DO PREGNANCY TEST KITS WORK?

Pregnancy test kits require you to test a sample of your urine. The absorbent wand (below) reacts if a hormone called hCG (human chorionic gonadotrophin), which is produced by the embryo, is present in your urine. As a backup, many kits include a second test.

Results windows   Cartridge   Absorbent pad

HOW TO USE A TEST KIT

Not all kits look like the one shown here, but they work in basically the same way. Remove the test wand from the cap or cartridge. Hold the absorbent sampler in your urine stream for a few seconds. Replace the wand into the cartridge. Wait as directed. If you are pregnant, both windows will show a color.

Results windows

Pregnant   Not pregnant

Q WHAT SHOULD I DO WHEN MY PREGNANCY HAS BEEN CONFIRMED?

A It's probably a good idea to see your general practitioner or gynecologist for a checkup as soon as your pregnancy has been confirmed, just to be sure that all is going well, and to discuss your pregnancy care (see p. 22). If you do not have a relationship with an obstetrician, ask your physician as well as family and friends for a referral. Midwives offer women another option in pregnancy care; ask your doctor for a reputable, hospital-affiliated practice. You may wish to interview a few doctors and/or midwives before you settle on someone you feel comfortable with to manage your prenatal care. Don't be afraid to ask any questions that will help you to decide.

Q WHY IS MY DOCTOR RECOMMENDING ULTRASOUND TO CONFIRM A DUE DATE?

A If your periods are infrequent or irregular, if you were on birth control pills when you got pregnant, or if you have a long cycle, your doctor will find it more accurate to date your pregnancy by looking at the size of the fetus on a scan.

Q I'VE MISSED MY PERIOD. WHY IS THE PREGNANCY TEST NEGATIVE?

A First, your period may, for a variety of reasons, simply be late, or perhaps you haven't ovulated. On the other hand, you may be pregnant, but your urine may not have contained enough hCG (see box, opposite) to show on the test. Wait a few days and try again.

WHEN IS MY BABY DUE?

If your periods are regular (28 days apart) and you haven't taken birth control pills, your pregnancy is dated 40 weeks after the first day of your last menstrual period (LMP). There are a few days around ovulation when fertilization could have occurred so pregnancy is not dated from the time of fertility or sexual intercourse. You are thought to be four weeks pregnant when you miss your first period.

HOW TO USE THE CHART
Look up the first day of your last period in the light-colored line next to the months that are in bold type. The date below is your estimated date of delivery (EDD). For example, if your last period began on April 15, then your EDD is January 20. In a leap year add one day to any date after February 29.

JANUARY	1	2	3	4	5	6	7	8	9	10	11	12	13	14	15	16	17	18	19	20	21	22	23	24	25	26	27	28	29	30	31
OCT/NOV	8	9	10	11	12	13	14	15	16	17	18	19	20	21	22	23	24	25	26	27	28	29	30	31	1	2	3	4	5	6	7
FEBRUARY	1	2	3	4	5	6	7	8	9	10	11	12	13	14	15	16	17	18	19	20	21	22	23	24	25	26	27	28			
NOV/DEC	8	9	10	11	12	13	14	15	16	17	18	19	20	21	22	23	24	25	26	27	28	29	30	1	2	3	4	5			
MARCH	1	2	3	4	5	6	7	8	9	10	11	12	13	14	15	16	17	18	19	20	21	22	23	24	25	26	27	28	29	30	31
DEC/JAN	6	7	8	9	10	11	12	13	14	15	16	17	18	19	20	21	22	23	24	25	26	27	28	29	30	31	1	2	3	4	5
APRIL	1	2	3	4	5	6	7	8	9	10	11	12	13	14	15	16	17	18	19	20	21	22	23	24	25	26	27	28	29	30	
JAN/FEB	6	7	8	9	10	11	12	13	14	15	16	17	18	19	20	21	22	23	24	25	26	27	28	29	30	31	1	2	3	4	
MAY	1	2	3	4	5	6	7	8	9	10	11	12	13	14	15	16	17	18	19	20	21	22	23	24	25	26	27	28	29	30	31
FEB/MARCH	5	6	7	8	9	10	11	12	13	14	15	16	17	18	19	20	21	22	23	24	25	26	27	28	1	2	3	4	5	6	7
JUNE	1	2	3	4	5	6	7	8	9	10	11	12	13	14	15	16	17	18	19	20	21	22	23	24	25	26	27	28	29	30	
MARCH/APRIL	8	9	10	11	12	13	14	15	16	17	18	19	20	21	22	23	24	25	26	27	28	29	30	31	1	2	3	4	5	6	
JULY	1	2	3	4	5	6	7	8	9	10	11	12	13	14	15	16	17	18	19	20	21	22	23	24	25	26	27	28	29	30	31
APRIL/MAY	7	8	9	10	11	12	13	14	15	16	17	18	19	20	21	22	23	24	25	26	27	28	29	30	1	2	3	4	5	6	7
AUGUST	1	2	3	4	5	6	7	8	9	10	11	12	13	14	15	16	17	18	19	20	21	22	23	24	25	26	27	28	29	30	31
MAY/JUNE	8	9	10	11	12	13	14	15	16	17	18	19	20	21	22	23	24	25	26	27	28	29	30	31	1	2	3	4	5	6	7
SEPTEMBER	1	2	3	4	5	6	7	8	9	10	11	12	13	14	15	16	17	18	19	20	21	22	23	24	25	26	27	28	29	30	
JUNE/JULY	8	9	10	11	12	13	14	15	16	17	18	19	20	21	22	23	24	25	26	27	28	29	30	1	2	3	4	5	6	7	
OCTOBER	1	2	3	4	5	6	7	8	9	10	11	12	13	14	15	16	17	18	19	20	21	22	23	24	25	26	27	28	29	30	31
JULY/AUGUST	8	9	10	11	12	13	14	15	16	17	18	19	20	21	22	23	24	25	26	27	28	29	30	31	1	2	3	4	5	6	7
NOVEMBER	1	2	3	4	5	6	7	8	9	10	11	12	13	14	15	16	17	18	19	20	21	22	23	24	25	26	27	28	29	30	
AUGUST/SEPT	8	9	10	11	12	13	14	15	16	17	18	19	20	21	22	23	24	25	26	27	28	29	30	31	1	2	3	4	5	6	
DECEMBER	1	2	3	4	5	6	7	8	9	10	11	12	13	14	15	16	17	18	19	20	21	22	23	24	25	26	27	28	29	30	31
SEPT/OCT	7	8	9	10	11	12	13	14	15	16	17	18	19	20	21	22	23	24	25	26	27	28	29	30	1	2	3	4	5	6	7

CONCERNS IN EARLY PREGNANCY

Q WE WANT A BABY SO MUCH. WHY AM I UPSET AND CONFUSED?

A It takes time to adjust to the idea of being pregnant. It is not unusual to feel confused about your feelings, or to feel ecstatic one minute and scared the next. Once you accept that the coming baby is a reality, you should be able to enjoy your pregnancy to the full.

Q I DRANK ALCOHOL BEFORE I KNEW I WAS PREGNANT. IS THIS BAD FOR MY BABY?

A Although regular, excessive drinking during pregnancy is a bad practice, the likelihood of your baby being affected by a bit of over-indulgence very early in gestation is very small. Whether you are planning a pregnancy or have recently discovered that you are pregnant, it is best to avoid alcohol.

Q MY PAP SMEAR SHOWED A CERVICAL ABNORMALITY. IS IT IMPORTANT?

A There are different degrees of seriousness of Pap smear abnormalities. However, irrespective of the degree of the abnormality, it is unlikely that you will need or receive treatment for this during your pregnancy. Nevertheless, you should not ignore a smear abnormality during your pregnancy and should still seek medical advice during this time, to best plan a course of action after you give birth.

Q WILL PRIOR TREATMENT OF MY CERVIX AFFECT MY PREGNANCY?

A Modern treatments for an abnormal smear are very unlikely to affect your pregnancy but if you have had abnormalities treated, be sure to mention this to your doctor or midwife at your first prenatal visit. Also, if you have had a cone biopsy (the removal of a cone-shaped area of cervical tissue) there is a slightly increased risk of a late miscarriage or premature labor. Most women who have had cone biopsies have normal pregnancies.

Q DO I NEED GENETIC COUNSELING?

A You may need advice if you are older than 35; if you or your partner has been or is a carrier of a genetic or chromosomal disorder; if you have previously had a child with a chromosomal or genetic problem; or if early tests show problems in this pregnancy (see p. 34).

Q WILL MY SECOND PREGNANCY BE LIKE MY FIRST?

A No two pregnancies are the same, but many women report that their subsequent pregnancies and labors are physically and psychologically easier than their first. This may be because you know what to expect and are not so worried by minor problems. You may also be more distracted by daily demands and lack the time to focus on minor discomforts.

I HAVE DISCOVERED THAT I AM PREGNANT ACCIDENTALLY...

... while taking birth control pills. Will this affect the fetus?
The hormones in oral contraceptives are similar to the estrogen and progesterone that occur naturally in your body. The amount of hormones in oral contraceptives is actually very small. Once you stop, they will clear very rapidly from your body, so it is very unlikely to cause any harm to the developing pregnancy. Stop taking them once the pregnancy is confirmed.

...while I have an IUD in place. Should it be removed?
It is important to establish first that the pregnancy is in your womb rather than in a fallopian tube, which can be established by ultrasound. If the pregnancy is at an early stage, the IUD is usually removed, but there is a small risk of miscarriage. It is more difficult to remove the IUD later in pregnancy; it may be left in place, and the baby is usually born unharmed.

... after taking "morning-after" contraception. Has this harmed the fetus?
"Morning-after" contraceptives – most commonly, birth control pills – act by preventing the survival of a fertilized egg. They are strong treatments and are generally very effective in early pregnancy. However, when the pregnancy is more established, morning-after pills significantly increase the risk of fetal abnormalities.

What could harm my baby?

	RISK TO FETUS	ADVICE
Alcohol	Fetal development can be harmed by alcohol because alcohol crosses the placenta and enters the fetus' bloodstream.	It is probably best to avoid alcohol during your pregnancy, especially hard liquor or spirits. Binge drinking can be particularly harmful (see p. 103).
Animals and pet litter	Toxoplasmosis is an infection that may cause blindness, mental retardation, and deafness (see p. 30).	Avoid direct skin contact with cat litter and use gloves while gardening.
Chemicals: hair dyes, permanents; chlorine in pools	There is no evidence of any harm, but hair dyes contain small amounts of potentially toxic chemicals.	There is no reason to avoid swimming pools. Avoid hair dyes and permanents.
Cigarettes	Smoking more than ten cigarettes a day can reduce the baby's birth weight and cause problems during pregnancy, labor, and your baby's first weeks of life (see p. 102).	Smoking should be stopped completely during pregnancy – not only does it affect the blood supply to the womb and oxygen to the baby, but it harms the mother's lungs and circulation.
Particular foods	Listeria bacteria found in some foods can cause miscarriage or stillbirth. Excess vitamin A may cause birth defects. Salmonella can cause miscarriage.	Avoid pâtés and unpasteurized dairy products such as soft cheeses. Avoid all undercooked meats, especially pork and raw fish (sushi). Do not eat liver or liver pâté. Avoid raw or partially cooked eggs (see p. 102).
Infectious illnesses	Chickenpox, mumps, and measles are all potentially harmful to the developing baby (see p. 121). Rubella (German measles) may cause severe abnormalities, but most women are vaccinated against this.	Avoid contact with young children who may have an infection. If you contract rubella, you might elect to consider termination. If you are worried, talk to your doctor.
	Genital herpes may cause severe infection in the baby after delivery.	Contact your doctor if you have herpes or develop genital blisters or ulcers (see p. 120).
Strenuous physical activity	Exercise in moderation will not harm you or your pregnancy.	It is sensible to avoid heavy lifting and any activity that involves the risk of injury. Don't take up any new strenuous physical activity.
Stress	There is no evidence of any harm.	Getting very stressed adds to your fatigue and can reduce your enjoyment of your pregnancy. Try to take time to relax and reduce stress.
VDTs, microwaves, and photocopiers	There is no evidence of any harm.	Use them as you would normally.
X-rays	It is possible that X-rays during the first 13 weeks may harm the development of fetal main organ systems.	X-rays (medical and dental) aren't usually done in the first 13 weeks. If an X-ray is necessary, make sure the doctor or X-ray technician knows you are pregnant, so that a low dose of X-rays will be used.

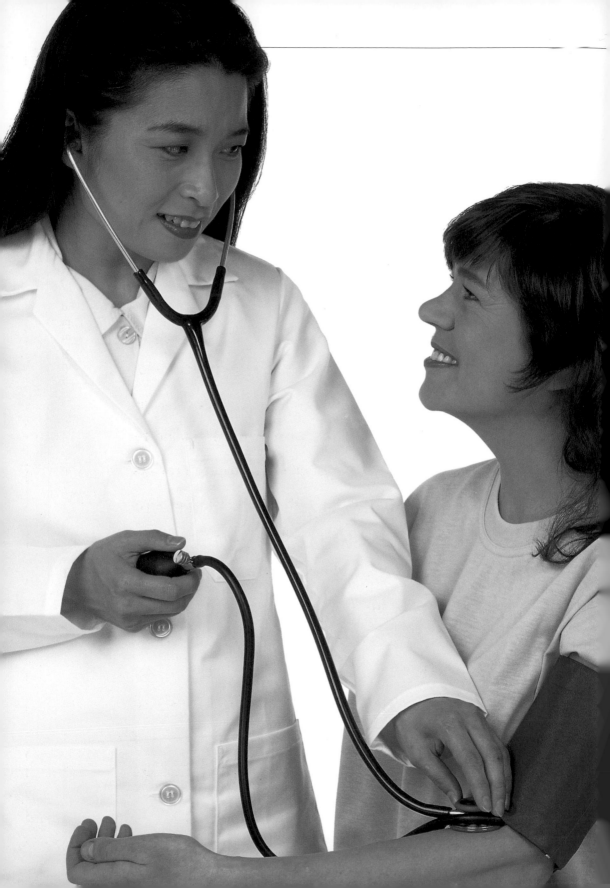

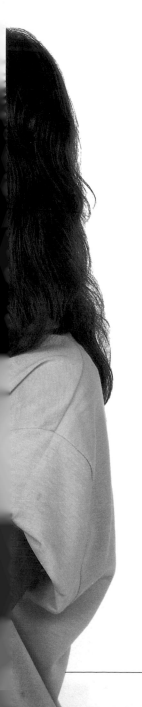

YOUR PRENATAL CARE

Now that you know that you are pregnant, you will want to find out as much as possible about your physical condition, what to expect in the coming months, and what plans you should be making for your labor. This chapter provides detailed information about the prenatal tests you may have, as well as your choices in prenatal care and labor so that you can decide what would suit you and your partner. To help you choose between a home birth and a hospital birth, your options are discussed. These pages also explain where you could get your prenatal care, what professionals are likely to take care of you, and what happens at your first checkup.

CHOOSING PRENATAL CARE

Q WHEN CHOOSING PRENATAL CARE, WHAT SHOULD I THINK ABOUT FIRST?

A Before you choose what kind of care you would like, think about what kind of birth you would, ideally, like. Your options include traditional hospital birth, a freestanding or hospital-affiliated birthing center, and home birth. You may be attended by physicians, midwives, or a combination of caregivers. All of these have pros and cons and you and your partner may wish to explore more than one option before deciding.

Q I FEEL GREAT. DO I REALLY NEED PRENATAL CARE?

A Even if you are feeling terrific, you should not miss your prenatal visits. The goal of prenatal care is to monitor your general well-being and identify potential problems for both the mother and fetus before they become serious. This may involve simple interventions such as iron supplements for anemia, or regular ultrasound scans for twins; some women experience a range of medical and psychological problems. Often, mothers-to-be welcome the regular reassurance that everything is going well and progressing normally.

Q WHAT CAN I EXPECT PRENATAL CARE TO INCLUDE?

A You will probably visit your doctor or midwife once a month for the first seven months of your pregnancy, then every two weeks until the last month, when you will be seen weekly. After your initial pregnancy examination, visits are likely to include urine testing, measuring your weight, and measuring fetal growth.

Q I KNOW I WANT TO HAVE A HOME BIRTH. HOW DO I ARRANGE IT?

A Discuss the options with your doctor or midwife as soon as you can. The possibility of a home birth will depend largely on whether your pregnancy is considered low-risk or high-risk (see p. 28). Women with high-risk pregnancies are usually advised to have a hospital birth. If you are told that you have a low-risk pregnancy, and no complications develop during the course of your pregnancy, home birth may be an option to consider (see opposite).

Q CAN I HAVE THE SAME DOCTOR OR MIDWIFE THROUGHOUT?

A In group practices, several doctors or midwives will see you in rotation. When you go into labor, one will be on call and will deliver your baby; you will know him or her from your office visits. If you choose a solo practitioner, you will see him or her at every office visit, but the practitioner may be unavailable when you go into labor. No one can be on call 24 hours a day so discuss the options together.

Q WILL MY OWN DOCTOR BE ABLE TO DELIVER MY BABY?

A Many general practitioners have had training in obstetrics and can therefore provide prenatal care throughout your pregnancy, but few get involved in the delivery itself. Your own doctor may agree to attend you if the obstetrician or midwife, and hospital, consent.

Q I HAVE SPECIAL NEEDS. HOW DO I FIND OUT IF THERE ARE FACILITIES FOR ME?

A Most hospitals in Canada provide facilities and staff with extra training for people with special needs during pregnancy. Today, midwifery and obstetrical training usually includes instruction on helping women with special needs. Check with your caregiver.

QUESTIONS TO ASK

What is the reputation of the hospital according to parents, midwives, and doctors?

Is there any particular specialty of the maternity department?

What kinds of birth and delivery options are available?

Is there a 24-hour anesthetic service available for late-night labors and birth?

How long will I stay in the hospital after giving birth under normal circumstances?

What level of neonatal emergency care is available?

WHAT IS BEST FOR ME?

In general, doctors recommend that first babies and high-risk pregnancies be delivered in a hospital, either in a traditional delivery room or a hospital birthing room. Some midwives also deliver in hospital birthing centers; others will attend a home birth.

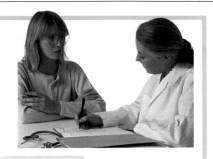

HOSPITAL

Advantages
- Provides a good, comfortable environment.
- Full medical backup is available.
- You have contact with other mothers and their babies.
- If you need help, 24-hour support is available.

Disadvantages
- Possible lack of privacy and intimacy.
- Medical intervention is more likely.
- Restricted access to visitors, family.

How do I choose a hospital?
Your doctor may be affiliated with more than one hospital. If so, it is worth comparing their facilities and asking questions about their procedures (see below, opposite). If you choose to use a midwife, she will usually be based at one hospital.

HOME

Advantages
- Freedom from hospital rules and strict routines.
- A more private and intimate birth is possible.
- There is no need to travel or be moved around during labor and afterward.
- Your partner and family share more in the birth.

Disadvantages
- If complications develop, medical help involves emergency transfer to a hospital.
- You may not get as much rest afterward if you have to take care of your family.

What should I consider?
- Is my home suitable (warm, comfortable, quiet, with adequate space and a telephone)?
- Will I worry that medical support is not on hand?
- Would I appreciate extra help with my baby?

CHOICES IN CHILDBIRTH

There are plenty of options, depending on how you want to give birth, the caregivers in your community, and how far you want to travel. Talk to friends, family, and neighbors for referrals.

1 Obstetrician These doctors work alone or in a group. An obstetrician in solo practice provides continuity of care, attending each prenatal visit and the birth. A possible drawback is the doctor's potential absence. In a group practice, doctors share responsibility for prenatal visits and deliveries.

2 Midwife This is a healthcare provider trained in low-risk pregnancy, labour and post-partum care. Midwives are regulated in two Canadian provinces where they must meet certain requirements to maintain registration. Midwives attend births at home or in hospital. She counsels the mother and refers her for specialized medical care if required.

The focus is on childbirth as a natural process and the use of preventive measures, such as nutrition, before, during and after birth.

3 Traditional hospital setting The most popular choice, this also gives doctors the most control. It can involve fetal monitoring and intravenous hydration. Women usually stay in bed during labor and move to a delivery room for the birth.

4 Birthing center This is a suite of rooms located in or annexed to a hospital, designed to provide a home-like environment, while having access to emergency care. They are usually furnished in a less institutional style and provide a bath, shower and other amenities that increase the mother's comfort. Birthing partners can stay overnight and family can visit. The centers are often located only in large cities, but are increasing in popularity.

PRENATAL VISITS

Q HOW OFTEN WILL I HAVE CHECKUPS?

A The first and longest checkup is the first visit, usually between the sixth and eighth week of your pregnancy. Routine checkups are at monthly intervals thereafter until 28 weeks, then every other week until 36 weeks; finally, they are once a week until your delivery. You may need more checkups if you are expecting twins or if a complication develops. Be sure you have telephone access to your caregivers between visits.

Q DO I HAVE TO GO TO EVERY APPOINTMENT?

A Comprehensive prenatal care is meant to insure your well-being and that of your baby. You may have to miss a visit for unavoidable reasons, which is unlikely to cause harm, but it is best to go even if you feel well.

Q CAN MY PARTNER COME WITH ME?

A It's a good idea to involve your partner as much as possible, both to resolve any medical issues and to ask any questions of concern. Perhaps most importantly, your partner will feel more involved with the pregnancy.

Q DO I NEED TO DO ANYTHING BEFORE MY FIRST VISIT?

A You may find it helpful to read a few books or get other information about pregnancy, just to learn what to expect. Check if there are any inherited abnormalities or diseases in either family. Make a note of the date of your last period, and the dates of any previous pregnancies and/or miscarriages. Write down any questions you wish to raise. If you have any health problems or religious concerns, now is an ideal time to discuss them.

WHAT DO THE NOTES IN MY RECORD MEAN?

Your caregiver will open a new file for you at your first visit, where all notes, records, test results, and comments will be stored. Although you will not usually see this file (unless you ask to see it), it can be helpful to know some of the abbreviations that are always used; the list below tells you what these abbreviations stand for.

BP Your blood pressure.
NAD Nothing abnormal detected, usually in your urine.
Hb Hemoglobin levels that indicate anemia if low.
Fe Iron tablets.
FHH/NH Fetal heart heard or not heard, usually from about 14 weeks. Also FHHR, which means fetal heart heard and regular.
FMF Fetal movements felt, usually from 16–20 weeks.
Ceph Cephalic. Means baby is head down in the womb.
Vx Vertex; also means baby is head down.

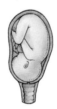 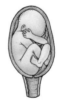

Cephalic or vertex   Breech

Br Breech. Your baby is bottom down in the womb.
Eng/E Engaged. The baby's head has dropped into the pelvic cavity ready for delivery.
NE Not engaged (see above).
SFH Symphysis fundal height is the measurement of the length of the womb (in centimeters)

from the top of the pubic bone. Indicates growth of pregnancy.
PP Presenting part, which refers to that part of the baby that is lying lowest.
Primagravida A woman who is in her first pregnancy.
Multigravida A woman who has been pregnant before.
EDC Estimated date of confinement (delivery).
Ed Edema, which means swelling of the hands, feet, and face.
CS/LSCS Cesarean section or lower segment cesarean section.
TCA To come again.

Q WHAT WILL HAPPEN AT MY FIRST PRENATAL APPOINTMENT?

A At your first prenatal visit you will probably be weighed and measured by office nurses, who will also collect a urine sample from you. Either a midwife or an obstetrician, depending on your choice of caregiver, will carry out a physical (and possibly an internal) examination. Should there be any complications, you may also wish to see a consultant obstetrician, neonatologist, or another specialist.

Q WHAT HAPPENS AT LATER PRENATAL APPOINTMENTS?

A Later appointments are less comprehensive and therefore shorter. There are several procedures that are routinely carried out at each checkup. Your weight is noted, your urine tested, and your blood pressure checked. Fetal position and stage of growth are established and the heartbeat heard. You will be asked about the fetal movements after about 18 weeks. Blood tests are taken intermittently to check for any problems like gestational diabetes.

WHO'S WHO IN PREGNANCY CARE

During your pregnancy, labor, birth, and after, you will encounter a number of health professionals. Your doctor or midwife will probably be the professional that you see most often during this time. You may not necessarily see anyone other than your own midwife. Usually you will need to speak to a medical specialist only if you have a complication and (apart from your first prenatal checkup) you will need to see a pediatrician or neonatologist only if your baby has a problem.

Doctor, internist, general practitioner (GP)

Your doctor is your first point of contact when you wish to find out about your pregnancy and your options. During your pregnancy, your obstetrician and staff may refer back to your doctor's initial contact and notes. General practitioners occasionally deliver their patients' babies, but most will refer you to a midwife or obstetrician. Some doctors are able to be involved with the delivery itself, with your obstetrician's or midwife's approval.

Midwife

A midwife is a highly trained and independent provider of comprehensive care to women throughout childbearing. Where regulated in Canada, a registered midwife is required to obtain a professional degree and pass examinations. To maintain her registration status, she must continually upgrade her skills and attend a minimum number of births each year, including home births. A midwife generally attends on low-risk pregnancies, referring high-risk or problematic pregnancies to an obstetrician. She will have privileges with at least one hospital and often works with a group of midwives whom back each other in order to provide continuous care. Birth can take place at the expectant woman's home, in a hospital or, where available, a birthing center.

Obstetrician/gynecologist

A doctor who specializes in the care of pregnant women; obstetricians are often also trained as gynecologists. Many women have a gynecologist, so when they get pregnant they have established a relationship. A few gynecologists do not practice obstetrics; in this case, your gynecologist will refer you to an obstetrician with similar opinions and experience, possibly in the same practice.

Consultant obstetrician

If there are special considerations, or your pregnancy is high-risk, your obstetrician or midwife may refer you to a consultant obstetrician who specializes in problems like gestational diabetes or preeclampsia.

Pediatrician

A doctor who specializes in the health of babies and children, a pediatrican attends all unusual deliveries and multiple births, assisted deliveries, or cesarean sections. All newborn babies are checked by a pediatrician after the birth. You should select a pediatrician several weeks before your due date.

Public Health nurse

This is a registered nurse with specialized training in family health. She is usually referred to a mother by the hospital and may contact you after delivery to check on you and your baby. She can also be contacted through your local Public Health office.

WHAT HAPPENS AT A PRENATAL VISIT?

Your first visit may seem daunting, but the procedures are neither lengthy nor distressing, although some waiting may be involved. The main purpose of the visit is to allow the doctors or midwives to gain a complete picture of your pregnancy, to troubleshoot for potential problems, and for you to get to know the caregivers in your practice and familiarize yourself with their routine.

HISTORY TAKING

An obstetrician, midwife, or nurse asks you about your partner and your families; your personal details, medical history, and the date of your last period are included in your file. You have to mention previous pregnancies, miscarriages, or terminations.

Weighing in

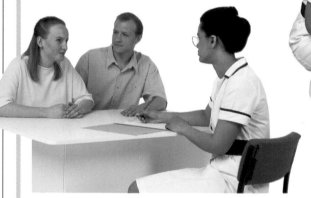

PERSONAL HISTORY
Your weight and height are recorded. You will also be asked about smoking, drinking, and street drug use, and given the chance to raise any problems or concerns.

URINE TESTS

You will be asked to provide a urine specimen, which is tested by a nurse or midwife to check for possible irregularities.

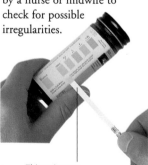
This strip test instantly shows any problems

Glucose (sugar)
More than a trace of glucose may be a sign of diabetes. You may need a blood test (see right).

Protein
When this is found in quantity in the urine, it may signal a kidney or bladder infection, or preeclampsia (see p. 127).

Ketones
These are substances, that if present, mean that the body's metabolic system is upset, probably because you haven't eaten enough or have vomited.

BLOOD TESTS

To establish your blood group and to screen for certain diseases and conditions, a series of routine blood tests is taken on the first prenatal visit (see p. 28). Blood is taken again at regular intervals thereafter to check on your hemoglobin (red cell) levels, which indicate whether you are anemic and require supplemental iron. Other routine blood tests include those that check your blood sugar level. If you are Rhesus (Rh) negative, you'll need a blood test that detects the presence of antibodies.

PHYSICAL EXAMINATION

At the first checkup, the doctor or midwife checks your heart, lungs, and general health, and that the fetus is developing normally.

Checking your womb

At each visit, your abdomen is measured to check the height of the top of your womb (fundus) to see the size of the fetus. On some visits, you may be examined internally (see right), which shouldn't be painful, but may be a bit uncomfortable. The fetal heartbeat will also be listened to.

Checking your breasts

Your breasts are checked to make sure there are no unusual lumps.

Pap smear and cervical check

If your pap smear is not up to date, it should be done at your first prenatal visit. This routine test involves a painless scraping of the cells of the cervix, which are then sent to be checked that they are healthy. Your cervix will also be examined visually.

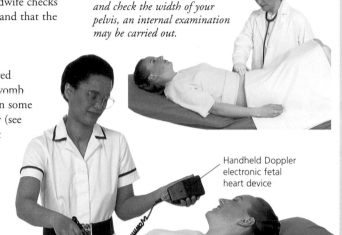

INTERNAL EXAMINATION
To find out the size of the fetus and check the width of your pelvis, an internal examination may be carried out.

Handheld Doppler electronic fetal heart device

The baby's heart rate should be 110–150 beats per minute

LISTENING TO THE HEART
The midwife or obstetrician listens to the baby's heart. This can be an enormous thrill for the expectant mom, her partner, and prospective siblings.

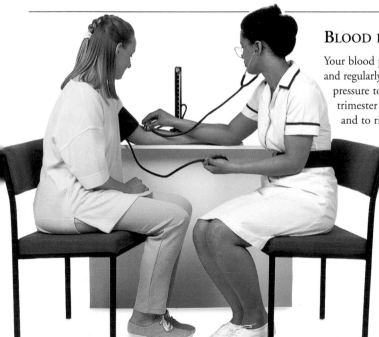

BLOOD PRESSURE

Your blood pressure is taken at your first visit and regularly thereafter. It is normal for blood pressure to drop slightly in the middle trimester of pregnancy (13 to 26 weeks), and to rise slightly in the last trimester (27 to 40 weeks). Abnormal rises in blood pressure may signal preeclampsia (see p. 127) and need attention. The doctor or midwife checks your legs and ankles for swelling which, if severe, can also be a sign of preeclampsia. Normal adult blood pressure is between $^{100}/_{60}$ and $^{120}/_{80}$ mm Hg.

BLOOD PRESSURE
Your blood pressure is a good way to assess how your body is coping with pregnancy.

PRENATAL MONITORING

Q WHAT MAKES A PREGNANCY LOW- OR HIGH-RISK?

A Certain factors constitute a risk to you and/or your baby. Some of these you can do something about, such as stopping smoking or not taking medicines or street drugs. Other factors, such as twins or a very large fetus, you cannot anticipate or affect, but careful prenatal monitoring should reduce the likelihood of unexpected complications. Should something unforeseen happen, your caregivers will be well prepared. In pregnancy care "the best predictor of the future is the past," meaning that, if you had a problem in a previous pregnancy, the same problem may recur. Be sure to give your caregiver details of any such difficulties.

General risk factors that may affect your pregnancy
- Alcohol abuse.
- Smoking.
- You are very thin or very large.
- You have a restrictive diet or are malnourished.
- You take street drugs such as heroin or cocaine.
- You have a medical condition requiring drugs.

Risks that mean you need close prenatal care
- Previous preterm delivery (before 37 weeks).
- Baby in previous pregnancy had an abnormality.
- You have diabetes and/or high blood pressure.
- Previous thrombosis (blood clot).

Risks that mean you need extra care in delivery
- Very large baby (estimated weight over 8½lb/4 kg).
- Very small baby (estimated weight less than 5½lb/2.5 kg).
- Twins.
- Breech baby.
- A previous delivery by cesarean section.
- Previous problems in delivery such as hemorrhage (excessive bleeding).
- High blood pressure in pregnancy (preeclampsia).
- Diabetes.

Low-risk pregnancies
If none of the factors listed above applies to you, and any previous pregnancy and delivery were normal and uneventful, it is unlikely that you will have a problem that needs special care or intensive testing. It is nevertheless essential to keep all your prenatal appointments so that your health and the progress of your pregnancy can be regularly monitored.

WHAT DO THE ROUTINE BLOOD TESTS SHOW?

- **Your blood group and Rhesus (Rh) status**
It is important to know which blood group you belong to in case you need a blood transfusion during pregnancy or labor. The most common is group O; A, B, and AB are much less common. Your Rh status is either positive or negative, so that you may be O negative or A positive and so on. Rh-positive simply means that there is a special identifying label on your blood cells, which is not there if you are Rh-negative. If you are Rh-negative, another test will be done to check if any antibodies are present; the tests will be repeated at intervals during your pregnancy. If there are antibodies present, your partner will also need to give blood for testing.

- **Your hemoglobin (red blood cells) levels**
Red cells contain iron and carry oxygen; if the test shows that your hemoglobin is low then you are anemic, and you will be advised to eat high-iron foods. You will probably have to take iron tablets. Anemia can make you feel very tired (see p. 125), and it will also be a problem if you bleed excessively during your pregnancy or at delivery.

- **Rubella (German measles)** A blood test shows whether you are immune to the disease. If you aren't and you contract rubella in early pregnancy, this could cause fetal blindness, deafness, and heart defects (see p. 121).

- **Syphilis** Because it is now fairly easy to cure, this sexually transmitted disease is rare these days. However, if the disease is present and untreated in pregnancy, it could cause congenital and developmental problems.

- **Hepatitis B** This liver disease, caused by a virus, can be passed to the baby, where it could cause serious liver damage.

- **Other blood tests** You may be offered other blood tests (see p. 30).

SPECIAL TESTS

Q WHY MIGHT I NEED SPECIAL TESTS?

A You will normally be offered extra tests if there is a significant reason to suspect your fetus might be suffering from a disease or an abnormality. The decision may be made on the basis of your age (over 35); if a routine ultrasound shows a problem; if you and/or your partner have a hereditary disease; or if you have previously had a baby with an abnormality.

Q WHAT TESTS WILL I HAVE?

A There are several kinds of tests that detect or rule out problems. Initially, tests on your blood may detect the possibility of problems in the baby such as Down syndrome or spina bifida (see AFP, p. 30), or a medical problem you may have, such as diabetes. An ultrasound may reassure you that the fetus seems to be normal and is growing well; it may also reveal any major defects. If the blood tests or ultrasound detect a problem, further tests, such as amniocentesis, may be offered to you (see p. 36).

Q WHAT ABNORMALITIES CAN BE DETECTED?

A Three kinds of abnormalities can occur: congenital, chromosomal, and genetic. Congenital abnormalities can usually be detected on ultrasound at 18 to 22 weeks (see p. 32). Chromosomal and genetic abnormalities are detected by invasive tests such as amniocentesis and CVS (see p. 36).

Q WHAT ARE CONGENITAL ABNORMALITIES?

A This term means that the fetus has developed a physical abnormality, such as cleft palate, heart and brain defects, spina bifida, absent limbs, or extra digits, in the womb. There is no genetic or chromosomal reason for this, and often no cause is found. Rarely, congenital abnormalities result from maternal toxoplasmosis or rubella infection. Congenital abnormalities can also be the result of dietary imbalances (such as a lack of folic acid) or linked to a harmful drug taken in early pregnancy.

Q WHAT HAPPENS IF A CONGENITAL ABNORMALITY IS DISCOVERED?

A The less severe abnormalities, such as cleft palate, club foot, and extra digits, can usually be dealt with surgically after the baby is born; often the baby is otherwise completely normal. Severe abnormalities such as major heart and central nervous system (brain and spinal cord) malformations often result in miscarriage or fetal death before 24 weeks. In either situation you may be referred to a specialist to discuss all the options.

DISCUSSION POINT

DO I HAVE TO HAVE SPECIAL TESTS?

The most difficult aspect of medical intervention is that it tells you facts about your pregnancy that you might prefer not to know. For this reason, you may not wish to proceed with further tests.

Positive results

There is little point in having screening for any abnormality unless you have carefully thought through what you would do if the results were positive. Once you know there is a problem, and realize the severity of the condition, you will have to decide whether or not to continue with the pregnancy.

Difficult decisions

Whether to terminate the pregnancy on the basis of test results is a question about which medical and popular opinions are divided. Some couples want only a completely "normal" baby and so would wish to have a termination. Others are prepared to continue with the pregnancy and raise a child with special needs; some cannot consider a termination. Knowing how you feel about this issue will help you and your medical advisors should a difficult decision be necessary.

SPECIAL BLOOD TESTS

Q WHY MIGHT I NEED TO HAVE A SPECIAL BLOOD TEST?

A Special blood tests are the tools of diagnosis. Each test reveals specific insights. There are the tests that detect existing diseases that might affect the pregnancy – these include diabetes and HIV; the tests that detect problem genes that you may be unaware of but could pass on to the baby – these include tests for thalassemia, and sickle cell anemia (see below); the tests that measure substances in your blood that indicate possible fetal abnormalities, such as an alpha fetoprotein test (AFP) to screen for neural tube defects.

Q IS THE AFP3 – OR TRIPLE TEST – DEFINITIVE?

A The AFP3 is a screening test generally done in your midwife's or doctor's office. The result of the test is not absolute, but indicates the risk of your fetus being affected with Down syndrome or neural tube defect. Carried out at 15 to 16 weeks, with ultrasound, this test measures the hormones in your blood. The test predicts Down syndrome and other chromosomal abnormalities 65 percent of the time. If the AFP3 results are positive, you will be offered an invasive test such as amniocentesis to answer any questions more definitively (see p. 36).

WHAT ARE THE SPECIAL BLOOD TESTS?

TEST	WHO IS TESTED	WHAT IT TESTS FOR
AFP3 (for spina bifida, hydrocephaly, Down syndrome)	Depends on local practice; is usually offered to women over the age of 35 or those at higher risk of Down syndrome.	It shows the level of three substances that are found in the blood stream of the mother: alpha fetoprotein (AFP), estriol, and human chorionic gonadotrophin (hCG).
Glucose tolerance test (for diabetes)	Women at risk of diabetes, including women who are known to have high blood sugar, sugar in the urine, diabetes in a previous pregnancy, or a previous large baby.	After a sugary drink, blood samples are taken over the next few hours. A blood sugar level that remains high can indicate the presence of diabetes.
HIV test (for human immunodeficiency virus)	Anyone who is at risk may ask to be tested. This is done only with your consent.*	It detects the presence of antibodies for the HIV virus.
Sickle cell test (for sickle cell anemia)	If you or one of your ancestors originate from an area where this trait is widespread, especially Africa and the West Indies.	It looks at the shape of hemoglobin in your red blood cells and detects the sickle cells.
Hemoglobin electrophoresis test (for thalassemia)	If you, or one of your ancestors originate from an area where this trait is widespread, especially Asia, parts of Africa, and the Mediterranean.	It identifies in red blood cells the different hemoglobins that denote the presence of thalassemia disease.
Toxoplasmosis test	If you have had a recent flulike illness, especially if you have been in regular contact with pets or farm animals.	It looks for antibodies to toxoplasma in your blood, which suggest that you have been infected.

*Anonymous HIV testing is carried out in many hospitals. Contact your local hospital or a nearby teaching hospital for more information.

Q WHEN DO I NEED TO HAVE THE TEST FOR TOXOPLASMOSIS?

A Toxoplasmosis is a parasitic disease passed on to humans by domestic cats, and, more rarely, by sheep and pigs. If this disease is contracted in pregnancy, it can cross the placenta, causing blindness, epilepsy, and learning difficulties in the baby. It can also cause fetal death. A blood test shows if you are immune to this disease. You will not usually be offered this test unless there is a high risk that you have been exposed to the illness, and it is your responsibility to report any exposure. If the test shows you have contracted the disease, you may need ultrasound to discover if fetal growth has been affected. Do not change cat litter when pregnant, and wear gloves when doing yard work.

WHAT HAPPENS IF A TEST IS POSITIVE

This test screens only. If it is positive, your fetus is at increased risk of Down syndrome. To diagnose this absolutely, you need an additional test such as an amniocentesis (see p. 36).

You are treated for diabetes, which means close control of your diet, possibly with insulin injections as well, and extra checkups. You may also have to have extra ultrasound scans.

Any infections that you develop must be carefully treated. The risk of transmitting HIV to the baby can be reduced by certain measures at delivery (see p. 124).

If sickle cell trait or disease is detected, your partner should be tested as well. If both are positive, the baby is at risk of being born with the disease. Amniocentesis will confirm this (see p. 36).

If this trait is detected, the fetus may develop the disease. Also, you may become anemic and require iron and folic acid supplements.

You may need to have antibiotics to treat the fetus, and ultrasound may be indicated to see if fetal growth is being affected by the illness (see p. 32).

Q WHY DOES MY DOCTOR WANT TO TEST ME FOR DIABETES?

A Your doctor is probably suggesting this because sugar has been found in your urine after several tests, your blood sugar level is high, or your baby is very large – all of which may indicate diabetes.

Q WHY IS UNTREATED DIABETES A PROBLEM IN PREGNANCY?

A Diabetes occurs when your body is not producing sufficient insulin. When diabetes develops because of the demands of pregnancy on your body it is called "gestational diabetes," which is usually not as serious as preexisting diabetes (see p. 125). Insulin is essential for regulating sugar conversion and the metabolism of fats and protein. If diabetes is not correctly treated by a carefully controlled diet or regular insulin, this condition can make you feel thirsty, weak, and very unwell, and may cause serious problems for the baby.

Q I HAD DIABETES IN MY LAST PREGNANCY. WILL I GET IT AGAIN?

A If you developed diabetes in a previous pregnancy, even if it subsequently got better after you gave birth, you are at a higher risk of developing it again. This means you will automatically be given an extra blood test for glucose between 20 to 26 weeks, or a glucose tolerance test (see chart, left).

Q WHEN SHOULD I HAVE AN HIV TEST?

A HIV stands for Human Immunodeficiency Virus. It is a retrovirus, which means that it incorporates itself into the genetic material of the cells in your body, especially those white blood cells that are important for fighting infections. There is as yet no known cure. You should think about having a test if you or your partner are from an area where HIV is most prevalent; if a past or present partner was a possible carrier of HIV; or if you have injected drugs and shared needles. Some doctors test for HIV automatically, with the initial blood tests.

Q IF I AM HIV-POSITIVE, WILL IT AFFECT MY BABY?

A If you are otherwise well, your pregnancy will not necessarily be affected. However, the disease can be transmitted to the baby, but there are ways of reducing this risk at or after delivery. Some women opt for a termination.

ULTRASOUND SCANS

Q WHAT IS AN ULTRASOUND SCAN?

A A scanner is placed on your skin (see box, opposite) and high frequency sound waves, inaudible to the human ear, are passed into your body. They are called ultrasounds because of the ultra-high frequency sound waves used; they are also called sonograms. As sound waves pass over objects in fluid, they give a pattern of echoes, which are converted into electrical signals, processed, and displayed on a screen as a two-dimensional image.

Q DOES IT HURT?

A Not at all. As the scanner travels across your abdomen, you will feel only the cold plastic. If your pregnancy is at a very early stage, you may need to have a full bladder and this may cause you slight discomfort.

Q WHY DO I NEED AN ULTRASOUND?

A There are several possible reasons: to measure the fetus and so give an accurate delivery date; to investigate possible multiple pregnancies; to check for any complications by looking at fetal limbs, organs, brain, and spine; to check that the placenta is not lying over your cervix (see placenta previa, p. 128); or to see the position of the fetus.

Q CAN I SAY NO TO HAVING ULTRASOUND?

A Yes, you can. You shouldn't feel forced into anything. Ultrasound is often offered as routine, but if you feel that this is unnecessary interference and you don't need extra reassurance, you can decline (see panel, below).

Q WHEN WILL I HAVE ULTRASOUND?

A This depends on your caregiver, but an early scan may be offered 8 to12 weeks after your last period, to accurately date the pregnancy. You may also have a scan at about 18 to 22 weeks to check fetal growth and development, or earlier, to guide amniocentesis (see p. 37).

Q WHY MIGHT I NEED MORE ULTRASOUNDS?

A Further scans may be recommended if it was not possible to see everything clearly because of the position of the baby, if there is a possible risk to the pregnancy, or if there is more than one fetus. More detailed scans that investigate particular problems, such as slow growth or chromosomal abnormalities, may be required (see p. 34). Some women have ultrasound during the last six weeks of pregnancy to check on the position of the placenta or the baby.

DISCUSSION POINT

DECIDING TO HAVE ULTRASOUND

Although the safety of ultrasound scans has never been seriously cast into doubt, there are differing views about whether pregnant women should routinely accept ultrasound scans.

Routine scanning
Many doctors support a routine early scan at 8 to 12 weeks to date a pregnancy and another at 18 to 22 weeks to check the baby's organs and limbs. You will be offered "serial" scans every 2 to 3 weeks if there is a possible problem with fetal growth or if other routine tests (see p. 26–8)

detect potential difficulties. Through close monitoring, your caregivers can anticipate any special circumstances, such as the need for an early delivery. Ultrasound is thought to provide reassurance – whether you have a "normal" pregnancy or one that carries risks (see p. 34). Certainly, if there is any suspicion that you may have a fetus with an abnormality that can be helped by intervention, then scanning is valuable.

Making an informed choice
Midwives agree that ultrasound scans should be available, however, you have a right to accept or decline them.

Q WILL ULTRASOUND HARM MY BABY?

A The most recent research indicates that ultrasound does not harm the fetus, but repeat scans are offered if they will add substantively to your prenatal care.

Q CAN I FIND OUT MY BABY'S SEX FROM AN ULTRASOUND?

A Accurate detection of the baby's sex is not always possible, as the cord, closed legs, or moving limbs can all contribute to a misreading of the gender. Many doctors or midwives prefer not to disclose the sex of the baby in case they are not absolutely correct. However, doctors will try to establish the sex if there is a risk of an hereditary disorder affecting one or other of the sexes. If you really want to know the sex, ask the ultrasound technician for a good look.

Q WHAT HAPPENS IF A DEFECT IS FOUND?

A You will probably be referred for more conclusive tests (see p. 36) before any further discussions take place regarding the pregnancy. At every stage, make sure you understand the doctors' explanations. If you need to decide about continuing with the pregnancy, it can help to get in touch with a counseling service or support group (see p. 232).

QUESTIONS TO ASK

What does the ultrasound show?

Does it confirm my expected delivery date?

Can I have a photograph of the scan?

What will you be looking for in further scans?

YOUR PRENATAL CARE

WHAT HAPPENS WHEN I HAVE ULTRASOUND?

If you have ultrasound in the early weeks of pregnancy, you may be asked to drink plenty of fluid; an enlarged bladder makes it easier to scan the tiny fetus. You will lie on a bed beside the machine and lift up your clothes – wear something loose. The procedure takes about 20 minutes.

THE SCREEN IMAGE
The image is not always clear. The technician will point out the head, heart, and limbs. This scan shows an 18-week fetus.

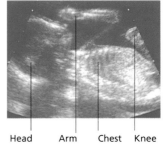

Head   Arm   Chest   Knee

THE MACHINE
The screen shows an image of the fetus from which the necessary measurements are taken.

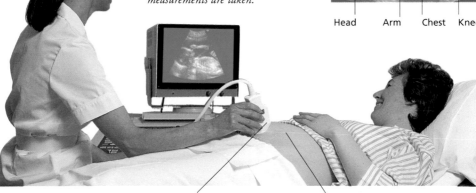

THE SCAN OPERATOR
Ultrasound may be done by a radiographer, an ultrasonographer, or a doctor or midwife.

The scanner is moved over the gel on your stomach to produce an image on the screen.

Gel is rubbed over your stomach to help conduct the sound waves. The gel is water-based and nonstaining.

DOPPLER AND NUCHAL SCANS

Q WHAT ARE THESE SCANS FOR?

A Doppler and nuchal scans are painless, noninvasive, special ultrasound scans that detect specific problems. As with all relatively new diagnostic resources, they are not widely available.

Q WHEN IS A DOPPLER SCAN OFFERED?

A A Doppler scan will be suggested if your doctor wishes to examine the blood flow in the fetus or in the placenta. It is used to check fetuses who are small in relation to their due date, to pinpoint congenital heart defects, and to identify women at risk of developing high blood pressure (preeclampsia) (see p. 127).

Q HOW DOES A DOPPLER SCAN WORK?

A A Doppler scan uses a different form of high-frequency sound waves which are processed to show special wave forms. These sound waves reflect off moving objects, particularly off red blood cells moving through your arteries and veins. A Doppler scan shows how fast these cells are traveling, which in turn tells your doctor about the flow of blood through your blood vessels.

Q IS A DOPPLER SCAN SAFE?

A The Doppler scan has been used in obstetrics, gynecology, and many other areas of medicine for at least ten years. It has never caused any safety concerns. To be on the safe side, however, it is not used in very early pregnancy. It is available at larger hospitals and medical centers. Ask your doctor for the latest safety information before having the test.

Q WHAT IS A NUCHAL SCAN AND IS IT SAFE?

A A nuchal scan is an ultrasound scan in which the baby's neck is examined closely (see below). It is a fairly new method of early prenatal screening for Down syndrome and is available primarily at large hospitals and teaching hospitals. Although it is not definitive, it gives a risk estimate of the chance that the fetus has Down syndrome. Be sure that your doctor is familiar with the procedure.

WHAT DOES A NUCHAL SCAN SHOW?

"Nuchal" means neck; nuchal ultrasound is carried out at 11 to 14 weeks to look at the thickness of a certain area of the back of the fetus' neck. A particularly thick nuchal pad has been linked with a higher risk of suffering from heart defects, Down syndrome, or some other chromosomal problem. A nuchal scan may follow or be followed by an AFP3, or Triple test, to gain more insight into possible problems. Subsequent amniocentesis, or another invasive diagnostic procedure (see p. 36) will help confirm or rule out these problems. Ask your doctor for a complete explanation of all procedures.

WHAT THE SCAN SHOWS
The picture (right) shows a normal fetus. The dotted lines indicate where the nuchal pad would be thicker, as in Down syndrome.

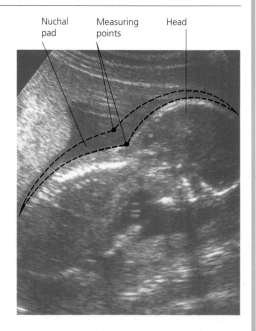

Nuchal pad   Measuring points   Head

CONFIRMING THE DIAGNOSIS

Q HOW IS A DIAGNOSIS CONFIRMED?

A If the special blood tests and/or ultrasound show a reason to suspect that the fetus may be suffering from a disease or a genetic or chromosomal abnormality, further invasive tests will then be suggested (see p. 36) to confirm or rule out these problems.

Q WHAT ARE GENETIC ABNORMALITIES?

A Genetic abnormalities include diseases that occur usually because of a defective gene that you are or your partner is carrying. You may or may not be aware of these genes.

Q WHAT ARE THE MOST COMMON GENETIC DISEASES?

A Examples of these are: cystic fibrosis, a rare disease of the lung and digestive systems that occurs in around 1 in 2,000 pregnancies; Tay-Sachs syndrome, sickle cell anemia, and thalassemia, which are common in certain populations. Fetuses suffering from these conditions are usually healthy in the womb, and the illness reveals itself only after birth. There are also some sex-linked conditions, such as muscular dystrophy and hemophilia, carried by the mother and passed to male children; you will almost certainly know if you have these genes.

Q HOW COULD MY BABY HAVE A GENETIC DISEASE IF I DON'T HAVE ANY DISEASES?

A The genes for some diseases are recessive, or hidden, so that you can be a carrier of a disease without actually suffering from it. If both parents have the same gene, the two sets of genes may match up in the fetus and yield the full condition. Some genes are passed directly from one or other parent. Occasionally, diseases occur due to a spontaneous genetic mutation.

Q WHAT ARE CHROMOSOMAL ABNORMALITIES?

A Chromosomal abnormalities include Down syndrome and other, usually fatal but very rare, chromosomal syndromes. In Down syndrome an extra chromosome 21 is present, which results in a child with physical abnormalities and learning difficulties (see p. 132). It occurs more frequently in babies of older mothers (see right).

HOW LIKELY IS IT THAT MY BABY WILL HAVE DOWN SYNDROME?

The risk of having a baby with Down syndrome is related to your age, although parents of any age can have a Down child. It is not related to how many children you have had, whether you have a new partner, or to drugs that you might have taken at or around the time of conception.

YOUR RISK INCREASES

IN YOUR TWENTIES
You have a 1 in 1,000 chance.

IN YOUR THIRTIES
You have a 1 in 900 chance at 30. At 35, this increases to 1 in 400. At 37, it becomes 1 in 250.

IN YOUR FORTIES
You begin with a 1 in 100 chance and by the time you are 45 it has increased to 1 in 25.

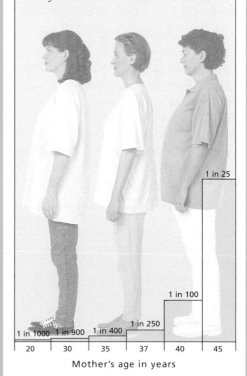

1 in 1000	1 in 900	1 in 400	1 in 250	1 in 100	1 in 25
20	30	35	37	40	45

Mother's age in years

INVASIVE TESTS

Q WHAT ARE INVASIVE TESTS?

A These are special procedures where small samples are taken from fluid and/or tissues in the womb. They are invasive because they involve piercing your skin and uterus with a fine needle.

Q WHAT EXACTLY ARE THESE TESTS FOR?

A Invasive tests detect chromosomal problems, such as Down syndrome, or neural tube defects, such as spina bifida, and genetic conditions, such as cystic fibrosis, hemophilia, or sickle cell anemia. They also show fetal sex and genetic makeup.

Q ARE THERE DIFFERENT KINDS OF INVASIVE TESTS?

A There are a few major tests. When a sample of the placenta is taken, it is called chorionic villus sampling (CVS). Taking a sample of amniotic fluid is called amniocentesis. CVS is done vaginally or by abdominal puncture. Amniocentesis is always performed with abdominal and uterine puncture. Cordocentesis is less common and involves taking a sample of fetal blood from the umbilical cord.

Q WHO PERFORMS THESE TESTS?

A These tests are normally performed by a doctor who is experienced in this area – it may be an obstetrician or, more rarely, a radiologist. In specialist centers, difficult cases may be referred to an expert in fetal medicine.

Q ARE THESE PROCEDURES SAFE?

A Any procedure that involves puncturing the womb carries a risk, albeit a small one. This risk is minimized in expert hands; however, do discuss this with your caregiver. At present, fewer than five percent of women have amniocentesis-related miscarriages. The loss rate for CVS ranges from about two to five percent, depending on the experience of the practitioner.

Q DOES IT HURT?

A It may feel a little uncomfortable when the needle enters the womb. You may be offered a local anesthetic to numb the area.

Q WHY WOULD I BE OFFERED ONE TEST AND NOT ANOTHER?

A Whichever test you are offered will depend on the stage of your pregnancy. CVS is best performed between the ninth and eleventh week of pregnancy; amniocentesis is carried out between 15 and 18 weeks.

Q HOW LONG DOES IT TAKE TO GET THE RESULTS?

A The results from CVS can be available after a few days because the cells obtained do not need to be cultured over a period of time in a laboratory. Amniocentesis results, however, take up to two weeks because the fetal cells contained in the amniotic fluid must be cultured.

Q CAN THE RESULTS EVER BE WRONG OR INCONCLUSIVE?

A Very rarely, the cells that are obtained in the samples are found to be your own instead of the fetus'; this is known as maternal contamination. Also, the cells can simply fail to grow in the laboratory and cannot be analysed. The procedure may then have to be repeated. These situations are very unusual but you should not worry if you learn that this has happened; it does not imply additional risk to the fetus.

Q DO I NEED ANY SPECIAL CARE AFTER THESE PROCEDURES?

A You may be advised to avoid any strenuous exercise for a day or two. You may feel drained, but unless you have any fever you need not worry. After a vaginal CVS, a small amount of vaginal bleeding is common. This blood should become dark brown and stop after a couple of days. If you bleed for longer than a day or two, or heavily with clots and pain, you should seek urgent medical attention. (If you are Rh-negative you will be automatically offered a protective injection after any test.)

QUESTIONS TO ASK

Are the results essential
in deciding the course of my care?

If I decide not to have the test, how would
this affect my pregnancy?

How accurate are the tests?

WHAT HAPPENS IN AN INVASIVE TEST?

Invasive tests are not routine, because genetic and chromosomal problems affecting the fetus are rare. You will be offered such tests if there is a specific concern, perhaps because of your age, or if you or your partner have a disease that can be passed on to your baby, or if an ultrasound scan suggests further investigation. The most common reason is to rule out the possibility of Down syndrome.

AMNIOCENTESIS

Amniocentesis can be carried out from 15 to 18 weeks. A doctor inserts a fine needle into your womb and extracts a few milliliters of amniotic fluid. The procedure should take from 10 to 20 minutes. The cells are then cultured in a laboratory – a process that can take up to two weeks.

GUIDING THE NEEDLE
First, to help the doctor be absolutely precise when inserting the needle, an ultrasound scanner is used to establish the exact position of the fetus and the placenta. Second, a fine needle is inserted into the womb and into a pool of amniotic fluid.

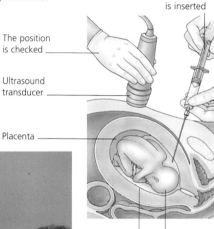

The needle is inserted

The position is checked

Ultrasound transducer

Placenta

Amniotic fluid

The fetus is head down

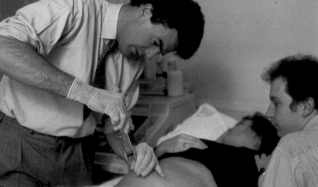

HAVING AMNIOCENTESIS
You are made comfortable on an examining table and a doctor takes a sample of amniotic fluid from your womb. Your partner may be present during the procedure.

OTHER INVASIVE TESTS

Amniocentesis is the most common invasive test, but you may also be offered CVS. Whichever test you are offered will depend on how advanced you are in your pregnancy.

CVS (Chorionic Villus Sampling)
The advantage of CVS is that it can be carried out as early as nine weeks. The basic procedure for this test is similar to amniocentesis (above), except that the doctor extracts a few fragments of the placenta through the needle. These cells are then sent off to a laboratory for detailed analysis, and the results are available a few days later.

Cordocentesis
This test can be carried out relatively late in pregnancy (from 18 to 24 weeks), when the umbilical cord has developed. A syringe is inserted into your womb, guided by ultrasound, and into one of the cord's blood vessels. A tiny sample of fetal blood is taken for analysis.

REMEMBER
These procedures carry a small risk of miscarriage. You will be advised about your options and the possible outcome of your decision. You shouldn't feel hurried into an invasive test if you don't want one. Usually there is time to consider it and discuss it with your partner.

APPROACHING PARENTHOOD

Q **WE WANT TO BE GOOD PARENTS. HOW DO WE BEGIN?**

A There is no short answer to this question. But the fact that you want to do the best for your child is a good start. Most parents, if asked, would tell you that it takes a lifetime of learning to be a good parent. You will grow with your child. And no matter how much you read about child care, you will always be learning something new. This is what makes parenting such a challenge.

Q **WE'RE IN OUR LATE THIRTIES; WILL WE BE UP TO SUCH A CHANGE IN OUR LIFE?**

A Physically, things may be harder in terms of sleepless nights and the energy that a new baby requires. Mentally and emotionally, however, you may be better prepared and more resilient than your younger counterparts. A baby can also broaden your horizons as you rediscover things you thought you had given up long ago. Don't worry about age. The important thing is your willingness to give your child all the requisite love and support.

Q **HOW DO WE LEARN ABOUT THIS DEMANDING JOB?**

A Very few people approach parenthood without some fears. This is natural, however, there's no need to panic! There are several ways in which both of you can prepare yourselves for what will be a demanding, challenging, and yet hugely rewarding part of your lives.

■ You and your partner could both attend prenatal classes, which will give both of you practical information about the birth itself and baby care (see p. 40) and answer any queries you may have.
■ Discuss the coming change in your lives; think positively, and focus on the probable high points of bringing up a baby, but be realistic about coping with the lows.
■ If you can, talk to your parents and other parents who have young babies and children; although they may tell you about the difficulties, usually they will also admit that they could not imagine their life without their child or children because of the richness the experience of parenthood brings.

WHAT ABOUT SINGLE PARENTHOOD?

Will I have to go through labor alone?
Contemplating pregnancy without the father of your child does not mean that you have to go through the birth on your own. Family or friends are often only too pleased to become involved. You can decide to choose an alternative labor partner such as a close friend or a sister who can be with you at the prenatal classes and during the delivery of your baby.

What practical support do I need?
If you are about to become a single mother, it will help greatly if you have good, reliable friends and/or family around you to assist you with baby-sitting, morale-boosting, and general all-round backup. If you don't have this support yet, it is probably a good idea to locate or develop a network of other single parents in your area with whom you can share your problems – and your solutions. There are several organizations and

support groups for single parents, perhaps with a local group in your area (see p. 232). Make contact as soon as you can.

Will I be able to cope?
You are not the only one in your situation. Although being a single parent is not easy, more and more women are becoming single parents, whether by choice or because of the death or absence of a partner. You can't predict how you will cope with the stresses and demands of single parenthood, but the same demands exist in two-parent families. All families find their own solutions, and you will, too.

Are there any advantages?
If you are a single mother, your relationship with your child may be closer, and you will be able to exert total autonomy in parenting and child-rearing practices.

FEARS ABOUT PARENTHOOD

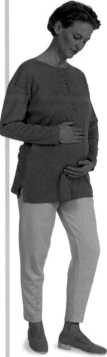

YOU

Since becoming pregnant I have changed so much; will I ever feel like "me" again?
You will probably not be quite your old self again because you are changing both physically and emotionally. Childbirth makes a woman mature very rapidly. Once you have been through the pregnancy and birth and have a child to care for, you may find that your priorities have shifted dramatically. Having a baby is probably one of the most difficult and yet, at the same time, one of the most rewarding experiences in life – go with it and enjoy your achievement!

I worry that I will become more and more like my mother.
Many women share this fear: you want to be a mother in your own unique way and not simply follow your mother's example. Of course, this also depends on the relationship you have or had with your mother. The relationship with your child, however, will be an entirely new one, although certain parallels may exist. You may find yourself taking pointers and examples from the good things you remember in your mother, and develop your own skills at the same time.

I find it hard to think of myself as a mother; when will this transformation take place?
This cannot be predicted. You may find the moment when you first hold your baby is so magical that it is no longer difficult to see yourself as a mother, but it is equally possible that this will not be the case. It should not be a question of transforming yourself, but rather of experiencing a natural feeling of love towards your baby. Being a good mother, however, takes time and practice, patience, and commitment, and love. It is a learning process that takes a lifetime.

YOUR PARTNER

What can I contribute as a partner and father?
There is a great deal to learn about childbirth and your role as a labor "coach." You can make time to attend prenatal visits and parent education sessions together. Often, these classes offer a dads-only session, giving you a chance to raise questions. You will also meet other fathers-to-be.

Will I be able to live up to my partner's expectations?
What are your partner's expectations? Explore them together and see if they are realistic and achievable. At the very least, plan to provide emotional support for her at prenatal visits, during the delivery, and after the birth; you can also provide practical help with the baby, especially in the first months after the baby is born. As long as you are willing and happy to do this, you are probably on your way to meeting her expectations.

I'm worried that I won't make a good father.
The fact that you are worrying is probably a good sign that you want to do your best. No amount of books or classes can ever fully prepare you for this experience. You can learn how to change diapers and care for the baby, but this is merely the beginning. Remember that fathers are made, not born. You and your partner will both be learning how to be good parents, and learning takes time and effort. Talk to your partner about your worries. Realize, too, that instant perfection is impossible; you will learn with time and practice.

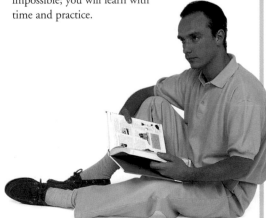

PRENATAL CLASSES

Q WHAT ARE PRENATAL CLASSES?

A Prenatal simply means before birth. These classes prepare you for childbirth. The best prenatal classes cover all aspects of having a baby, from exercises before the birth to labor, breastfeeding, and baby care. Special classes may also be held for partners to encourage them to rehearse the role they will play during the labor, as well as showing them how they can help to look after the new baby.

Q WHO GIVES PRENATAL CLASSES?

A The classes are run by midwives and childbirth educators. Ask your doctor or midwife for a referral to an accredited prenatal class in your community or inquire at the hospital where you will give birth.

Q ARE PRENATAL CLASSES USEFUL?

A Yes, because they provide a relaxed and informal setting in which you can learn about and discuss the techniques of childbirth with other parents-to-be. If you are thoroughly prepared for your delivery you will be less apprehensive and therefore less tense when you go into labor, which may result in a less painful and certainly less frightening experience. The classes also offer an opportunity to meet other prospective parents.

Q WHEN SHOULD I START GOING TO PRENATAL CLASSES?

A The classes are usually held once a week over a period of six to eight weeks. It is best to begin going to the classes around the 31st or 32nd week of your pregnancy. Ask your caregiver for a recommendation. Different schedules are available, but many classes are offered in the evening to accommodate working parents.

Q HOW DO I FIND OUT WHERE MY NEAREST CLASSES ARE?

A Ask your doctor or midwife for information about the health authority classes at your hospital, or for contact numbers for the private classes in your area (see p. 232). You could attend both if you wish to have a broader perspective.

Q SHOULD I RESERVE CLASSES?

A Private classes run by independent organizations may limit their numbers, so it is best to reserve a space early. Enrolling in other classes may only involve finding out when and where they take place.

Q I WILL BE GOING ALONE. WILL I BE THE ONLY ONE WITHOUT A PARTNER?

A You will almost certainly not be the only solo expectant mother at the classes. There will be single mothers and women whose partners cannot attend because of work or because there are other children to look after. Some women have partners who just don't want to go to classes.

Q I HAVE HAD A BABY BEFORE, IS IT WORTH GOING TO CLASSES AGAIN?

A "Refresher" classes are especially useful. It will also be more than a year or so since your last baby, and you may find that the classes can update you on changes that have occurred in certain procedures. Sometimes you can receive reassurance or education about a particular aspect of your previous labor that worried you. Equally important, you will meet other women who are expecting around the same time, and they could be a great source of friendship and support.

Q WHAT ARE PRENATAL EXERCISE CLASSES?

A Prenatal exercise classes offer soon-to-be mothers a chance to stretch in a safe, comfortable atmosphere, as well as introduce specific exercises to ease labor and recovery after you give birth. They can be a valuable source for new friendships, too.

QUESTIONS TO ASK

What is the emphasis of the class?

Who normally takes the class?

Is the teacher a professional caregiver or childbirth educator?

Can I contact anyone in your previous class?

What is the fee for the course?

WHAT SUBJECTS ARE COVERED?

The exact content of the classes varies according to the educators and participants. Before you sign up for a course, it is worth telephoning to be sure that the approach is consistent with your ideas. Also, many teachers ask at the first class which topics you wish to discuss. In general, topics include your health and any minor problems; exercises; labor (the mechanics, how to recognize its start, types of delivery); relaxation techniques; pain relief in labor; baby care, and so on. Your hospital usually offers a tour of the delivery room – and nursery!

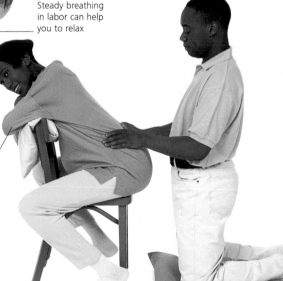

HOW TO LOOK AFTER YOUR NEW BABY
Diaper-changing may seem basic, but it often strikes panic into the minds of first-time parents. Practicing on a model in prenatal classes will give you the know-how and confidence to undertake this task when your new baby arrives.

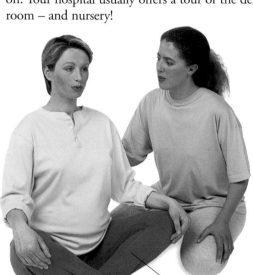

Steady breathing in labor can help you to relax

PAIN RELIEF IN LABOR
Classes will discuss the merits of various methods of pain relief during labor, including relaxation techniques. These can be practiced under the teacher's supervision in a calm atmosphere.

Leaning over a chair back can be a comfortable position in early labor

MASSAGE
Many women find that lower backache is a feature of the early stage of labor and it can be relieved by massage. This is something your partner can learn and practice on you in the stress-free environment of prenatal classes.

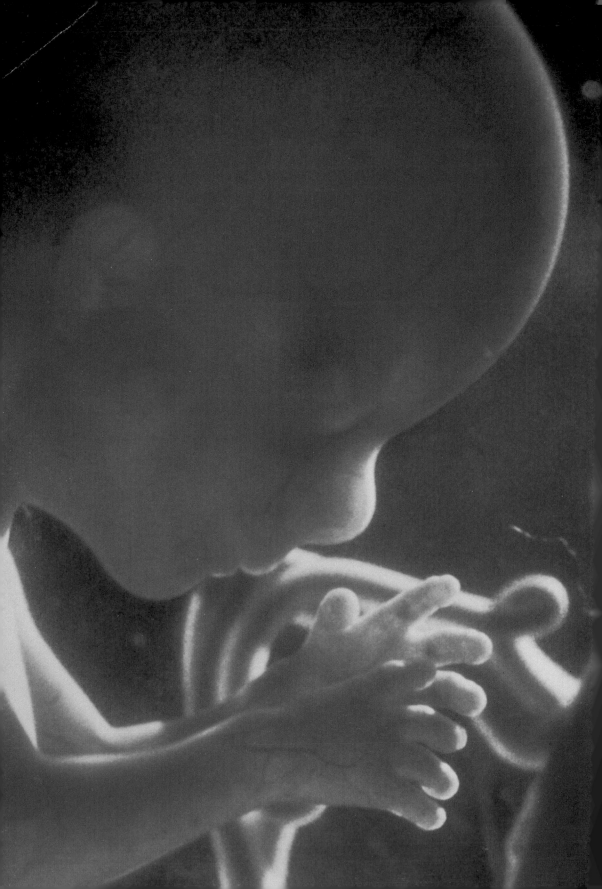

YOUR
DEVELOPING
BABY

Inside your expanding womb your baby is growing, taking from you all the nourishment he or she needs to become a unique human being. What started as a microscopic two-celled egg will, by only 12 weeks, have developed into a tiny but perfectly formed baby. Although at this stage, you cannot detect any movements, as the weeks pass you will be able to feel his or her presence in your body. This chapter explores the miracle of this new life in detail, showing exactly how your baby develops from conception to term – month by month – and gives you a complete and fascinating picture of what is happening to you and your baby.

HOW YOUR BABY GROWS

AT THE MOMENT OF conception, when the sperm penetrates the egg, the genes from both parents join to make a new combination, and your child, a unique human being, is created. Below is a visual summary of this achievement. Pregnancy is looked at in three stages. The first 12 weeks – the first trimester – are crucial to fetal development. You may be unaware of it, but the cluster of cells is multiplying into a fully formed (but immature) human shape. From 13–25 weeks – the

second trimester – the fetus grows rapidly, about 2 in (5 cm) a month, and forms facial expressions, swallows, hears, and kicks. By 26 weeks – the third trimester – the fetus could survive if born. In the last three months, he or she should double in weight, weighing an average 7 lb 7 oz (3.4 kg) at birth.

STAGES OF DEVELOPMENT

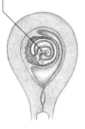
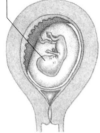
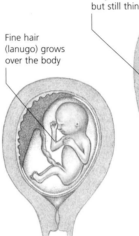
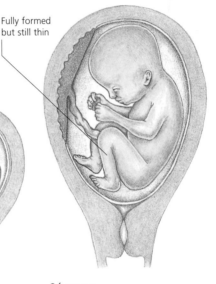

The fetus begins to look human

The head grows faster than the rest of the body

Fine hair (lanugo) grows over the body

Fully formed but still thin

8 WEEKS
The limbs are developing and major organs are forming.

12 WEEKS
The facial features are apparent, but there is no layer of fat yet and the skin is translucent.

16 WEEKS
The fetus now resembles a tiny human being; nails are starting to grow on the fingers and toes.

24 WEEKS
Much larger now and very active, all of the major organs are working, but the lungs and digestive system need more time to mature.

HOW IS THE AGE OF THE FETUS CALCULATED?

The length of your pregnancy is calculated by an old convention that began when it was thought that conception occurred during the menstrual period. Although it is now known that conception usually occurs just after ovulation – between nine to 18 days after the start of your last period – the old system is still used when your date of delivery (due date) is being calculated. Therefore, the number of weeks you are pregnant will always

be worked out from the first day of your last period (see p. 17). Throughout this book, when discussing the age of the fetus, we give the gestational (development) age as dated from the first day of your last menstrual period – not the age of the fetus. The dates in this book will therefore correspond with the dates that are given to you by your doctor or your midwife and should help to avoid any confusion.

There is not much
room to move in
the womb

By this stage,
most babies lie
head down in
the womb

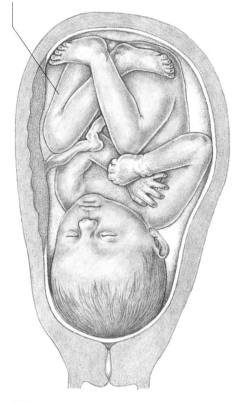

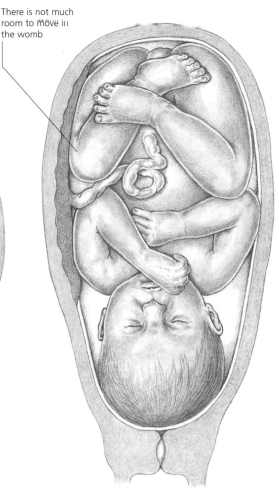

32 WEEKS
*The head is now more in proportion
to the body. Fat is accumulating under the
skin. Babies born at this stage stand a good
chance of survival.*

40 WEEKS
*Now fully mature, much plumper, and
ready to emerge, your baby moves less and
less as the surrounding fluid reduces and the
womb expands to its limits.*

Are there different stages of development?
Pregnancy is divided into three stages, called
trimesters. Your pregnancy has three trimesters
of 12 or 13 weeks. Each trimester is distinctly
different as regards your experience of pregnancy
and the development of your child.

PREGNANCY TIMELINE
*To help you find information about the precise
developmental stage for both you and your baby, this
chapter and the next one feature a timeline running
across the bottom of each page. The shaded area
indicates which trimester you are reading about.*

Pregnancy timeline

■ First day of last period   ■ Likely date of conception   WEEKS IN PREGNANCY

1	2	3	4	5	6	7	8	9	10	11	12	13	14	15	16	17	18	19	20	21	22	23	24	25	26	27	28	29	30	31	32	33	34	35	36	37	38	39	40
			FIRST TRIMESTER											SECOND TRIMESTER												THIRD TRIMESTER													

CONCEPTION

Q WHEN DOES CONCEPTION TAKE PLACE?

A You are most likely to conceive if sexual intercourse takes place when you are at your most fertile – just after an egg has been released from a follicle in one of your ovaries. This usually happens around the middle of your menstrual cycle (see p. 12).

Q WHAT HAPPENS TO THE EGG WHEN IT IS RELEASED?

A Once the egg has been released from your ovaries, it is swept into the fallopian tube and then slowly carried down the tube by fine hairs (called cilia) that line the inside of the tube. These cilia act like a moving carpet, brushing the egg towards the womb.

HOW IS THE BABY'S SEX DETERMINED?

Chromosomes contain all the information needed to determine the genetic structure of the new baby. All human beings normally have two sex chromosomes – a combination of either an X and a Y (male) or an X and an X (female). The woman's egg always has an X chromosome, but sperm can have an X or a Y. The sex of the baby depends on whether an X or a Y sperm penetrates the X egg.

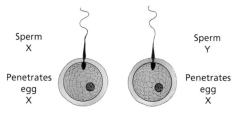

Sperm X		Sperm Y
Penetrates egg X		Penetrates egg X
and produces		and produces
Girl XX		Boy XY

X AND Y SPERM
The diagram above shows the penetration of two eggs by sperm containing either an X or a Y chromosome. The egg always has an X chromosome, so an X sperm produces a girl; a Y sperm, a boy.

Q HOW DOES FERTILIZATION TAKE PLACE?

A Once sperm are inside the vagina, they use their long tails to swim very rapidly up through the cervix, inside the womb, into the fallopian tubes and then toward the released egg. The sperm are attracted to chemicals that the egg produces. Although several sperm may meet the egg at more or less the same time and cling to its surface, only one sperm actually penetrates the egg's membrane. Fertilization takes place when a sperm enters the egg.

Q WHERE DO THE SPERM AND EGG MEET?

A The sperm and egg normally meet in a fallopian tube, where fertilization takes place. Occasionally, the sperm and egg meet and fertilize in other places, for example, at the ovary where the egg is released. This can cause an ectopic pregnancy (see p. 134), which is a pregnancy that develops outside the womb. Fertilization usually takes place within 36 hours of the egg's release from the ovary; after this time the egg is too old, and conception is unlikely to occur. Sperm can survive for up to three days in the womb.

Q WHAT HAPPENS AFTER FERTILIZATION?

A Once the sperm has penetrated the egg, the two cells fuse. The egg's outer membrane prevents any other sperm from entering the egg. The fertilized egg then moves down the fallopian tube into the womb and within a few days of fertilization becomes a cluster (called a blastocyst) of about 60 cells. At around the time you miss your period, the blastocyst starts to embed itself in the inside wall of your womb; this is called implantation (see right).

Q WHAT IF THE FERTILIZED EGG DOES NOT IMPLANT?

A Sometimes, in the complex events of fertilization and cell division, something goes wrong and a "nonviable" embryo (one that is unlikely to survive) is produced. When this occurs, the fertilized egg does not implant properly in the wall of the womb but continues on out of the womb. The only clue that this has happened may be a slightly late and heavy period.

WHAT HAPPENS AT CONCEPTION?

Conception is that singular moment when one sperm penetrates an egg's outer membrane and fuses with the egg. When the sperm and the egg (each of which has 23 chromosomes) fuse, the fertilized egg then has the full 46 chromosomes necessary to form a human being. Twins or multiple births occur when two or more eggs are fertilized at the same time. Identical twins occur when one fertilized egg divides into two and becomes two babies (see p. 66).

THE JOURNEY OF THE EGG

When the egg is first fertilized, as it journeys down the fallopian tube to the womb, it is like a self-contained space capsule that survives on its own energy stores. At this stage, the egg is still microscopically small and can only just be seen by the human eye. After six days, just as it begins to exhaust its supply of energy, it attaches itself to the wall of the womb.

The beginning
The fertilized egg divides rapidly into two cells, then four, then eight, and so on. These early cells, when the fertilized egg (morula) is fewer than 32 cells, have the ability to form any part of the human body and are known as "totipotential" cells.

Two cells

Four cells

Eight cells

Multicelled

THE MOMENT OF CONCEPTION
Normally, only one sperm can break through the tough outer membrane of the egg; once the sperm enters the egg, the sperm loses its tail.

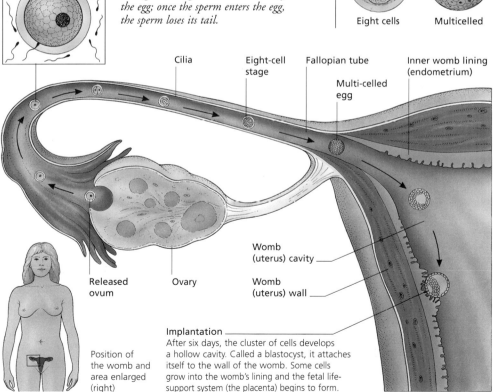

Cilia

Eight-cell stage

Fallopian tube

Multi-celled egg

Inner womb lining (endometrium)

Released ovum

Ovary

Womb (uterus) cavity

Womb (uterus) wall

Position of the womb and area enlarged (right)

Implantation
After six days, the cluster of cells develops a hollow cavity. Called a blastocyst, it attaches itself to the wall of the womb. Some cells grow into the womb's lining and the fetal life-support system (the placenta) begins to form.

YOUR DEVELOPING BABY

THE FIRST SIX WEEKS

VITAL STATISTICS

Length (crown to rump)
¾ in (4 mm)
Weight Less than ⅓₃ oz (1 g)

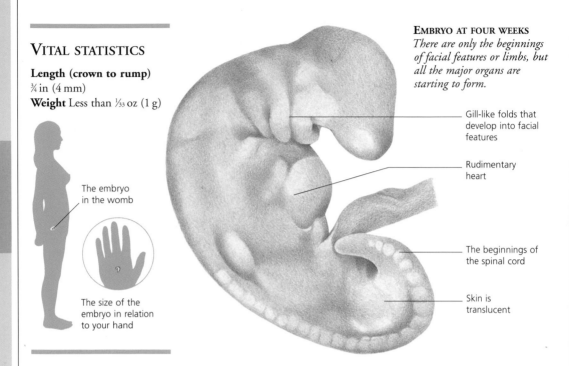

EMBRYO AT FOUR WEEKS
There are only the beginnings of facial features or limbs, but all the major organs are starting to form.

The embryo in the womb

The size of the embryo in relation to your hand

Gill-like folds that develop into facial features

Rudimentary heart

The beginnings of the spinal cord

Skin is translucent

HOW IS THE BABY GROWING?

What does the embryo look like?
When you are six weeks pregnant, the cluster of cells (blastocyst) that will become your baby has developed into what is called an embryo. Around ¾ in (4 mm) in length (crown to rump) and weighing less than ⅓₃ oz (1 g) the embryo looks more like a tadpole than a baby.
■ **Head and face** A "bloblike" head curves down towards the tip of a pointed tail. At the head's base there are gill-like folds that develop into facial features.
■ **Limbs** Little buds appear at each side of the embryo; these are the beginnings of arms and legs, and will develop nodules that will become hands and feet.
■ **Skin** The skin, a thin layer of cells, is translucent and permeable to fluids. The follicles that produce hair develop later.

What is happening inside the body?
At six weeks, although the embryo is only about the size of your fingertip, the beginnings of all the major organs will have formed.

■ **Heart** The embryo has its own tiny heart, which circulates blood through new blood vessels.
■ **Nervous system and brain** A "row" of darker cells runs down the embryo's back – this is the basis of the spinal cord and nervous system. These cells form a lengthwise fold which, when it closes, becomes the neural tube and the brain. At the top of this row of cells are two large lobes for the brain, which is out of proportion to the rest of the body.
■ **Digestive system** The beginnings of a system are in place; there is a tube that runs from the mouth to the tail, from which the stomach and bowels will develop. However, it will be many weeks before it begins to function as a digestive system.

The embryo's life-support system
The cells of the fertilized egg burrow into the womb lining where little "fingers," or villi, form with tiny blood vessels to provide a blood supply for the embryo. The embryo's needs are simple at first, requiring just energy and protein obtained from its yolk sac (see opposite) as its cells rapidly divide.

WEEKS IN PREGNANCY

1	2	3	4	5	6	7	8	9	10	11	12	13	14	15	16	17	18	19	20
				FIRST TRIMESTER														SECOND	

YOUR DEVELOPING BABY

Q WHAT HAPPENS AFTER THE CELL CLUSTER REACHES THE WOMB?

A Once the blastocyst has implanted itself in the womb wall, it releases chemicals that send signals to stop your menstrual cycle and let your body start to prepare itself for the pregnancy. These chemicals also send messages to your immune system to ensure that the blastocyst is not rejected by your body but is allowed to develop.

Q HOW DOES THE CLUSTER OF CELLS DEVELOP INTO AN EMBRYO?

A The rapidly dividing cells eventually develop different functions, probably around the time of the thirty-second cell division, and just before the cluster of cells (blastocyst) imbeds itself in the wall of the womb. The cells can then be divided into three different types: endoderm (forming the lining of the bowel, digestive system, and organs); ectoderm (forming the skin, nervous system, and brain); and mesoderm (forming the bones, muscle, and cartilage). Once a cell has a specific function, it cannot change to become another cell type.

Q WHEN DOES THE EMBRYO START TO TAKE A HUMAN FORM?

A In the fifth to sixth weeks of pregnancy, the embryo grows quickly and can be seen on ultrasound. After the sixth week, the head, chest, limbs, and spinal cord begin to form. By week eight, the embryo has a recognizable human form.

Q WHEN DOES THE HEART START TO BEAT?

A The heart starts to form in the fifth week of pregnancy and begins to "flutter" or beat. An early scan, at around six weeks, may show the heart fluttering. Initially, the heart is simply a tube, and throughout the following six weeks this develops into the complicated structure that is the definitive four-chambered human heart.

Q DO EARLY DEVELOPMENTAL STAGES FOLLOW ANY PARTICULAR PATTERN?

A In the first 12 weeks, all embryos develop at the same rate. In fact, their growth rate is so predictable that your pregnancy can be dated precisely by measuring the embryo's exact length from crown to rump. Differences in growth appear in the second trimester.

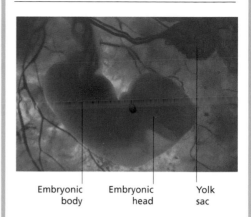

WHAT YOU CAN SEE

| Embryonic body | Embryonic head | Yolk sac |

AT SIX WEEKS
At this early stage, the embryo floats in a fluid-filled bubble that will develop into the amniotic sac. This sac is covered by a protective layer of cells, called the chorion. The yolk sac, which looks rather like a balloon attached to the embryo, supplies the embryo with all its nutrients until the placenta is fully developed and takes over at around the twelfth week.

Q HOW CAN I AVOID HARMING MY BABY IN THE WOMB?

A During its first 12 weeks, the embryo will develop all the features and major organs of a human being and be particularly susceptible to harmful environmental influences. You can help the embryo to develop healthily in this vital time by, for example, taking supplements of folic acid, avoiding certain foods (see p. 98), and completely cutting out alcohol, cigarettes, and any unnecessary drugs or medicines (see p. 102).

Q CAN THE EMBRYO EXPERIENCE PHYSICAL SENSATIONS?

A It is unlikely that the embryo can feel anything until the nervous system is fully developed and the nerves and muscles are connected, which occurs at around the thirteenth week. Even then, physical sensations are unlikely to be experienced until the brain is sufficiently developed to process information from the nerves.

see p. 98 ... see p. 102

WEEKS IN PREGNANCY

21	22	23	24	25	26	27	28	29	30	31	32	33	34	35	36	37	38	39	40
TRIMESTER										THIRD TRIMESTER									

49

UP TO NINE WEEKS

VITAL STATISTICS

Length (crown to rump)
1¼ in (3 cm)
Weight ⅒ oz (3 g)

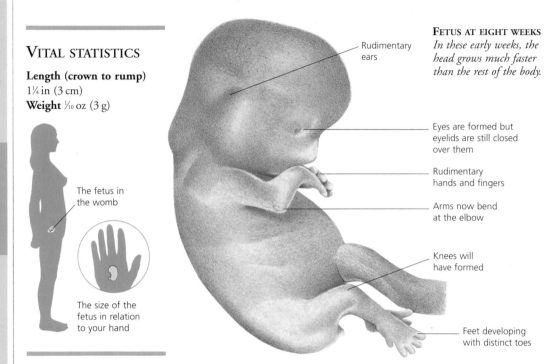

The fetus in
the womb

The size of the
fetus in relation
to your hand

Rudimentary
ears

FETUS AT EIGHT WEEKS
*In these early weeks, the
head grows much faster
than the rest of the body.*

Eyes are formed but
eyelids are still closed
over them

Rudimentary
hands and fingers

Arms now bend
at the elbow

Knees will
have formed

Feet developing
with distinct toes

HOW IS THE BABY GROWING?

What does the fetus look like?

By nine weeks the fetus is about 1¼ in (3 cm) long
(crown to rump) and weighs about ⅒ oz (3 g). The
body has begun to straighten and the head has a more
defined shape, but it is tucked forward over the chest.
Limbs have developed and the little tail has almost
disappeared. Now four times the size it was at six
weeks, it is known as a fetus, meaning "young one."

■ **Head and face** There is a high forehead and you can
see ears, nose, and mouth, as primitive bones form the
framework of facial features. Even now, tooth buds for
all the teeth are in place, and tastebuds are developing.

■ **Arms and legs** The arm buds first sprout wrists and
fingers, and then grow longer to form arms, complete
with a bend for each elbow. Little touchpads appear at
the end of each stubby finger. The same process takes
place with the legs, feet, and toes.

■ **Skin and hair** The skin is still fine and transparent,
but is now in two layers. Sweat glands have started to
develop, and light downy hair has begun to sprout.

What is happening inside the body?

By nine weeks the basic structure of all the major
organs is in place.

■ **Heart** This is now a four-chambered and fully
formed organ; it beats about 180 times per minute –
twice the speed of the average adult heart.

■ **Brain and nervous system** The brain is four times
the size it was at six weeks. Specialized glial (glue) cells
are being formed within the neural tube; these are vital
because they allow nerve cells to be joined so that
messages can be transmitted from the brain to the body.

■ **Digestive system** The mouth, intestine, and stomach
are developing very rapidly, but do not yet function.
The middle part of the intestine grows so quickly that
it briefly protrudes out of the fetal stomach.

The fetal life-support system

The placental tissue that initially surrounds the fetus
and the amniotic sac is becoming concentrated in one
circular area on the womb wall to form the placenta.
It does not yet perform all the placental functions of
respiration, digestion, and excretion.

WEEKS IN PREGNANCY

1	2	3	4	5	6	7	8	9	10	11	12	13	14	15	16	17	18	19	20
FIRST TRIMESTER												SECOND							

Q WHY IS THE HEAD SO LARGE IN RELATION TO THE BODY?

A The developing fetus appears to have a small body dominated by a large head; this is simply because the brain and head of the fetus grow much faster than the rest of the body in the first few weeks after conception. The back portion of the head grows even faster than the front, and so the head can appear to be nodding forward or curled around over the body.

Q WHEN WILL THE LIMBS DEVELOP?

A These grow more slowly than the brain and other internal organs. At about five weeks the limbs begin as little buds, or folds of skin. These buds begin to condense into cartilage (the origin of bone) until, at about eight to nine weeks, distinct fingers and toes have formed. Gradually (by about 12 weeks) the cartilage develops ossification centers, where calcium is deposited. These eventually become hard bone, a process that continues long after birth. At this stage, the hands and feet look quite similar and it is only after about 12 weeks that they are distinguishable from each other.

Q DO THE ARMS AND LEGS GROW AT THE SAME RATE?

A At first the arms develop more rapidly than the legs; this is a natural progression that carries on into babyhood when a baby can grasp things long before learning to crawl or to walk.

Q WHEN WILL THE FETUS BE ABLE TO SEE AND HEAR?

A At six weeks, very primitive eyes and ears appear as little swellings on the head. They look more recognizable at about nine weeks when the development of the eyes and inner ears is complete, but the eyes are still hidden behind sealed eyelids and they won't function until the nervous system is fully formed, later in the second trimester.

Q IS IT POSSIBLE TO TELL THE SEX AT THIS STAGE?

A No, this is not possible because the vagina and male organs are not yet visible externally. There is some swelling in the genital area. After 12 weeks, this swelling becomes the penis in a boy or the clitoris in a girl.

WHAT ULTRASOUND SHOWS

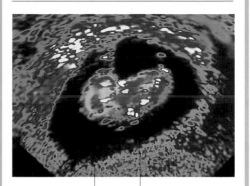

Lining of the womb — Fetus

AT NINE WEEKS
This ultrasound shows that by nine weeks the fetus is beginning to resemble a person. The facial features are becoming more distinct, and the "tail" has disappeared. The muscles are also developing, so movement may be visible.

Q HOW IS THE BABY'S BLOOD MADE?

A In the first few weeks, the blood is formed from cells in the yolk sac (see p. 48). Toward the end of the first trimester, at around 10 to 12 weeks of pregnancy, the liver is formed and takes over the manufacture of blood cells. The liver does this until the bone marrow (the final site of blood production) starts to produce blood cells, later in the second trimester.

Q HOW DOES THE HEART DEVELOP?

A At six weeks, the heart is a single tube bent in an S-shape. Over the next few weeks this tube divides into four chambers, two of which are called atria and receive blood; the other two are called ventricles, which pump blood out to the lungs and the rest of the body. At around nine to ten weeks, special valves have developed at the outflow of each atrium and ventricle; these ensure that the blood is only pumped in one direction and does not leak back into the heart. Fetal circulation is separate from the mother's circulation.

(see p. 48)

WEEKS IN PREGNANCY

21	22	23	24	25	26	27	28	29	30	31	32	33	34	35	36	37	38	39	40
TRIMESTER											THIRD TRIMESTER								

YOUR DEVELOPING BABY

UP TO TWELVE WEEKS

VITAL STATISTICS

Length (crown to rump)
2½ in (6 cm)
Weight ½ oz (15 g)

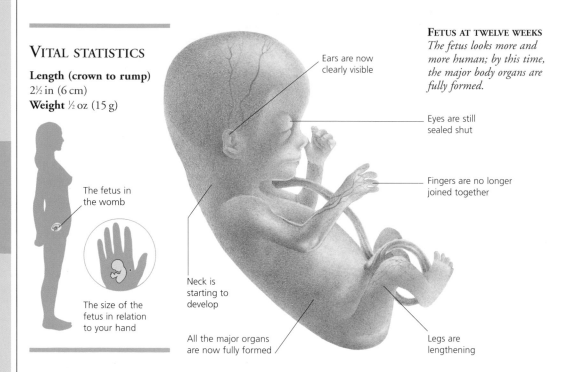

The fetus in the womb

The size of the fetus in relation to your hand

Ears are now clearly visible

Eyes are still sealed shut

Fingers are no longer joined together

Neck is starting to develop

All the major organs are now fully formed

Legs are lengthening

FETUS AT TWELVE WEEKS
The fetus looks more and more human; by this time, the major body organs are fully formed.

HOW IS THE BABY GROWING?

What does the fetus look like?
At twelve weeks the fetus looks like a tiny human. It is about 2½ in (6 cm) long (crown to rump) and weighs about ½ oz (15 g). It has miniature arms and legs, with fingers, toes, and more defined facial features. The body is straighter and the first bone tissue appears. The head is still relatively large (about one third of the entire length of the body), but it is now supported by the suggestion of a neck.

■ **Face** The face is completely formed, with a chin, high forehead, and the small button nose of a young baby. The eyes are further developed and are at the front of the face, rather than the sides, but they are still widely spaced and shut tight by sealed eyelids. The ears are now higher on the sides of the head.
■ **Arms and legs** These are now beginning to move.
■ **Skin and hair** The fetus' skin is red, translucent, and permeable to amniotic fluid.
■ **Feet and hands** The fingers and toes are by now more defined, and nails are starting to grow.

What is happening inside the body?
By the end of the eleventh week of pregnancy, the main organs are completely formed but not all are fully functional.

■ **Heart** The heart is now complete and working, pumping blood to all parts of the body.
■ **Digestive system** The stomach has formed and is linked to the mouth and the intestines.
■ **Sexual organs** Ovaries or testes have formed inside the body, but although external sexual organs are developing, the baby's sex cannot yet be established visually on ultrasound.

The fetal life-support system
At around 12 weeks, the placenta has achieved its final shape and takes over from the yolk sac to become the fetal life-support system (see opposite). Much larger than the fetus at this stage, the placenta is a thick disc-shaped organ attached to one area of the womb. After its initial rapid enlargement, the placenta's growth slows; by the time the baby is born, it weighs about one sixth of the baby's weight.

WEEKS IN PREGNANCY

1	2	3	4	5	6	7	8	9	10	11	12	13	14	15	16	17	18	19	20
					FIRST TRIMESTER													SECOND	

Q WHAT IS THE UMBILICAL CORD?

A The cord, which connects the placenta to the fetus' navel, consists of three blood vessels wound around each other. Two of the vessels are arteries taking blood from the fetus to the placenta and one is a vein returning blood from the placenta to the fetus. These vessels are surrounded by a thick protective substance called Wharton's jelly and are encased in a further covering.

Q CAN KNOTS OCCUR IN MY BABY'S CORD?

A Yes, the cord can occasionally become knotted, but because the cord is very rubbery and slippery, the knot or knots are usually loose and cause no problem. However, should a knot become tight during the delivery, it can cause great fetal distress by cutting off the supply of oxygen and nutrients. This is a rare occurrence but it can be linked to stillbirth.

Q WHEN CAN I HEAR A HEARTBEAT?

A The heart can be heard by ten weeks with a device called a sonicaid. This uses Doppler ultrasound waves (see p. 34), which are high-frequency sound waves and quite harmless to you and the fetus. At this early stage, the fetal heart rate is very rapid, around 160 beats per minute. This rate slows as the fetus grows.

Q WHEN DO THE BONES DEVELOP?

A The cartilage foundations are laid down in the body at about six weeks. Although the joints and bones are all formed in outline by 12 weeks, the process by which cartilage turns into hardened bone (ossification) takes far longer than this. Centers of hard bone are created while your baby is in the womb but the bones are still forming at and after the birth and will not be complete until adolescence.

WHAT IS THE PLACENTA AND WHAT DOES IT DO?

The placenta is a marvelous piece of biological engineering. Attached to your womb wall and connected to the fetus by the umbilical cord, it has several functions. It produces hormones that are vital to maintain the pregnancy and it acts as a filtering membrane, rather like the lungs, to breathe, digest, and excrete for your baby. Without ever mixing maternal and fetal blood, it takes in oxygen and nutrients from your blood, and expels fetal carbon dioxide and waste products.

HOW THE PLACENTA WORKS
Where the placenta adheres to the womb wall, it consists of very fine blood vessels that contain fetal blood. These are enveloped by pools of the mother's blood and this is where fluids, nutrients, and gases are exchanged.

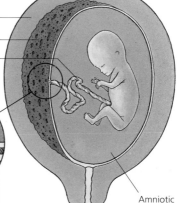

Womb wall

Placenta

Umbilical cord

Fetal blood vessels

Maternal blood vessels

Pool of mother's blood

Umbilical arteries and vein

Amniotic fluid

21	22	23	24	25	26	27	28	29	30	31	32	33	34	35	36	37	38	39	40

WEEKS IN PREGNANCY

TRIMESTER — THIRD TRIMESTER

UP TO SIXTEEN WEEKS

VITAL STATISTICS

Length (crown to rump)
4¾ in (12 cm)
Weight 4½ oz (130 g)

The fetus in the womb

The size of the fetus' hand in relation to your hand

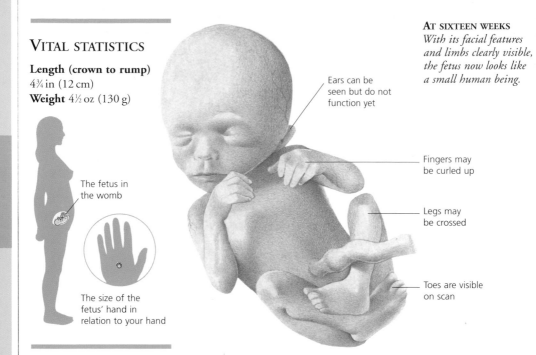

Ears can be seen but do not function yet

AT SIXTEEN WEEKS
With its facial features and limbs clearly visible, the fetus now looks like a small human being.

Fingers may be curled up

Legs may be crossed

Toes are visible on scan

HOW IS THE BABY GROWING?

What does the fetus look like?
By 16 weeks, the fetus is about 4¾ in (12 cm) long from crown to rump, and weighs about 4½ oz (130 g). Although it is still very small, all the limbs and features are formed, and are more in proportion. Because there is no layer of fat, the fetus looks thin; the skin is so fine and translucent that underlying blood vessels can be clearly seen. It is also very active and can make a fist, suck its thumb, swallow fluid, and excrete into the amniotic fluid.
■ **Head** The facial bones have formed, so ultrasound at this stage may reveal more delicate features, such as the nose or mouth. Because the facial muscles have developed, the fetus can make – but not control – expressions. The eyes are becoming sensitive to changes in light, even though they are still shut tight. Very fine eyebrows and eyelashes have started to grow; tastebuds appear on the tongue. By 16 weeks, the small bones in the ear harden and some first sounds are audible.

■ **Arms and legs** The legs have now caught up with arm development, and become longer than the arms. Tiny fingernails are appearing at the end of delicate fingers, but toenails begin to grow later.

What is happening inside the body?
The range of movements greatly increases due to the development of the nervous system.
■ **Nervous system** A layer of fat (myelin) is beginning to coat the nerves that link muscles to the brain. This is important because once the connections are complete, messages can be passed to and from the brain, allowing coordinated movement.

The fetal life-support system
Inside the sac of membranes, the fetus is surrounded by protective amniotic fluid, which means that it can move about freely and develop muscle tone. Head down one minute and feet down the next, you are unlikely to feel any of the fetus' movements at this stage of the pregnancy because the fluid cushions you from these tiny sensations.

WEEKS IN PREGNANCY

1	2	3	4	5	6	7	8	9	10	11	12	13	14	15	16	17	18	19	20
FIRST TRIMESTER																		SECOND	

Q WHY IS MY BABY SURROUNDED BY FLUID?

A The amniotic fluid protects the fetus from knocks, and keeps the temperature in your womb steady. Until 14 weeks the amniotic fluid is absorbed through the fetus' delicate skin. After this time, as the kidneys start to work, it swallows and excretes the fluid back into the amniotic cavity. Although the amount of fluid around the fetus is relatively stable, it is constantly absorbed and replaced and never becomes stale. Until around the thirtieth week there is enough to allow your baby to move around and develop the muscles.

Q WHY DOESN'T A FETUS DROWN IN THE SURROUNDING FLUID?

A The fetus cannot actually breathe yet and instead obtains all its oxygen from the blood in the placenta. Imagine the fetus as a diver immersed in water, using the placenta as an oxygen tank; the only difference between the fetus and a diver is that the fetus' oxygen is passed directly into the circulatory system via the placenta, bypassing the lungs.

Q WHAT CAN THE FETUS DO AT THIS STAGE?

A All the connections between the brain, the nervous system, and the muscles are established by now, allowing for a far more intricate range of movements. The fetus will be able to flex and extend its fingers, arms, and legs. If you have ultrasound, you may even be able to see the fetus sucking his or her thumb, or appearing to grasp the umbilical cord. The bladder is filling and emptying with amniotic fluid as a rehearsal for its eventual role.

Q CAN I FEEL FETAL MOVEMENTS THIS EARLY?

A It is rare to feel any movement as early as this; even though the fetus can move in a reasonably coordinated way from about 13 weeks, the surrounding amniotic fluid cushions these small movements. Some women say that they can feel very light sensations like "butterflies" in their lower abdomen at around 16 weeks, but this is unusual. As the fetus grows, you will be able to feel the movements become more and more definite.

DISCUSSION POINT

WHAT AFFECTS A BABY'S SIZE?

Family and medical reasons

A baby's size depends on many different factors, although genetics usually determine the size of a baby, which is related to the size of the mother. Therefore, if you are small in stature, your baby is also likely to be small, and if you are tall, you are likely to have a larger baby. You will probably have a small baby if you yourself are small but your partner is very tall. If you have already had a baby, subsequent babies will tend to be heavier than the earlier one. Boys tend to weigh more than girls at delivery. However, the birthweight does not necessarily relate to the eventual size of the adult. Medical conditions can also have a major effect on your baby's size; preeclampsia, for example (see p. 127), can result in a small baby, and diabetes can cause a baby to be overly large at birth (see p. 125).

Other factors

Your lifestyle and environment can also affect the size of your baby. What and how you eat is important for your baby's welfare. If you eat a balanced diet, your baby should receive all the necessary nutrients to grow to the optimum size. However, if you are malnourished, you can have a low birthweight baby, which can lead to problems with the baby's health. Regular heavy smoking can cause small babies because smoking reduces the amount of oxygen and nutrients reaching the baby. For each cigarette smoked per day, the baby's weight will be reduced on average by ½oz (13 g). Your ethnic origin can also influence the size of your baby; for example, for genetic and dietary reasons, women from Asia tend to have smaller babies than those of Scandinavian and American origin.

WEEKS IN PREGNANCY

21	22	23	24	25	26	27	28	29	30	31	32	33	34	35	36	37	38	39	40

TRIMESTER | THIRD TRIMESTER

UP TO TWENTY WEEKS

VITAL STATISTICS

Length (crown to rump)
6⅓ in (16 cm)
Weight 12 oz (340 g)

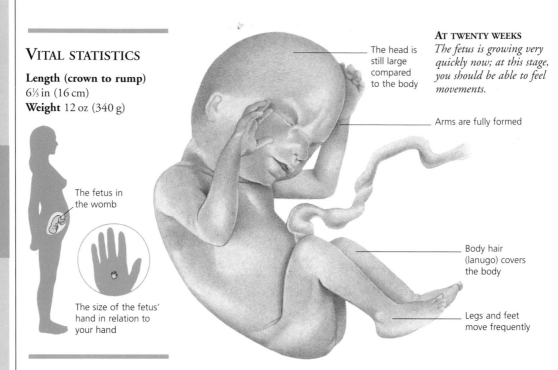

The fetus in the womb

The size of the fetus' hand in relation to your hand

The head is still large compared to the body

AT TWENTY WEEKS
The fetus is growing very quickly now; at this stage, you should be able to feel movements.

Arms are fully formed

Body hair (lanugo) covers the body

Legs and feet move frequently

HOW IS THE BABY GROWING?

What does the fetus look like?
By 20 weeks, the fetus will be about 6⅓ in (16 cm) long (crown to rump), and weigh approximately 12 oz (340 g). The growth rate of the fetus, which has previously been very rapid, now slows down to allow the lungs, digestive system, and immune system time to mature. It can now hear acutely and loud bangs will make the fetus startle. You should feel these movements very clearly.

■ **Head and face** The eyes are still shut but eye movements have developed enabling the eyes to move slowly from side to side. The taste buds are very well developed and the first teeth have now formed within the gums.

■ **Body** The fetus is not quite as thin as last month because it has developed a layer of fat. Some of this is brownish-colored (brown fat) and appears around the nape of the neck, the kidneys, and behind the breastbone. Layers of ordinary (white) fat are also building up on the rest of the body.

■ **Skin and hair** The skin is covered by fine downy hair, known as lanugo, and a protective waxy coating of thick white cream known as the vernix (see p. 63).

What is happening inside the body?
Movements are far more coordinated and the fetal reproductive organs are developing rapidly.

■ **Movements** The fetus will be much more active and have far greater control because the muscles and nervous system are more developed. Most of the major organs are now functioning.

■ **Sexual organs** These are now well developed and are usually visible on ultrasound. In a girl, the ovaries will now hold all her eggs (about seven million at this stage) and the nipples and mammary glands appear.

The fetal life-support system
From now on, the fully developed placenta will provide all the fetus' needs until birth; in addition to providing oxygen, nutrients, and protective antibodies, it disposes of waste products. Although the placenta continues to grow, it is now smaller than the fetus.

WEEKS IN PREGNANCY

1	2	3	4	5	6	7	8	9	10	11	12	13	14	15	16	17	18	19	20
			FIRST TRIMESTER															SECOND	

Q WHEN WILL I BE ABLE TO FEEL FETAL MOVEMENT?

A You may not be able to feel movement properly before 22 weeks, although you may sometimes detect occasional "flutterings" from about 16 weeks. If you have had a baby before, you may be more aware of these light movements. However, you will not notice any regular movements until 24 weeks. Try not to worry about movement at this stage.

Q WHEN DOES THE BABY START TO GROW ANY HAIR?

A The first hairs appear around the fetus' eyebrows and upper lip from about 14 weeks. By around 20 weeks, the fetus is covered all over by fine hair. This hair, called lanugo, is usually shed at or before birth. Both lanugo and the head hair (which may be scarce or plentiful at birth) are entirely replaced by new, coarser hair that grows out of new hair follicles within the first three months of life.

Q WHEN WILL I KNOW WHETHER THE BABY IS NORMAL OR NOT?

A Most babies are born perfectly normal and healthy. An ultrasound scan at 18 to 20 weeks is usually detailed enough to allow detection of many major abnormalities; this scan will also allow your doctor to check the major organs such as the brain and heart. If there is any question of a chromosomal or genetic problem (see p. 35), further tests are usually done during this trimester. If all these tests are clear, it is very likely that your baby is normal. However, it is important to understand that no test can guarantee a perfect baby, as some minor defects cannot be detected before birth (see p. 132).

QUESTIONS TO ASK

Is the fetus the right size for my dates?

Is it moving enough?

Where is the placenta situated?

Are the major organs developing well?

Is there enough amniotic fluid?

WHAT YOU CAN SEE

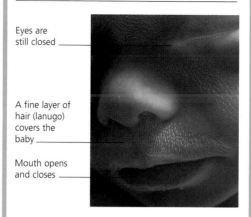

Eyes are still closed

A fine layer of hair (lanugo) covers the baby

Mouth opens and closes

AT TWENTY WEEKS
If you were to see a photograph or have a scan of your baby at around 18 to 20 weeks, you would see that the facial features are very clear. It may be possible to see the baby's tongue poking out through parted lips.

Q CAN THE BABY FEEL COLD IN THE WOMB?

A This is unlikely, because it is protected by your body, and also bathed in warm amniotic fluid to maintain a consistent, temperature-controlled environment.

Q IS THE BABY AWARE OF ANYTHING OUTSIDE THE WOMB?

A Fetuses can hear, and respond, to acoustic (sound) stimulation from the end of the first trimester. They respond by moving, or their heartbeats can change. Some mothers report that their babies change the pattern of their movements in response to different kinds of music.

Q CAN THE BABY SEE ANYTHING?

A Until about 22 weeks, the fetus' eyelids are shut. After this time, the fetus can't see much, partly because it is very dark, and also because babies have a limited visual range until a few weeks after birth. However, it is thought that babies are aware of light and darkness in the womb.

WEEKS IN PREGNANCY

21	22	23	24	25	26	27	28	29	30	31	32	33	34	35	36	37	38	39	40
TRIMESTER											THIRD TRIMESTER								

UP TO TWENTY-FOUR WEEKS

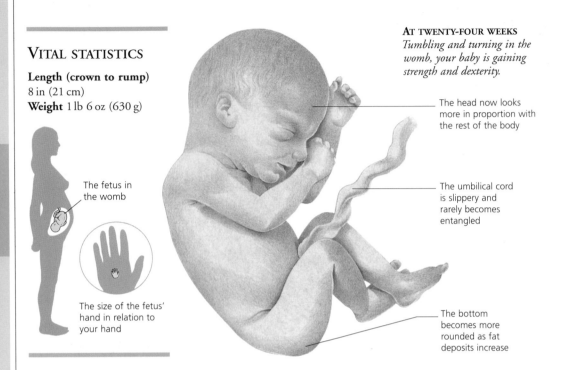

VITAL STATISTICS

Length (crown to rump)
8 in (21 cm)
Weight 1 lb 6 oz (630 g)

The fetus in
the womb

The size of the fetus'
hand in relation to
your hand

AT TWENTY-FOUR WEEKS
*Tumbling and turning in the
womb, your baby is gaining
strength and dexterity.*

The head now looks
more in proportion with
the rest of the body

The umbilical cord
is slippery and
rarely becomes
entangled

The bottom
becomes more
rounded as fat
deposits increase

HOW IS THE BABY GROWING?

What does the fetus look like?

By 24 weeks, the fetus has become less delicate and
has probably gained about 1 lb (500 g) in weight
in the last month; it is now about 8 in (21 cm) long
(crown to rump) and weighs about 1 lb 6 oz (630 g).
■ **Skin** Still fine but no longer translucent, the baby's
skin is now reddish in color and, because layers of fat
have yet to form, rather wrinkled.
■ **Eyes** At 22 to 24 weeks, the eyes open.

What is happening inside the body?

Surrounded by about 18 fl oz (500 ml) of amniotic
fluid, the baby can move around inside your womb
with great mobility. He or she can kick, suck its thumb,
open and close its mouth, and will respond to
movement or loud noises. The heart rate has dropped
to about 140–150 beats per minute, and it is now
possible to get a printout of your baby's heart rate on
an external fetal monitor (see p. 158). All the major
organs, except the lungs, are now functioning.

■ **Brain and nervous system** If the brainwaves
of your 24-week-old baby are viewed on a special
monitoring machine called an EEG (electro-
encephalogram), they would resemble those of a
newborn infant. The cells that control conscious
thought are developing, and the baby becomes much
more sensitive to sound and movement and, by this
stage, is also thought to have developed a cycle of
sleeping and waking.
■ **Lungs** The lungs, which are still full of amniotic
fluid, are the least mature organs and still have several
weeks before all the small air exchange sacs (alveoli)
are completely formed.
■ **Digestive system** Your baby is constantly swallowing
and excreting amniotic fluid.

The fetal life-support system

The walls of the tiny blood vessels (villi) of the
placental tissue become thinner and more permeable
as pregnancy progresses, so that the amount of
nutrients passed to the baby increases and greater
quantities of waste are eliminated.

WEEKS IN PREGNANCY

1	2	3	4	5	6	7	8	9	10	11	12	13	14	15	16	17	18	19	20

FIRST TRIMESTER　　　　　　　　　　　　　　　　　　　SECOND

WHAT IS THE EARLIEST AGE AT WHICH BABIES CAN SURVIVE?

The legal definition of viability (the age at which a baby can survive) is 24 weeks and after. A baby born before this time is unlikely to survive and the mother will be considered to have had a miscarriage. At 24 weeks, there is a possibility of damage to the baby's internal organs during labor and the baby may be physically or mentally disabled. If you give birth after 24 weeks, you are considered to have had a premature labor and your baby may be placed in an incubator in a neonatal intensive-care unit (see p. 214). After 28 weeks, the risks decrease and the prospects for the baby's survival are very good (over 90 percent).

CAN THE BABY DEVELOP IMMUNITY TO INFECTIONS WHILE IN THE WOMB?

Your body provides certain antibodies that cross the placenta and provide your baby with immunity during the pregnancy and for several months after delivery. (Breastfeeding augments this protection.) Your baby can produce antibodies while in the womb, but this usually happens only if you contract an infection to which you and your baby have no immunity.

IS IT QUIET IN THE WOMB?

On the contrary, evidence suggests that the womb is very noisy. With the sound of your blood whooshing through your arteries and the placenta, the continuous humming of blood along major veins, as well as the gurgling of your bowels, it is probably comparable to being underwater in a busy swimming pool. Your baby can also hear voices, and learns to identify your voice and that of your partner or older children.

WHY IS MY BELLY BIGGER/SMALLER THAN MY FRIEND'S?

Some women have a large bulge at 24 weeks, others seem to hide the pregnancy completely until 30 weeks or later! It all depends on your body shape, how thin or heavy you are, the strength of your abdominal wall muscles, and the size of your baby – or babies. If your doctor or midwife confirms that your baby is growing normally, don't worry about comparisons with other bellies – it really does not matter.

WHAT YOU CAN SEE

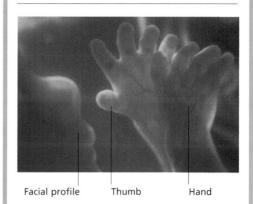

Facial profile   Thumb   Hand

AT TWENTY-ONE WEEKS
An ultrasound photograph of your baby in the womb at this time (like the one above) would show that the fingers are now fully formed and can grasp. This baby seems to be holding on to the umbilical cord.

WILL MY BABY GROW BIGGER AND HEALTHIER IF I EAT MORE?

Unless you have been severely malnourished and you suddenly start eating a tremendous amount of food, the answer is no. As long as your diet is providing the basic nutrients, your baby will continue to grow at a steady rate regardless of what you actually eat (see p. 100). However, it is important not to eat too much during your pregnancy; if you become seriously overweight, you increase the risk of developing a condition such as gestational diabetes (see p. 125). Also, if your baby has to be delivered by cesarean section, being very overweight can make the operation more complicated.

WHY ARE SOME BABIES MORE ACTIVE IN THE WOMB THAN OTHERS?

This is a difficult question to answer. Some babies do seem to move more than others, but the reason for this is not clear. However, it is also true that some women simply feel their babies moving more. Other women do not feel their babies moving, even when the baby has done a complete somersault in the womb.

WEEKS IN PREGNANCY

21	22	23	24	25	26	27	28	29	30	31	32	33	34	35	36	37	38	39	40

| TRIMESTER | | | | | THIRD TRIMESTER | | | | | | | | | | | | | | |

YOUR DEVELOPING BABY

UP TO TWENTY-NINE WEEKS

VITAL STATISTICS

Length (crown to rump)
10 in (26 cm)
Weight 2 lb 7 oz (1.1 kg)

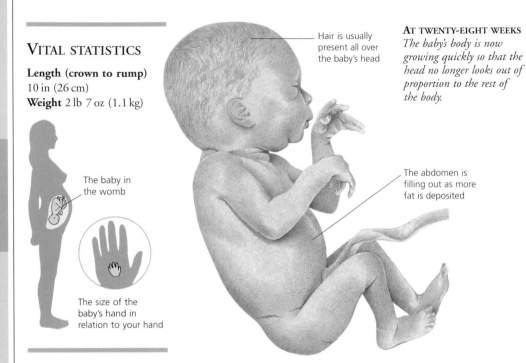

The baby in the womb

The size of the baby's hand in relation to your hand

Hair is usually present all over the baby's head

AT TWENTY-EIGHT WEEKS
The baby's body is now growing quickly so that the head no longer looks out of proportion to the rest of the body.

The abdomen is filling out as more fat is deposited

HOW IS THE BABY GROWING?

What does the baby look like?
By 29 weeks your baby is about 10 in (26 cm) long (crown to rump) and weighs about 2 lb 7 oz (1.1 kg). A greasy substance called vernix covers and insulates the baby's skin (see p. 63). If born now, your baby should be physically developed enough to survive, but could need special care.

What is happening inside the body?
Your baby moves around regularly in the womb.
■ **Brain** This grows much larger, and a fatty protective sheath covers the nerve fibers; this important development allows brain impulses to travel faster, enhancing the ability to learn.
■ **Movements** Your baby is now more cramped in the womb due to the increase in length and weight. However, your baby can still change position. Less cushioning fluid means that you will begin to feel these movements more; they may even be visible from outside your body.

■ **Lungs** At 29 weeks, the lungs have developed most of their smaller airways and tiny air sacs (alveoli). Equally important is the development of a substance called surfactant, which is produced by cells in the lungs. Surfactant assists with breathing by reducing the surface tension of the lining of the lungs; this prevents the airways in the lungs from collapsing when breath is exhaled. A premature baby may have problems with breathing because this substance has not been produced. In a premature birth, either a steroid injection is given to the mother to stimulate the baby's lungs to produce surfactant, or the baby is given artificial surfactant at birth.

The baby's life-support system
At this stage the placenta grows at a slower rate than your baby. It receives about 14 fl oz (400 ml) of blood from your circulation every minute and exchanges nutrients, gases, and waste products. The placenta is quite selective in what it allows to pass from the mother to the baby's blood, stopping some harmful substances, such as certain drugs, from crossing over.

WEEKS IN PREGNANCY

1	2	3	4	5	6	7	8	9	10	11	12	13	14	15	16	17	18	19	20
			FIRST TRIMESTER															SECOND	

Q SHOULD THE BABY STILL BE MOVING?

A Yes, at 29 weeks your baby should feel very active. It is only after 36 weeks that your baby will quiet down because, by this stage, there will be less space and therefore less amniotic fluid to move around in. You may see your baby move if your belly heaves and bulges, and you can often feel movement under your hand.

Q CAN THE BABY DAMAGE ME BY KICKING AND MOVING?

A Although vigorous movement is common after about 28 weeks, your baby cannot injure you because the amniotic fluid will absorb any kicks, and the thick muscular wall of the womb protects your stomach, liver, and bowels.

Q I SOMETIMES FEEL A SHARP PAIN UNDER MY RIBS. SHOULD I BE CONCERNED?

A If the baby is head down (cephalic) and he or she kicks, it can sometimes hurt you just below the ribs. Occasionally, pain beneath your ribs can be caused by your baby's head bobbing around in the breech position (see p. 63). This isn't dangerous but it can be uncomfortable. Sometimes a sharp pain under the ribs is the only sign that your baby is breech.

Q IF THE BABY'S HEAD IS DOWN AT THIS STAGE, WILL IT STAY THAT WAY?

A No, not necessarily. At this stage, the baby can still move around and will continue to move until about 35 to 36 weeks; after this time, the baby is too big to move easily and usually settles into one position, ready for labor.

Q WHY DO BABIES GET HICCUPS?

A Babies do have occasional short, jerky "hiccups" which you can sometimes feel. They are probably caused by the baby moving the chest in an attempt to practice breathing. These movements can be seen on ultrasound, and are thought to allow the baby's lungs to expand and develop properly. However, the baby doesn't need to breathe in the conventional sense until after the birth because oxygen is carried through the placenta into the baby's blood system via the umbilical cord.

WHAT ULTRASOUND SHOWS

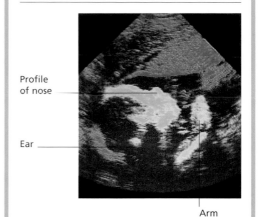

Profile of nose

Ear

Arm

AT TWENTY-FOUR WEEKS
This ultrasound scan shows the profile of a baby around six months. By this stage, all facial features are formed, so that he or she will look much the same now as at birth, only smaller. The eyes are still shut, but will open in the next few weeks.

Q DO BOYS AND GIRLS WEIGH THE SAME?

A Boy babies during the third trimester of pregnancy usually weigh slightly more than girls at the same number of weeks.

Q WHAT DOES IT MEAN IF MY BABY IS SAID TO BE SMALL FOR DATES?

A This means that your baby is smaller than is typical for his or her number of weeks. The most common reason for this is genetic: your baby was never meant to be large in the first place, especially if you and/or your partner are short or underweight. Another possible cause for a baby being small for dates is that the placenta isn't functioning properly, therefore the baby is not getting enough nutrients and oxygen. This is called "placental insufficiency" and is sometimes, but not always, linked to the development of preeclampsia (see p. 127). A possible but less likely reason is that your dates are wrong and you are, in fact, less far advanced in your pregnancy than everyone thinks. Rarely, an infection or a chromosomal or genetic problem can hinder growth (see p. 52).

WEEKS IN PREGNANCY

21	22	23	24	25	26	27	28	29	30	31	32	33	34	35	36	37	38	39	40

TRIMESTER   THIRD TRIMESTER

UP TO THIRTY-FIVE WEEKS

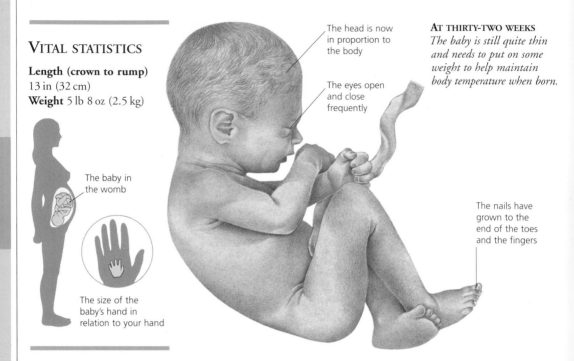

VITAL STATISTICS

Length (crown to rump)
13 in (32 cm)
Weight 5 lb 8 oz (2.5 kg)

The baby in the womb

The size of the baby's hand in relation to your hand

The head is now in proportion to the body

The eyes open and close frequently

AT THIRTY-TWO WEEKS
The baby is still quite thin and needs to put on some weight to help maintain body temperature when born.

The nails have grown to the end of the toes and the fingers

HOW IS THE BABY GROWING?

What does the baby look like?
At this stage of the pregnancy the baby is 13 in (32 cm) long (crown to rump), weighs 5 lb 8 oz (2.5 kg), and is fully formed; the head is more in proportion with the body. More fat has accumulated under the skin, which helps to regulate body temperature after birth, although the skin is still quite thin.
■ **Face** The skin on your baby's face is much smoother, having lost many of its wrinkles. If you have an ultrasound scan around this time, the structure of the baby's face should have formed sufficiently for you to see its profile quite clearly. The baby's eyes now open and close often and can sense changes in light through the wall of the abdomen; if you were to give birth now, the baby's eyes would open and close automatically.
■ **Arms and legs** These are developed and the muscles and nerves are linked, allowing relatively coordinated movements. The baby tends to rest with its arms and legs drawn up and can now grip with its fingers.

■ **Skin and hair** The skin loses its transparent quality as fat is deposited, taking on color as the blood vessels become harder to see. The vernix increases and there may be some hair on the baby's head.

What is happening inside the body?
Most of the major organs have developed and your baby starts gaining weight in preparation for birth.
■ **Lungs** These are still developing. However, if your baby was born now, there would be a very good chance of survival with assisted breathing.
■ **Brain and nervous system** These are now fully developed although, if born now, the reflexes, such as the sucking reflex, and coordination would be poor.
■ **Digestive system** Meconium, a dark green, thick, substance made up of dead cells and secretions from the bowel and liver, fills the intestine. Your baby may pass meconium (the first feces) if distressed during labor.

The baby's life-support system
The placental supply of nutrients to the baby is at its most efficient as the placenta reaches maturity.

WEEKS IN PREGNANCY

1	2	3	4	5	6	7	8	9	10	11	12	13	14	15	16	17	18	19	20
				FIRST TRIMESTER															SECOND

Q WHY IS THE BABY'S SKIN NOT WATERLOGGED BY THE AMNIOTIC FLUID?

A During the third trimester your baby's skin is impermeable to the amniotic fluid that surrounds it, unlike the first and early second trimesters (see p. 55). This is because, at around 28 weeks, a thick, white, waxy covering called vernix develops, which is protective and stops the skin becoming thick and soggy – as yours would if you spent several hours in water. Also, the level of some salts and minerals in the amniotic fluid, which are not easily absorbed through a baby's skin, increases at this time.

Q HOW MUCH DOES A BABY SLEEP?

A As you have probably noticed, whenever you lie down, your baby often wakes up and starts to kick and move around. Babies may lie quietly in the womb or sleep for several hours and then be awake and move for several hours. Studies on babies' movements and heart rate changes reveal that they appear to have alternating sleep/waking cycles. This pattern of sleep can also persist in newborn babies until a more regular sleep pattern has been established.

Q CAN I INFLUENCE WHETHER MY BABY IS AWAKE OR ASLEEP?

A Your baby's sleep pattern is quite separate from your own. Often it is possible to wake a baby up by pressing gently on your abdomen, getting up and moving around, or even by eating a high carbohydrate meal. Loud noises can provoke some activity, and some mothers say that their babies wake up and/or react to certain types of music. Obstetric researchers use vibro-acoustic stimulation applied directly to the abdomen; this wakes a baby up so that changes in the heart rate when asleep and awake can be investigated.

Q MY BABY IS SITTING HEAD UP IN MY WOMB. IS THIS COMMON?

A Babies often lie head up (breech) until the last weeks of pregnancy, which is why premature babies are often born breech. About 30 percent of premature babies are breech but only about four percent of babies born at 37 weeks are in this position. The breech position is more common with very large or small babies. If you are expecting twins, one baby is often breech. It is possible for your baby to be in the breech position at a late stage, but to turn just before the birth.

HOW IS MY BABY POSITIONED IN THE WOMB?

How your baby's body is positioned within your womb is called the "lie" of your baby. The presentation of your baby is described in terms of the part of your baby – head or bottom – that lies closest to your pelvis.

How position can affect birth
The normal way for a baby to lie in the womb is "up and down" (longitudinally). However, very rarely, the lie may be across the womb (transverse) or angled between transverse and longitudinal (oblique). If your baby is in one of these positions or is breech (see right) when you start labor, you are more likely to need a cesarean delivery (see p. 182).

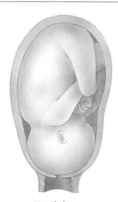

Head down

CEPHALIC PRESENTATION
This is the most common position for a baby at birth, with the head on the cervix.

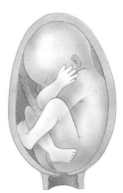

Bottom down

BREECH PRESENTATION
This is much less common; only about four percent of babies are breech at term.

WEEKS IN PREGNANCY

21	22	23	24	25	26	27	28	29	30	31	32	33	34	35	36	37	38	39	40

TRIMESTER | THIRD TRIMESTER

BY FORTY WEEKS

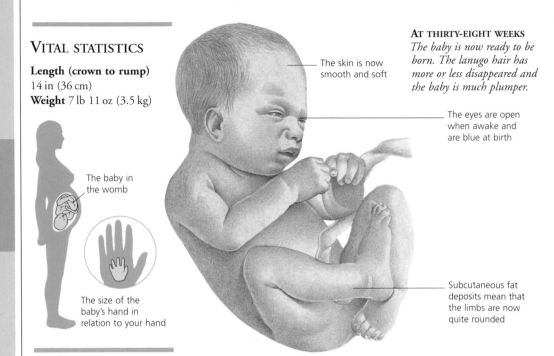

VITAL STATISTICS

Length (crown to rump)
14 in (36 cm)
Weight 7 lb 11 oz (3.5 kg)

The baby in
the womb

The size of the
baby's hand in
relation to your hand

The skin is now
smooth and soft

AT THIRTY-EIGHT WEEKS
*The baby is now ready to be
born. The lanugo hair has
more or less disappeared and
the baby is much plumper.*

The eyes are open
when awake and
are blue at birth

Subcutaneous fat
deposits mean that
the limbs are now
quite rounded

HOW IS THE BABY GROWING?

What does the baby look like?
The average baby is about 14 in (36 cm) in length
(crown to rump) and weighs about 7 lb 11 oz
(3.5 kg). At 36 weeks, your baby is almost fully
mature and would probably survive if born, without
needing to spend time in a neonatal unit. In the last
four weeks of pregnancy your baby puts on a lot of
weight and in particular, develops a thick layer of
subcutaneous fat, so is relatively plump at birth.
■ **Face** At birth, the face is quite rounded and the
eyes are always blue, although the color may change
up to six months or more after the birth.
■ **Arms and legs** These are fully developed and, by
week 36, your baby's fingernails and toenails should
also be fully grown.
■ **Skin and hair** The lanugo hair (see p. 57) has
almost completely disappeared by this stage, although
a few patches may remain at birth. The skin may be
pale, peeling, and cracked, and have deeply indented
creases, especially over the palm of the hand.

■ **Sexual organs** In girls, breast tissue is present and
the nipples are raised. In boys, the testicles have
usually descended into the scrotum.

What is happening inside the body?
Your baby is now plump and ready to be born; his or
her consciousness and coordination are well established.
■ **Lungs** These should be fully formed by now,
although they still need to mature; your baby is now
producing the hormone, cortisol, which helps the
lungs to develop in preparation for the birth.
■ **Heart** The heart is beating at a rate of 110–150
beats per minute. Once your baby is born, major
changes will occur in his or her circulation as the lungs
expand, allowing blood to flow into the lung tissue.

The baby's life-support system
The placenta, which has been providing your baby
with nourishment and oxygen during the pregnancy,
reaches maturity at around 34 weeks. It then stops
growing and starts to age. At birth, it weighs about
one sixth of your baby's weight.

WEEKS IN PREGNANCY

1	2	3	4	5	6	7	8	9	10	11	12	13	14	15	16	17	18	19	20
				FIRST TRIMESTER															SECOND

Q WHEN ARE MY BABY'S LUNGS FULLY MATURE?

A By 37 weeks the cells lining the airways of the lungs have developed, and the many dividing branches of the lungs are present; this insures that there is adequate gas exchange at birth. Crucially, at this stage, the lungs have produced enough surfactant and cortisol to allow the lungs to function normally.

Q IS MY BABY'S SKULL FULLY FORMED AT 40 WEEKS?

A A baby's brain is surrounded by a series of "flat" bones, but unlike an adult skull, they are not yet fused. The bones of a baby's skull are quite soft and can slide over each other and overlap, allowing the head to pass through the birth canal and vagina without damage. There are spaces called fontanelles at the top of the head where bones meet. Fontanelles remain soft until several months after the birth.

Q WHY DOES MY BABY MOVE LESS NOW THAT I AM 38 WEEKS PREGNANT?

A It is normal to feel less activity from your baby after 36 weeks. Now that your baby is mature enough to be born, there is less amniotic fluid and less room for big turns or kicks inside your womb, and you will be less aware of its smaller gestures.

Q SHOULD I BE CONCERNED IF MY BABY DOESN'T MOVE AT ALL?

A Although it is common for babies to move less vigorously around the time they are due (see above), if there are no movements at all, or suddenly much less than you are used to, you should contact your doctor or midwife. The baby's heart rate can be checked by an external fetal monitor (see p. 158).

Q HOW DO I KNOW IF THE BABY HAS ENGAGED?

A Some women experience a definite decrease in pressure around their diaphragm and stomach, which makes it easier to breathe deeply and eat a large meal. There is also an increase in discomfort in the bladder and perineal area, so you may urinate more frequently. Your doctor or midwife will confirm engagement by an internal examination (see box, right).

WHAT IS ENGAGEMENT, AND WHEN WILL IT TAKE PLACE?

When the head moves down from high in your abdomen and settles deeper into your pelvis in preparation for the birth, it is said to have engaged. Engagement is also referred to as the head "dropping."

When will my baby engage?

This can happen any time between 36 weeks and labor. It is more likely to engage early if this is a first baby. If the baby does engage, this doesn't mean that labor is about to begin; you may have several weeks to go. Also, if the baby does not engage, do not worry that you won't have a normal delivery because it can occur any time up to your labor. Indeed, with second or subsequent babies, the baby often doesn't engage until labor has started.

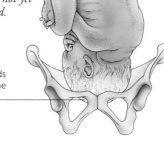

DESCENT TO PELVIS
The baby's head has settled down in the pelvis but is not yet fully engaged.

Baby's head settles towards the inlet of the pelvis

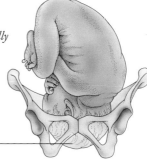

ENGAGEMENT POSITION
When engaged, the head is usually down, fitting in the hollow of the pelvis.

Soft skull bones compress to fit through the birth canal

WEEKS IN PREGNANCY

21	22	23	24	25	26	27	28	29	30	31	32	33	34	35	36	37	38	39	40
TRIMESTER											THIRD TRIMESTER								

TWINS AND MULTIPLE BIRTHS

Q AM I MORE LIKELY TO HAVE TWINS IF THERE ARE TWINS IN MY FAMILY?

A Yes, you are. Fraternal twins are more likely if a close relative has had twins or triplets, or if you are a fraternal twin. However, the incidence of identical twins is more random and not always linked to your family history.

Q HOW COMMON ARE TWINS?

A Twins are more common in women who conceive after the age of 35, or have had fertility treatments, such as IVF and GIFT (see p. 15); over half of triplets result from assisted conception techniques. Although the reason for this is not clear, multiple pregnancies are also more common in certain parts of the world such as Nigeria, where 45 per 1,000 births are twins. In the US, about 11 of every 1,000 births is a twin birth.

Q WHEN WILL MY DOCTOR OR MIDWIFE CONFIRM THAT I'M EXPECTING TWINS?

A It is possible to see twins on ultrasound at about eight weeks. However, because there is a higher risk of miscarriage (of one or both babies), a diagnosis of "viable" twins is rarely made until the beginning of the second trimester, at 12 to 14 weeks.

Q WHAT ARE THE RISKS INVOLVED IN HAVING TWINS?

A If you are expecting twins, you are considered to be a high-risk pregnancy. Extra demands are placed on the mother and the placental system on which the babies rely. In turn this can slow the growth of one or both the babies, and cause high blood pressure in the mother. There is also a strong chance of premature birth. These risks are further compounded with triplets or even higher multiple pregnancies (see p. 130).

HOW DO TWINS DEVELOP?

Twins develop at an early stage when, or just after, the egg and sperm meet. Twins are either fraternal (more common, accounting for about 80 percent of twins) or identical (less frequent, about 20 percent). The twins below are in a vertex (head down) position, but they can also occupy other positions in the womb (see p. 185).

IDENTICAL TWINS

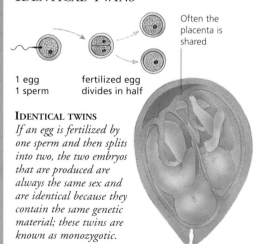

Often the placenta is shared

1 egg
1 sperm

fertilized egg divides in half

IDENTICAL TWINS
If an egg is fertilized by one sperm and then splits into two, the two embryos that are produced are always the same sex and are identical because they contain the same genetic material; these twins are known as monozygotic.

FRATERNAL TWINS

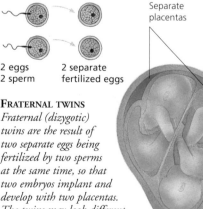

Separate placentas

2 eggs
2 sperm

2 separate fertilized eggs

FRATERNAL TWINS
Fraternal (dizygotic) twins are the result of two separate eggs being fertilized by two sperms at the same time, so that two embryos implant and develop with two placentas. The twins may look different and be different sexes.

Q HOW WILL I BE AFFECTED IF MY PREGNANCY IS HIGH-RISK?

A You will be under the very close care of an obstetrician, and have frequent ultrasounds and prenatal appointments. A nonhospital birth will not be recommended.

Q WILL TWO BABIES BE ABLE TO DEVELOP PROPERLY IN MY WOMB?

A The womb is amazingly elastic and it is quite possible for two, and sometimes three (or more) babies to grow and develop quite normally. There is usually no problem in their development as long as each is surrounded by a separate protective amniotic sac (see below). It is, however, much more likely that you will go into labor before 40 weeks because the amount of space in your womb is limited.

Q CAN THE TWINS BUMP INTO OR HURT EACH OTHER IN THE WOMB?

A Your twins can and will bump into each other in your womb, because they will be quite active. They may even seem to be playing with each other. However, they cannot hurt each other because they are cushioned by the amniotic fluid.

Q DOES IT MATTER IF MY TWINS ARE IDENTICAL OR NOT?

A Yes, it is important. If they are identical and share the same placenta and amniotic sac, they may encounter more problems with their development and delivery than fraternal twins (see p. 130). For this reason, if you are pregnant with identical twins, you will be closely monitored and you can expect frequent ultrasounds.

Q WHY DID MY EARLY SCAN SHOW TWINS, AND NOW ONLY ONE BABY SHOWS?

A Twin pregnancies may develop more often than we think, but at an early stage one twin dies or doesn't develop. As the surviving twin grows, the nonviable twin is "reabsorbed" and disappears, with almost no trace. In the first trimester this shouldn't cause problems, but if one fetus dies later in pregnancy, difficulties may occur (see p. 130).

Q DO TWINS AND TRIPLETS DEVELOP AT THE SAME RATE AS SINGLE BABIES?

A Yes, they develop in exactly the same way, at the same rate except that they may not grow quite as large as single babies, even taking into account the fact that they are usually born earlier.

Q DO TWINS SHARE THE SAME SAC OF AMNIOTIC FLUID?

A Fraternal twins, which result from two eggs fertilized by two separate sperm, and develop independently of each other, have separate umbilical cords, placentas, and amniotic sacs. Although identical twins, the result of one fertilized egg that has divided to form two embryos, share a placenta, they always have their own cord.

Q I'M TOLD THAT MY TWINS ARE GROWING AT DIFFERENT RATES. WHY IS THIS?

A Twins may be different sizes to start off with, and can also grow at different rates. This is why if you have twins, you are offered frequent ultrasounds. It isn't usually a problem if both babies start off at different sizes but grow at normal rates; however, it may become a problem if they were both the same size initially, and one suddenly starts to grow much slower than the other (see below).

Q WHAT HAPPENS IF ONE TWIN IS GROWING MORE SLOWLY?

A If there is "discrepant growth," you will have more frequent ultrasound scans and, depending on the well-being of the smaller, least healthy twin, the twins may be delivered early. A big difference in identical twins may suggest a rare condition called "twin-to-twin transfusion syndrome," caused by an abnormal blood vessel connection (see p. 131).

Q IS IT TRUE THAT I WILL BE ABLE TO FEEL MY TWINS MOVING SEPARATELY?

A Because of each baby's own specific patterns of movement and relative position in the womb, many mothers can identify which baby is moving at a particular time. Twins do move separately; often one can be fast asleep or not moving much while the other is bouncing around.

QUESTIONS TO ASK

Are my babies growing at the same rate?

Are my twins identical or fraternal?

Is there a normal amount of amniotic fluid around each twin?

Are they the same sex or different sexes?

Is there one or two placentas?

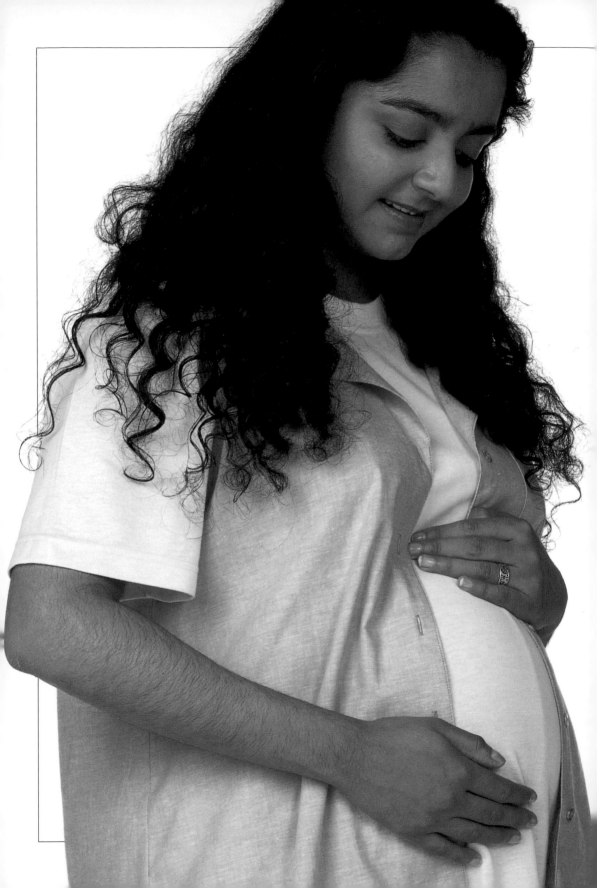

YOUR
CHANGING
BODY

In pregnancy, powerful forces are at work changing your body to allow your baby to grow and develop. You will experience new symptoms and feelings that may give you some discomfort even as you revel in the positive signs of your advancing pregnancy; or you may feel better than ever before – and look like the picture of health. To reassure you that all is progressing normally, this chapter discusses and explains the physical and emotional upheavals that you are undergoing, sometimes offering possible solutions and remedies; it also reminds you that these changes serve one purpose only – to benefit the new life inside you.

HOW YOUR BODY CHANGES

A S SOON AS YOU become pregnant, your body begins to change so that it can support you and your pregnancy over the coming weeks. Because your body will eventually be supporting two systems, all of your body functions start to work much harder. Your heart has to pump more blood around your body, in particular to and from your womb, placenta, and the fetus, so your pulse rate increases by about ten beats per minute; your breathing rate speeds up to take in more oxygen for your baby and to exhale more carbon dioxide; your metabolic rate accelerates in response to the increased workload. As well as these physical demands, pregnancy also causes a range of emotional reactions that varies from woman to woman. Below, you can see how much your body is likely to change; details of these changes are charted in the following pages.

STAGES OF DEVELOPMENT

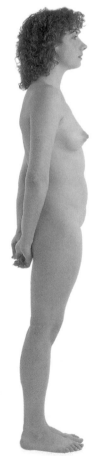
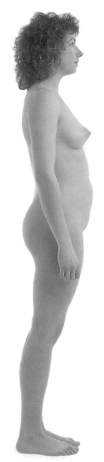
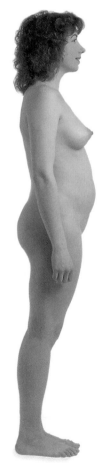
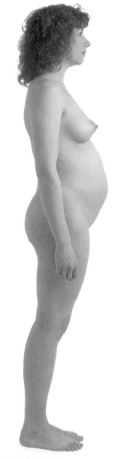

AT 12 WEEKS
Although the fetus is growing rapidly, you will not see a "belly" yet.

AT 16 WEEKS
Your nipples start to darken as your skin becomes more pigmented.

AT 20 WEEKS
Your belly is expanding quickly but you may have lots of energy.

AT 24 WEEKS
Your face, hands, and upper body may swell because of fluid retention.

THE STAGES OF PREGNANCY

The 40 weeks, or approximately nine months, of pregnancy are discussed by trimester because each three-month period has distinct characteristics. In the first trimester, the first 12 weeks, little is visible but a great deal is happening; the fetus' major organs are fully formed. The second trimester, weeks 13 to 25, is when your pregnancy becomes obvious and you begin to feel your baby move. In the third trimester, from 26 weeks until delivery, as your baby grows and matures, your belly expands enormously so that at term you find even simple tasks tiring and sleeping comfortably at night hard.

Pregnancy timeline

WEEKS IN PREGNANCY

1	2	3	4	5	6	7	8	9	10	11	12	13	14	15	16	17	18	19	20	21	22	23	24	25	26	27	28	29	30	31	32	33	34	35	36	37	38	39	40
FIRST TRIMESTER												SECOND TRIMESTER													THIRD TRIMESTER															

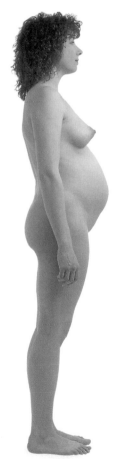
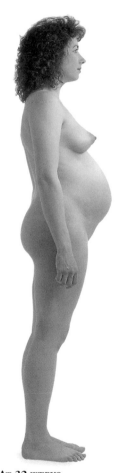
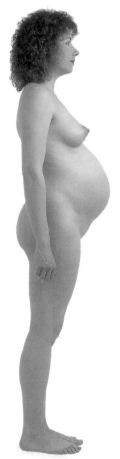
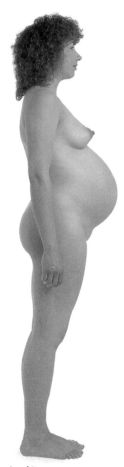

AT 28 WEEKS
The fetus is now very active with much kicking and turning.

AT 32 WEEKS
Your growing womb presses on internal organs and may cause discomfort.

AT 36 WEEKS
By this stage, the baby's head may have dropped down into your pelvis.

AT 40 WEEKS
Your belly is now so large that it is difficult to get comfortable at night.

YOUR CHANGING BODY

THE FIRST TRIMESTER

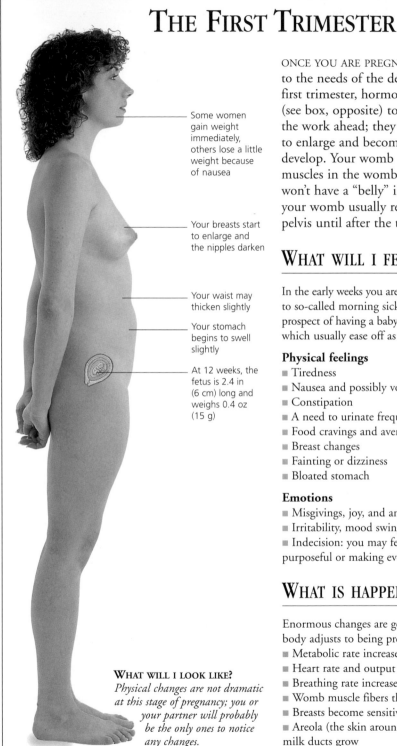

Some women gain weight immediately, others lose a little weight because of nausea

Your breasts start to enlarge and the nipples darken

Your waist may thicken slightly

Your stomach begins to swell slightly

At 12 weeks, the fetus is 2.4 in (6 cm) long and weighs 0.4 oz (15 g)

WHAT WILL I LOOK LIKE?
Physical changes are not dramatic at this stage of pregnancy; you or your partner will probably be the only ones to notice any changes.

ONCE YOU ARE PREGNANT your body responds to the needs of the developing fetus. In the first trimester, hormones are produced (see box, opposite) to prepare your body for the work ahead; they also cause your breasts to enlarge and become tender as milk ducts develop. Your womb begins to grow and the muscles in the womb wall thicken, but you won't have a "belly" in the first weeks because your womb usually remains tucked into the pelvis until after the third month.

WHAT WILL I FEEL?

In the early weeks you are likely to be tired and prone to so-called morning sickness. Excitement at the prospect of having a baby often offsets these symptoms, which usually ease off as the pregnancy progresses.

Physical feelings
- Tiredness
- Nausea and possibly vomiting
- Constipation
- A need to urinate frequently
- Food cravings and aversions
- Breast changes
- Fainting or dizziness
- Bloated stomach

Emotions
- Misgivings, joy, and anxiety (or a mixture)
- Irritability, mood swings, weepiness
- Indecision: you may feel incapable of being purposeful or making even simple decisions

WHAT IS HAPPENING TO MY BODY?

Enormous changes are going on inside you as your body adjusts to being pregnant.
- Metabolic rate increases by 10–25 percent
- Heart rate and output rise by up to 40 percent
- Breathing rate increases
- Womb muscle fibers thicken and lengthen
- Breasts become sensitive and increase in size
- Areola (the skin around your nipples) darken and milk ducts grow

WEEKS IN PREGNANCY

1	2	3	4	5	6	7	8	9	10	11	12	13	14	15	16	17	18	19	20
				FIRST TRIMESTER														SECOND	

How Will The Changes Affect Me?

Q I DON'T FEEL OR LOOK AT ALL PREGNANT YET. IS THIS NORMAL?

A This is perfectly normal. Some women breeze through the early weeks of their pregnancy without experiencing any nausea, tiredness, or other symptoms. If you are one of these lucky ones, relax and enjoy it. After about 12 weeks, at the start of the second trimester, when your womb has grown upward into your abdomen, you will start to see and feel that your fetus is growing.

Q WHY DO MY CLOTHES ALREADY FEEL TIGHT AROUND MY WAIST?

A Although this can happen early on, it is probably not caused by your growing womb. Unless you are expecting twins or triplets, your bowels rather than your baby are the reason. The increase in progesterone affects the bowels and causes gas and constipation, which can make you feel bloated. This condition should improve during pregnancy, but eating high-fiber foods and drinking plenty of fluids will help (see p. 100). However, do not overeat in the early weeks – the baby does not need it and you may put on unwanted weight.

What Part Do Hormones Play?

The production of some hormones greatly increases in pregnancy, and new hormones are produced. Some are controlled by the pituitary gland (at the base of the brain), others are produced by the ovaries, thyroid gland, and later the placenta; their purpose is to prepare your body for pregnancy. Hormonal changes can cause side effects, but they are a sign of the pregnancy's progress.

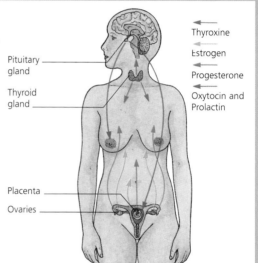

Progesterone

This hormone is important for the maintenance of your pregnancy and eventually for the onset of labor. Its most significant action is to relax certain muscles in your body. This has several effects: it prevents preterm labor; blood vessels dilate, which lowers blood pressure and can make you feel faint; the digestive system slows down, causing indigestion and constipation. Progesterone affects moods, raises body temperature, increases breathing rate, and can cause nausea. It also contributes to the preparation of the breasts for breastfeeding.

Estrogen

This hormone causes your nipples to enlarge and stimulates the development of milk glands. It strengthens the womb wall to cope with the powerful contractions of labor and softens body tissue, which allows the ligaments and joints to stretch. This can lead to varicose veins and backache.

HORMONAL INCREASES
The arrows show the origin of the major pregnancy hormones. Progesterone and estrogen are produced by the ovaries and later by the placenta. Oxytocin and prolactin are produced by the pituitary gland, and thyroxine is controlled by the thyroid gland.

Other hormonal changes

Human chorionic gonadotrophin (hCG) and human placental lactogen (hPL) are produced by the placenta and are unique to pregnancy. HPL is associated with breast enlargement while hCG stimulates your thyroid gland to produce extra thryoxine, which can affect your metabolism. Prolactin and oxytocin help produce breast milk. Oxytocin also stimulates contractions in labor.

YOUR CHANGING BODY

WEEKS IN PREGNANCY

21	22	23	24	25	26	27	28	29	30	31	32	33	34	35	36	37	38	39	40
TRIMESTER						THIRD TRIMESTER													

COMMON COMPLAINTS

Q WHY I AM HAVING HOT FLASHES?

A As your metabolism speeds up, it generates extra heat, and your blood vessels, especially those in the skin, dilate with extra blood. You may feel flushed and warm, particularly during the summer. It can be hard to prevent hot flashes but it helps to wear loose, layered clothing that you can take off when you need to cool down.

Q WHY DO I GET NOSEBLEEDS?

A An increased volume of blood and changes in the blood's ability to clot can cause nosebleeds. When your nose bleeds, sit down and pinch the soft part of your nose below the bridge until it stops.

Q WHY DO I NEED TO URINATE SO OFTEN, BUT ONLY A TINY AMOUNT?

A This happens because your womb expands and presses on your bladder. You should get some relief in the middle trimester, as the womb expands higher into the abdomen and eases the pressure on the bladder. However, in late pregnancy, the growing fetus presses on the bladder from above (see p. 122) and the need to urinate frequently returns.

Q I HAVE A STINGING FEELING WHEN I URINATE. WHY?

A A stinging feeling as you pass urine, low abdominal pain, or blood in your urine could mean that you have a urinary tract infection (UTI) (see p. 120). Such infections are common in pregnancy and you should see your doctor, or midwife as soon as you can. You may need antibiotics to clear the infection.

Q I SEEM TO BE BREATHING VERY QUICKLY THESE DAYS, IS THIS NORMAL?

A Your lungs are adapting to your body's extra energy needs. As your metabolism speeds up, more carbon dioxide is produced, which has to be cleared by your lungs. At the same time, your body takes in more oxygen, increasing your lung capacity by about 40 percent. Therefore, as well as a larger volume of air and gas exchanged per breath, your breathing rate speeds up.

HOW DO I COPE WITH TIREDNESS?

Why am I so tired?
Even though you may not be aware of it, your body is now working harder than it ever has before. To make this possible, your metabolic rate has increased by one fifth to support it. Your heart is pumping more blood more quickly around your body and your breathing rate has also increased. With this major increase in your body's workload, it is not surprising that you feel tired.

How tired should I feel?
Anything from mildly tired to absolutely drained is normal. As well as all the changes mentioned above, you may also be feeling sick and find it difficult to eat anything or to keep food down once you've eaten.

What can I do to reduce general fatigue?
Don't fight it, give in to it. As your pregnancy progresses, you should gradually feel more energetic; in the meantime, just take it easy and, if possible, try to get more rest during the day or early evening.

How can I get a good night's sleep?
Try to rest during the day so that you are not totally exhausted by bedtime or, if this is not possible, go to bed much earlier than usual. Get yourself into a pleasantly relaxed state by the end of the day, perhaps by having a warm bath and a mug of warm milk (unless you are feeling nauseous) (see p. 112). Getting a full night's undisturbed sleep is unlikely during the first and last trimesters as you may need to urinate in the night. You should therefore avoid drinking tea, coffee, and alcohol; also avoid taking sleeping pills, which may leave you feeling groggy.

Should I see a doctor about feeling tired?
If after several weeks you feel more and more exhausted, see your doctor or midwife to make sure that you are not anemic. Anemia is a blood condition that can usually be corrected by diet or taking iron supplements (see p. 122).

WEEKS IN PREGNANCY

1	2	3	4	5	6	7	8	9	10	11	12	13	14	15	16	17	18	19	20
			FIRST TRIMESTER															SECOND	

YOUR CHANGING BODY

Q WHAT ARE THE SPIDERY RED LINES ON MY LEGS, AND WILL THEY GO AWAY?

A These are called spider nevi and are small blood vessels in the skin that have expanded. Caused by the estrogen surge of pregnancy, they should (but don't always) fade after the pregnancy. They are not a sign that anything is wrong.

Q I USED TO LOVE THE TASTE OF COFFEE; WHY DOES IT TASTE BAD NOW?

A The change in hormones and blood chemicals that your body undergoes during pregnancy affects your saliva; this in turn can cause certain foods and drinks to taste odd, sometimes to the point where you no longer enjoy them. It has been suggested that this may be nature's way of steering you away from harmful substances, such as alcohol, during your pregnancy. Some women report that they suddenly want to drink tea or coffee when they never liked it before, which illustrates the contrary nature of cravings.

Q I CONSTANTLY FEEL SICK; IS SOMETHING WRONG WITH ME OR THE BABY?

A No, unpleasant though it is, morning sickness or nausea is one of the most common symptoms of early pregnancy. Despite its name, morning sickness can occur at any time and can last all day. It usually occurs during the first trimester (before 14 weeks) and is thought to be due to the presence of human chorionic gonadotrophin (hCG), a hormone that is only produced during pregnancy (see p. 73).

Q I AM VOMITING EVERY DAY AND CANNOT KEEP ANY FOOD DOWN. WHAT CAN I DO?

A If you are almost constantly sick and this stops you from keeping down fluids as well as solid foods, see your doctor or midwife; you may be given a medication to decrease your nausea and vomiting. You may also be advised to spend one or two days in hospital for observation, rehydration, and vitamin supplements.

WHAT CAN I DO TO STOP NAUSEA OR MORNING SICKNESS?

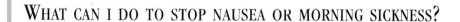

If you feel most ill in the morning, try to eat something plain, such as a saltine cracker or dry toast, before you get out of bed. If your nausea persists throughout the the day, try to eat and drink small amounts more often, and avoid fatty foods and milky drinks. Some women report that sodas or sweets reduce their nausea; others are soothed by herbal remedies such as ginger, peppermint, or camomile teas (see p. 105).

Recipe for ginger tea
Place one teaspoon of ground or grated fresh ginger into a teapot or small bowl. Pour boiling water over it, allow it to steep for a few minutes, then strain into a cup or a glass. Add brown sugar or honey to taste, if you like.

BEFORE YOU GET UP
Eating crackers or dry toast before you get up in the morning may help prevent or reduce morning sickness.

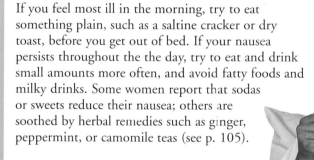

WEEKS IN PREGNANCY

21	22	23	24	25	26	27	28	29	30	31	32	33	34	35	36	37	38	39	40

TRIMESTER | THIRD TRIMESTER

THE SECOND TRIMESTER

THIS MAY BE THE most enjoyable part of your pregnancy. You will become more energetic and will feel fetal movements for the first time. The nausea and tiredness of the early weeks usually eases by this stage and, as your thickening waistline rapidly grows into a noticeable belly, you start to look pregnant.

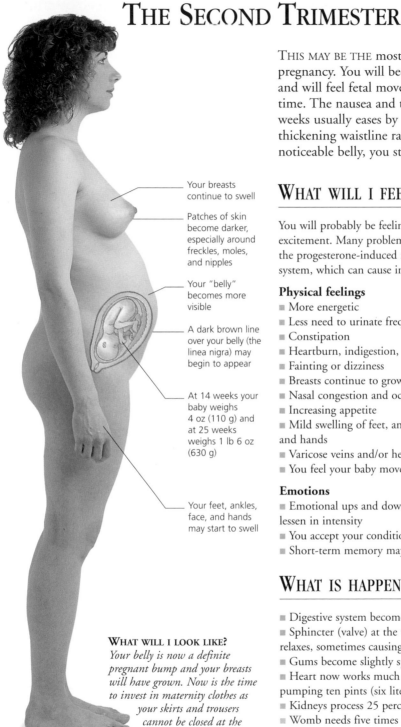

Your breasts continue to swell

Patches of skin become darker, especially around freckles, moles, and nipples

Your "belly" becomes more visible

A dark brown line over your belly (the linea nigra) may begin to appear

At 14 weeks your baby weighs 4 oz (110 g) and at 25 weeks weighs 1 lb 6 oz (630 g)

Your feet, ankles, face, and hands may start to swell

WHAT WILL I LOOK LIKE?
Your belly is now a definite pregnant bump and your breasts will have grown. Now is the time to invest in maternity clothes as your skirts and trousers cannot be closed at the waist (see p. 86).

WHAT WILL I FEEL?

You will probably be feeling full of vitality and excitement. Many problems at this stage are due to the progesterone-induced relaxation of the digestive system, which can cause indigestion and constipation.

Physical feelings
- More energetic
- Less need to urinate frequently
- Constipation
- Heartburn, indigestion, gas
- Fainting or dizziness
- Breasts continue to grow
- Nasal congestion and occasional nosebleeds
- Increasing appetite
- Mild swelling of feet, ankles, sometimes face and hands
- Varicose veins and/or hemorrhoids possible
- You feel your baby move by 22–24 weeks

Emotions
- Emotional ups and downs may be the same or may lessen in intensity
- You accept your condition – you feel pregnant now
- Short-term memory may be poor

WHAT IS HAPPENING TO MY BODY?

- Digestive system becomes sluggish
- Sphincter (valve) at the top of your stomach relaxes, sometimes causing heartburn
- Gums become slightly spongy and may bleed
- Heart now works much harder than normal, pumping ten pints (six liters) of blood a minute
- Kidneys process 25 percent more blood
- Womb needs five times more blood supplied to it than before pregnancy

WEEKS IN PREGNANCY

1	2	3	4	5	6	7	8	9	10	11	12	13	14	15	16	17	18	19	20
				FIRST TRIMESTER															SECOND

HOW WILL THE CHANGES AFFECT ME?

Q MY SKIN HAS CHANGED COLOR AND LOOKS SPLOTCHY; IS THIS NORMAL?

A Extra amounts of estrogen in pregnancy affect the melanin-producing cells of the skin, the cells that produce the pigment that darkens the skin. This can result in a color change where your skin is already darker, for example, where you have freckles or birthmarks. You may also develop a darker area around your forehead, nose, mouth, and chin, known as chloasma or "the mask of pregnancy." Some women also find that they tan more readily and unevenly in the sun. These color changes are normal and usually fade once the baby is born.

Q WHY AM I NOT FEELING THE NEED TO URINATE AS URGENTLY AS BEFORE?

A By the time you have reached the second trimester, your womb has expanded up into your abdomen, which means that the pressure on your bladder is reduced.

Q I FAINTED THIS MORNING. DOES THIS MEAN THERE'S SOMETHING WRONG?

A Fainting is quite common in the second trimester. Although disconcerting, it seldom means that there is anything wrong with you or your baby. It usually happens when you stand for a long time: blood vessels, especially in the legs, dilate, causing blood to pool in the lower parts of the body; as a result, your heart works harder to pump blood throughout your body. You are more likely to faint when you are tired and have not had enough to eat. Mention it to your doctor or midwife who can give you a blood test to exclude anemia (see p. 122).

Q IS THERE ANYTHING I CAN DO TO KEEP MYSELF FROM FAINTING?

A Yes, you could try to avoid standing for long periods of time. Remember not to stand up too quickly from your bed, a chair, or from the floor. Make sure you eat regularly or carry a supply of food such as plain crackers, nuts, or fruit with you. If you feel lightheaded, sit or lie down until you feel better. Take several deep breaths.

YOUR CHANGING BODY

WHY ARE MY BREASTS SO BIG AND SORE?

The hormones estrogen, progesterone, human placental lactogen, oxytocin, and prolactin prepare your body for feeding your baby and cause your breasts to enlarge, become tender, or painful. However, this tenderness may not continue for the entire pregnancy. It is important to wear a good bra to support your breasts.

What is happening
Visible dark blue veins appear as a result of the increased blood flow to the breast tissue, and new milk ducts grow. The dark skin around the nipple (areola) usually becomes larger and darker; the bumps around the nipple (called Montgomery's tubercles) also enlarge and secrete a fluid to lubricate the nipples. Your breasts may sometimes leak a clear fluid called colostrum, which is an early form of milk (see p. 203); this is nothing to worry about.

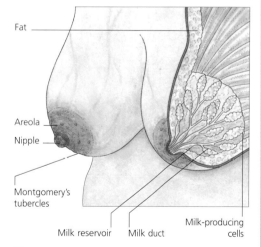

Fat

Areola

Nipple

Montgomery's tubercles

Milk reservoir   Milk duct

Milk-producing cells

BREAST CHANGES
Progesterone causes the main changes in your breasts in pregnancy, while estrogen is primarily responsible for the growth of milk ducts. Some women find that their breasts become very sensitive.

WEEKS IN PREGNANCY

21	22	23	24	25	26	27	28	29	30	31	32	33	34	35	36	37	38	39	40

TRIMESTER | THIRD TRIMESTER

COMMON COMPLAINTS

Q I OFTEN HAVE A BURNING PAIN IN MY STOMACH. IS THIS HEARTBURN?

A Very probably. Heartburn occurs in pregnancy when high levels of the hormone progesterone relax the valve that normally stops the contents of your stomach moving back into your esophagus (food pipe). The stomach contents irritate your esophagus and cause heartburn. Later in pregnancy, heartburn can occur because your enlarged womb squashes your stomach and gastric acids seep out.

Q WHAT CAN I DO TO PREVENT HEARTBURN?

A Try to eat little and often and preferably long before you go to bed. Some women find that a glass of milk eases acute heartburn (although it can cause nausea, see p. 75); there are also various herbal remedies (see p. 105). Sit up straight when you eat to prevent squashing your stomach. Also, avoid eating highly spiced food unless you are used to it. If you suffer from heartburn at night, do not lie completely flat in bed but prop up your upper body with pillows. If these solutions don't work, your doctor or midwife may recommend an antacid to neutralize the acidity of your stomach.

Q WHY DO I HAVE INDIGESTION ALL THE TIME?

A Indigestion is common in pregnancy because high progesterone levels slow the rate of digestion; food therefore remains in the stomach for longer. Try eating little and often; large heavy meals may cause an uncomfortable, heavy feeling in your stomach, and occasionally a burning pain, like heartburn.

Q HOW CAN I CURE MY CONSTIPATION?

A The hormones that slow down your digestive system also make your bowel action sluggish. Eat plenty of fruit, vegetables, and other high-fiber foods (see p. 100), and drink plenty of water (about 4 pints/2 liters a day). Some iron supplements cause constipation; if taken for a prolonged period they may cause hemorrhoids (see p. 82). If this is a problem, and you are anemic, ask your doctor or midwife about changing your iron tablets.

Q DO ALL PREGNANT WOMEN GET VARICOSE VEINS?

A The tendency to get varicose veins is hereditary. Varicose veins are caused by the weight of the womb pressing on the veins in the pelvis; this increases the pressure in the veins in your lower body. Progesterone also makes the veins dilate (open) so that blood pools in your legs, vulva, and anus. You may notice that your veins bulge out or your legs ache when you stand for a long time. Very rarely, redness, swelling, or pain in your calves may be a serious condition, called venous thrombosis (see p. 129). If you have these symptoms, you should seek prompt medical advice.

Q MY LEGS HAVE BECOME SWOLLEN AND UNCOMFORTABLE. IS THIS NORMAL?

A The same pressure that causes varicose veins can also cause your legs to swell with fluid, especially if you are carrying more than one baby. This is usually noticeable around 24 weeks and can be very uncomfortable near the end of pregnancy. Rarely, rapid leg swelling is a sign of preeclampsia (see p. 127); you should contact your midwife or doctor if you notice this.

Q WHAT CAN I DO TO HELP PREVENT VARICOSE VEINS AND SWOLLEN LEGS?

A Wear support tights or stockings and rest with your legs raised whenever possible. Try to avoid excessive salt intake and weight gain, and standing still for long periods. Gentle daily exercise (see p. 106) also improves the circulation.

Q MY VAGINAL DISCHARGE HAS BECOME HEAVY. HAVE I GOT AN INFECTION?

A Vaginal discharge does increase in the second trimester but it should be clear and mucus-like. If there are other symptoms, such as itching, soreness, or an unusually strong smell, you may have an infection that needs treatment (see p. 121).

Q MY GUMS BLEED AFTER I BRUSH MY TEETH. WHAT DOES THIS MEAN?

A Hormonal changes cause gums to thicken and soften; this makes you prone to gum injury from hard toothbrushes or sharp foods, which can cause bleeding and infection (gingivitis). Make sure you brush gently, and regularly use dental floss. It's a good idea to see your dentist for a checkup.

WEEKS IN PREGNANCY

1	2	3	4	5	6	7	8	9	10	11	12	13	14	15	16	17	18	19	20
				FIRST TRIMESTER															SECOND

WEIGHT GAIN

Q HOW MUCH WEIGHT GAIN IS NORMAL?

A This depends on your body type. A weight gain of between 24 and 35 lb (11 and 16 kg) by the end of pregnancy is normal. However, there are many variations and some women may gain very little weight in a normal pregnancy. With a multiple pregnancy your weight gain does not double; the average weight gain is around 40 lb (18 kg).

Q IF I GAIN A LOT OF WEIGHT WILL MY BABY BE LARGE AND HARDER TO DELIVER?

A Probably not, because it is you, not the baby who gains the excess weight. Whether you have a large or a small baby is usually determined by factors other than how much you eat (see p. 55).

Q IS IT EASY TO LOSE THE WEIGHT AFTER THE BIRTH?

A The time it takes to regain your figure varies. Some women are slim again within weeks of delivering, others find that it takes much longer (see p. 220). Following a healthy, balanced diet before, during, and after the birth, and doing postnatal exercises, should all help. You may also lose weight faster and more easily if you breastfeed.

Q HOW CAN I KEEP MY WEIGHT UNDER CONTROL DURING PREGNANCY?

A There is no magic formula, apart from eating a balanced, nutritious diet and doing regular exercise. This can be especially hard during pregnancy, when food cravings and a faster metabolic rate make you hungrier. If you gain weight gradually, you should find it easier to keep it to a minimum (see p. 100).

CAN MY WEIGHT GAIN CAUSE CONCERN?

Professional opinion is that an average gain of 25–28 lb (11.5–12.5 kg) by the time of the birth is ideal – but you may gain more or less weight than this. In fact, your doctor or midwife will probably show little concern about your weight unless you gain too little weight or far too much. A poor diet (resulting in low weight gain) can cause a low birthweight. Excessive weight gain during pregnancy can cause you back problems, varicose veins, or indicate preeclampsia. Ideally, your weight gain should be gradual until the third trimester, but there are no hard and fast rules.

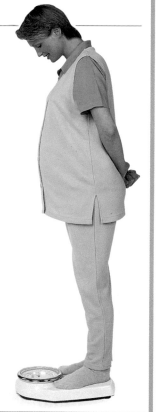

AVERAGE WEIGHT DISTRIBUTION

The fetus, placenta, and amniotic fluid account for just over a third of your weight gain. The remaining weight comes from your enlarged breasts and womb, extra body fat, increased blood volume, and fluid retention. You should experience your most dramatic weight gain in the third trimester (see p. 80).

AVERAGE WEIGHT GAIN

Blood volume	2 lb 15 oz	(1.3 kg)
Breasts	14 oz	(0.4 kg)
Womb	2 lb 3 oz	(1 kg)
Fetus	7 lb 8 oz	(3.4 kg)
Placenta	1 lb 8 oz	(0.7 kg)
Amniotic fluid	1 lb 13 oz	(0.8 kg)
Fat	7 lb 11 oz	(3.5 kg)
Retained water	3 lb 5 oz	(1.5 kg)
(This can be as much as 10 lb/4.5 kg.)		
TOTAL	27 lb 13 oz	(12.6 kg)

WEEKS IN PREGNANCY

21	22	23	24	25	26	27	28	29	30	31	32	33	34	35	36	37	38	39	40

TRIMESTER | THIRD TRIMESTER

THE THIRD TRIMESTER

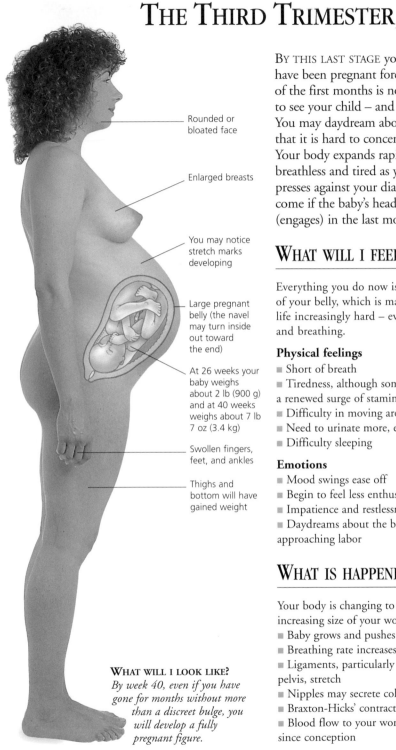

Rounded or bloated face

Enlarged breasts

You may notice stretch marks developing

Large pregnant belly (the navel may turn inside out toward the end)

At 26 weeks your baby weighs about 2 lb (900 g) and at 40 weeks weighs about 7 lb 7 oz (3.4 kg)

Swollen fingers, feet, and ankles

Thighs and bottom will have gained weight

WHAT WILL I LOOK LIKE?
By week 40, even if you have gone for months without more than a discreet bulge, you will develop a fully pregnant figure.

BY THIS LAST STAGE you probably feel as if you have been pregnant forever and the excitement of the first months is now an impatient desire to see your child – and get rid of your belly! You may daydream about your baby so much that it is hard to concentrate on other things. Your body expands rapidly and you may feel breathless and tired as your womb enlarges and presses against your diaphragm. Relief may come if the baby's head drops into the pelvis (engages) in the last month (see p. 65).

WHAT WILL I FEEL?

Everything you do now is affected by the sheer size of your belly, which is making the activities of daily life increasingly hard – even bending over, sleeping, and breathing.

Physical feelings
- Short of breath
- Tiredness, although some women experience a renewed surge of stamina just toward the end
- Difficulty in moving around
- Need to urinate more, especially if the head engages
- Difficulty sleeping

Emotions
- Mood swings ease off
- Begin to feel less enthusiastic about being pregnant
- Impatience and restlessness for the birth to be over
- Daydreams about the baby and anxiety about your approaching labor

WHAT IS HAPPENING TO MY BODY?

Your body is changing to cope with the ever increasing size of your womb and the baby in it.
- Baby grows and pushes out your lower ribs
- Breathing rate increases further
- Ligaments, particularly in the hips and pelvis, stretch
- Nipples may secrete colostrum
- Braxton-Hicks' contractions (see opposite) may begin
- Blood flow to your womb has increased tenfold since conception

WEEKS IN PREGNANCY

1	2	3	4	5	6	7	8	9	10	11	12	13	14	15	16	17	18	19	20
				FIRST TRIMESTER														SECOND	

How will the changes affect me?

Q CAN I DO ANYTHING TO PREVENT STRETCH MARKS?

A Unfortunately, there are no pills or creams that make any difference to whether or not – and how badly – you get stretch marks. Stretch marks are not directly related to how much your stomach has had to expand; they are probably connected with the collagen and elastin content of your skin. The marks can be red and bright in pregnancy, but in the weeks and months after the delivery, they lose their color, usually become silvery-white and less obvious.

Q MY BELLY TIGHTENS SEVERAL TIMES A DAY. WHAT DOES IT MEAN?

A You may feel your abdomen tightening for about 30 seconds, several times a day in the last trimester. This tightening, called Braxton-Hicks' contractions means that your womb is "practicing" for labor: the contractions don't mean that you are in – or about to go into – labor. Real labor contractions are very different; they are regular, usually more powerful and painful, and do not go away (see p. 156). As your due date approaches, you may experience Braxton-Hicks' contractions often: try to relax and use the contractions to practice your breathing (see p. 151).

Q MY FINGERS HAVE BECOME SWOLLEN. WILL THEY STAY LIKE THIS?

A Many women suffer from mild swelling of the fingers, hands, and ankles toward the end of their pregnancy. It's a good idea to remove your rings until after your baby is born, when the swelling will go down.

Q WHY HAS MY FACE BECOME SWOLLEN AND ROUND?

A This is caused by the effect of the hormone estrogen and a steroid hormone, cortisol, which change the distribution of fat in your body. Extra fluid also collects under the skin in a normal pregnancy. Occasionally, general but marked swelling of the legs, arms, and face are symptoms of preeclampsia (see p. 127), which is a serious condition that needs medical attention. Mention signs of swelling to your doctor or midwife.

Q WHAT IS THE FLUID LEAKING FROM MY BREASTS?

A This watery discharge is called colostrum and it is the first "milk" you produce, usually just after giving birth. Sometimes, in second and subsequent pregnancies, colostrum is produced well before you go into labor.

Q MY URINE LEAKS WHEN I LAUGH, SNEEZE, OR COUGH. HOW CAN I STOP THIS?

A The weight of the womb pressing on your bladder and pelvic floor means that a little urine may escape because of the extra pressure: this is called stress incontinence (see p. 120). Doing Kegel exercises to strengthen the muscles of the pelvic floor is important and of great benefit both during and after pregnancy (see p. 107). While this problem persists, you may feel more comfortable if you wear a sanitary pad or liner.

Is it safe to be active?

If you are enjoying a healthy pregnancy and have the energy, motivation, and willpower, it is certainly safe for you to be active, but you will find it harder to move fast. Mild exercise, such as walking or swimming, is beneficial and there is no reason why you shouldn't do household chores or go to work. However, don't overdo it or tackle difficult jobs such as climbing ladders or lifting heavy boxes on your own.

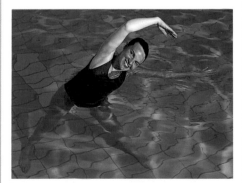

STAYING FIT AND ENJOYING LIFE
You can enjoy being physically active if you feel energetic – just rest whenever you feel the need.

WEEKS IN PREGNANCY

21	22	23	24	25	26	27	28	29	30	31	32	33	34	35	36	37	38	39	40
TRIMESTER											THIRD TRIMESTER								

COMMON COMPLAINTS

Q MY BELLY IS HUGE AND I AM VERY UNCOMFORTABLE – WHAT CAN I DO?

A There is little you can do about the discomfort in the final phase of your pregnancy because your baby is very large and takes up a lot of space in your abdomen. Lying on your back may no longer be possible or advisable because the weight of your womb presses on the main blood vessels. This causes your blood pressure to drop, which in turn can make you feel faint. By this stage of pregnancy, your baby is probably also pushing out your ribs, causing them to ache, too. There are positions you can adopt to ease some of the pressure (see p. 113). It may also help to know that if your baby engages, a few of these discomforts should ease.

HOW CAN I RELIEVE LEG CRAMPS?

Leg cramps are the excruciating pain of muscles in spasm. The causes of cramp are uncertain but may be linked to low calcium levels. Cramp often occurs in bed at night, and particularly if you point your toes.

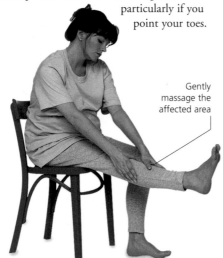

Gently massage the affected area

WHAT TO DO
To help relax the muscle that is in spasm, try extending the leg and then bringing the toes toward your body. Having a glass of milk (which contains calcium) can ease leg cramps.

Q IS IT NORMAL TO BE OUT OF BREATH ALL THE TIME?

A It is normal to feel that you are not breathing deeply enough. Also, as your womb continues to expand into your abdomen, it presses against your diaphragm and your lungs, making it more difficult for you to take deep breaths. The increase in the hormone progesterone may also speed up your breathing (see p. 73).

Q WHY ARE THE PALMS OF MY HANDS RED AND BURNING?

A You may have palmar erythema; this occurs because of the increased blood flow through the skin tissues. It is not serious, but is just a result of the changes in your blood vessels.

Q I SEEM TO BE CONSTANTLY ITCHING ALL OVER. IS THERE SOMETHING WRONG?

A As your belly expands, your skin stretches to accommodate the growing pregnancy; this stretching can make the skin itchy. Creams, calamine lotion, and bath oils can moisturize the skin, helping to reduce this itching. Rarely, severe generalized itching, especially late in pregnancy, needs medical attention, because it could indicate a liver disease (see p. 126).

Q I'VE DEVELOPED HEMORRHOIDS. CAN I DO ANYTHING TO RELIEVE THEM?

A Hemorrhoids are varicose veins in the anus that swell when the weight of the fetus puts pressure on the main veins in the pelvis; this pressure in turn reduces the return of blood from the pelvic organs to the heart. Hemorrhoids can be painful and delivery of your baby is really the only cure. Avoid constipation, as this will add to your discomfort. Your doctor can prescribe soothing ointments for hemorrhoids; if they ache, sit for ten minutes on an ice pack or bag of frozen peas wrapped in a towel. Pelvic floor exercises may also help to reduce them (see p. 107).

Q MY HEARTBEAT FEELS UNEVEN SOMETIMES – IS THIS UNUSUAL?

A "Missed" beats are also called palpitations, and normally they are nothing to worry about. However, if your heart starts missing beats very frequently, or you feel breathless or have chest pain with these palpitations, seek medical advice.

WEEKS IN PREGNANCY

1	2	3	4	5	6	7	8	9	10	11	12	13	14	15	16	17	18	19	20
				FIRST TRIMESTER															SECOND

Why do my back and hips ache?

Throughout your pregnancy, hormones relax the ligaments and joints, particularly those in the pelvis, causing the ligaments to soften and stretch to allow the baby an easier passage in labor. The weight of your growing baby can weaken your stomach muscles and put pressure on your lower back. As your center of gravity changes, you may also tend to lean backward, which can result in even more strain. If your back pain is constant or severe, consult your doctor or midwife: it may be necessary to see a physical therapist or a chiropractor for help with pain relief.

Types of back and joint ache

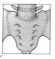

Sacroiliac joint
Steady pain in middle/low back
Where your pelvis meets the lower spine (the sacrum), there are joints on either side called sacroiliac joints. In pregnancy these can become unstable, which can be very painful, especially when walking, standing, or bending.

Treatment Wear low-heeled shoes and be sure of correct posture (see p. 110). If in severe pain, seek medical advice.

Coccyx
Pain in the lower spine
The coccyx can become slightly displaced from the sacrum, causing excruciating pain especially when sitting. This type of pain usually results from previous injury.

Treatment Ask your midwife or doctor about pain-relieving drugs. After the birth, a chiropractor may be able to help.

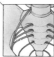

Pubic joint
Pain in the front of the pelvis
The pelvis is made up of fused bones, which form a ring-like structure; at the front, where the bones meet, is the symphysis pubis. If the ligaments around this joint loosen in late pregnancy, the pubic bones rub against each other, causing severe pain when you walk. Rarely, these bones separate: this is called diastasis of the symphysis pubis.

Treatment This usually requires consultation with a doctor or physical therapist. You may have to wear a special support belt to relieve the pressure, or you may need further treatment.

Sciatic nerves
Sharp/constant/intermittent pain in the back, buttocks, and legs
As your baby's head moves down into your pelvis, it often presses directly on the pelvic bones which in turn affects the sciatic nerves in your lower back and legs. This can cause severe back and leg pain, or your legs may feel weak and numb. This is called sciatic nerve pain (see p. 120).

Treatment The best way of dealing with this is to spend some time lying down on a firm mattress. Your baby's head may move and relieve the pressure on the nerves; the pelvic tilt exercise may help (see p. 108).

YOUR CHANGING BODY

WEEKS IN PREGNANCY

21	22	23	24	25	26	27	28	29	30	31	32	33	34	35	36	37	38	39	40

TRIMESTER	THIRD TRIMESTER

FAMILY CHANGES

Q HOW SHOULD I PREPARE MY CHILD FOR THE NEW BABY'S ARRIVAL?

A First, tell your child that a new baby is on the way and explain what this will mean; then prepare for changes in your child's routine. You need to handle these issues positively but with great care and sensitivity. What you say and how you say it will obviously depend on the age of your child (see opposite).

Q WHY IS IT IMPORTANT TO PREPARE MY CHILD FOR THE NEW BABY'S ARRIVAL?

A After the birth of your baby, your child will undergo a major change in his or her life. After all, your first child has been an only child for all of his life and has enjoyed not only all of your attention but also that of close family and friends. Whatever the age of your child, he or she has been your "baby" for some time and is now expected to relinquish that role to become a big brother or sister. This can seem like a very bad deal.

Q HOW IS MY CHILD LIKELY TO REACT?

A The chances are that you will be faced with mixed emotions, ranging from excitement at having a new playmate, to worry that the new baby will become your favorite. Your child may appear to be unaffected by the news but then go through a bout of naughtiness, or be unable to comprehend that a new baby is on its way and not react until after the birth. Or you may hear your child proudly tell friends that he or she is going to have a sister or brother. Whatever the reaction, your child will need reassurance and understanding from you.

Q HOW DO I CHANGE MY CHILD'S ROUTINE TO ADAPT TO THE NEW BABY?

A If you are planning any major changes in your child's routine, try to do this months before your baby is born. For instance, if you want your child to move from a crib to a bed, to start nursery school, or to go to bed earlier every night, try to establish these new routines months ahead of the birth or these changes will become inextricably linked with the baby's arrival. Alternatively, you could leave any changes in your child's routine until a few months after the birth.

Q I HAVE A TEENAGE CHILD – WILL A NEW BABY CAUSE PROBLEMS?

A Some teenagers will have no trouble coping with the fact that you are pregnant; others may feel deep embarrassment at seeing the proof that their mother or parents still have an intimate sexual relationship. There may be some resentment toward the baby because they see the newcomer as a definite rival for your time and attention. These reactions are very common. Try to discuss the situation with them as adults, confirm that you have no intention of remaining heavily pregnant for longer than is necessary, and remind them of the special place they occupy in the family.

Q CAN MY OTHER CHILD/CHILDREN BE PRESENT AT THE BIRTH?

A This depends on many factors. The first and most important consideration is whether you feel confident that your child could cope with seeing you in pain. Many children find this very upsetting and it may therefore be better not to put them through the experience. If you are having a hospital birth, it would also be difficult to have your child waiting around for many hours. Furthermore, should any complications develop during the birth, your partner would have to take the child outside when you may prefer that your partner stay with you. In a birthing center or at home, things are easier because you can call the child in at the appropriate moment to witness the actual birth (see p. 144).

Q HOW CAN I GET TIME ALONE WITH MY BABY WITHOUT UPSETTING MY CHILD?

A You could try to encourage a strong, loving attachment between your child and another adult who can occasionally stand in for you. This will not only give you more time for the baby but also enrich your child's emotional life. You can do this by making sure your partner, a grandparent, or another friend is part of your everyday routine. However, you must also make time to give your older child special attention without a demanding baby around. For instance, you could try asking your partner or another adult to take the baby out for walks so that you can establish a regular time alone with your older child.

PREPARING YOUR CHILD

The arrival of a new baby can be a difficult time for your existing child, who may feel left out and so demand more attention. Making plans and preparing your child for the new arrival could spare you the trauma of an unhappy older child. How you tell your child about the new baby can make a difference to how they view the event.

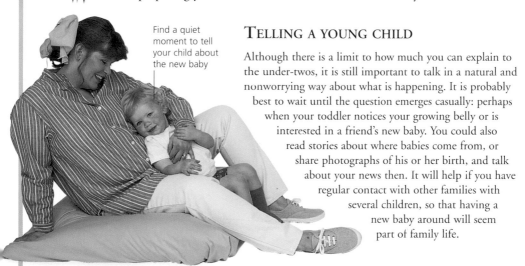

Find a quiet moment to tell your child about the new baby

TELLING A YOUNG CHILD

Although there is a limit to how much you can explain to the under-twos, it is still important to talk in a natural and nonworrying way about what is happening. It is probably best to wait until the question emerges casually: perhaps when your toddler notices your growing belly or is interested in a friend's new baby. You could also read stories about where babies come from, or share photographs of his or her birth, and talk about your news then. It will help if you have regular contact with other families with several children, so that having a new baby around will seem part of family life.

TELLING AN OLDER CHILD

The older the child, the more you can explain and the earlier you can share your news. An older child may be interested in what is happening to you and how the baby grows; encourage him or her to feel the baby move inside you. You could involve your child in choosing a name for the new baby. All this will help to make the coming birth an important family event.

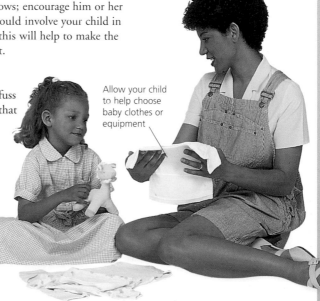

Allow your child to help choose baby clothes or equipment

Family and friends can help

Encourage family and friends to make a fuss of the older child. Discuss your concern that your child should not feel that all the attention is focused on the new baby.

Presents

Your new baby will receive plenty of presents, which may make your other child feel left out. When you pack for the hospital, wrap up a gift for your child from the new baby. Ask grandparents and close family to bring something for the older child when they come to see the new baby.

DRESSING FOR THE OCCASION

How you dress during your pregnancy obviously depends on your own personal taste and your lifestyle. When it comes to buying maternity clothes, you will find that there is a large choice available: department stores, specialist shops, mail order catalogs, and even some fashion chain stores now offer up-to-date and fashionable maternity wear. You may not wish or need to buy many special maternity outfits; a selection of large shirts or sweaters, a few loose-fitting dresses, and some maternity leggings could easily carry you through most of your pregnancy.

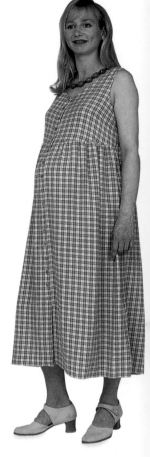

WHAT TO BUY

You don't need to spend a fortune on expensive maternity clothes. Instead, you can buy just a few basic items, like those listed below, and then treat yourself to a few special garments.

- Maternity trousers or leggings
- Maternity dresses
- Loose-fitting shirts
- Large sweaters or cardigans
- Support bras
- Maternity support tights or stockings
- Cotton socks
- Comfortable, low-heeled shoes
- Nightgowns (preferably with a front opening so that you can wear them for breastfeeding)

Optional extras
- Good jacket (especially if working during pregnancy)
- A dressy outfit
- Maternity swimsuit
- Maternity exercise leotard and leggings
- Sneakers

WHEN TO BUY

Most women start looking at looser clothing in the third or fourth month when their waistbands can no longer be fastened. However, don't buy everything at once: you'll need to buy clothes in stages to cope with your changing size and shape and different seasons.

SEASONAL CLOTHES
Bear in mind the changing seasons: you become pregnant in one season, but by the time you need big dresses, the weather will have changed.

WHY COMFORT COMES FIRST

Whatever style you prefer, make sure your clothes feel comfortable as well as look good. There is nothing worse than squeezing into a dress that binds under the arms and is tight across your breasts or belly. During pregnancy you are likely to feel much warmer and perspire more, so it is best to wear natural fibers, such as cotton, wool, or linen, that allow heat and moisture to escape.

BIG IS BEST
Large sweaters or shirts and layers of clothing work well in pregnancy, because they allow plenty of air to circulate and you can peel off a layer when you get too warm.

WHAT TO WEAR AT WORK

Your job may require more of a wardrobe than the casual clothes you can wear at home, particularly if there is a strict dress code, so that you may have to invest some money in more formal maternity wear. You will get the most value out of separates: build different outfits around a good basic jacket or suit, a skirt and/or trousers with elasticated waists, loose-fitting shirts, and a few dresses that can be mixed and matched.

FITTED ELEGANCE
You do not have to wear loose clothes. Fitted and tailored suits are fine, as long as you are comfortable.

SHOES

Low-heeled, comfortable shoes are best in pregnancy. Your feet, ankles, and calves need good support because the ligaments (like those in the pelvis) can easily become stretched. As you get bigger, your balance is altered; high heels can make you feel unsteady on your feet. Also, high heels encourage bad posture, which could cause back problems. In late pregnancy, feet and ankles can swell and you may temporarily need a larger shoe size. Choose shoes with a nonslip sole.

UNDERWEAR

The most important items in your maternity wardrobe should be new bras; be sure to invest in ones that are well-fitting and supporting.

Support Bras
Your breasts enlarge almost at once and can become very swollen and heavy; they will sag without support, especially after the baby is born or is weaned. A good support bra is essential but do not guess your size; measure yourself or have a fitting done at a lingerie shop or department store each time you buy. For comfort, choose cotton-rich maternity bras with wide shoulder straps and a deep band under the cups. Buy at least two at first, then more as your breasts grow. When you have had your baby, buy two or three nursing bras for breastfeeding. Some women like to wear a sleep bra for nighttime support.

Briefs
It is best to avoid briefs with a tight waistband and leg elastic that may feel constricting. Choose small minibriefs that fit under your belly, or maternity briefs; these have an expanding front panel in stretch fabric (see right).

Support tights and stockings
Support hosiery can help prevent or reduce tired, aching legs, swollen ankles, and varicose veins, particularly if you work through your pregnancy.

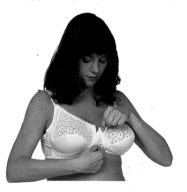

NURSING BRAS
An ordinary bra is awkward to undo at the back when breastfeeding, so a nursing bra with cups that can be opened individually at the front is essential. Some have cups that unzip, others unhook from the strap.

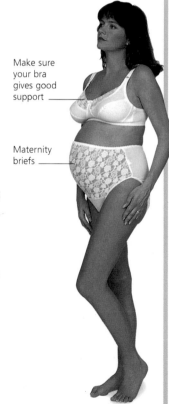

Make sure your bra gives good support

Maternity briefs

BASIC NEEDS
Well-fitting maternity underwear should support you and increase your comfort.

TWINS AND MULTIPLE BIRTHS

Q WILL I NEED TO TAKE EXTRA CARE OF MYSELF?

A Being told you are expecting twins or more can be a shock, particularly if you have no family history of twins. Although you will get more prenatal care (see p. 22), you will also need to take better care of yourself than if you were having one baby, but there is no reason to consider yourself an invalid. Making sure that you eat a healthy diet and have enough rest are important because your body has to work even harder. You probably won't go to full term; if you work, you might go on leave earlier than planned. If you have older children, try to arrange for help so that you don't feel exhausted.

WHEN WILL I FIND OUT?

Your doctor or midwife may suggest an early ultrasound if you look large for your due date or have a history of twins in your family. However, you are most likely to learn that you are having twins at a routine ultrasound, at 12 to 14 or 18 to 22 weeks. On rare occasions, the second baby is missed in an earlier scan as it is hidden behind the first. In the past, some mothers have been told they were expecting two babies as late as 24 weeks.

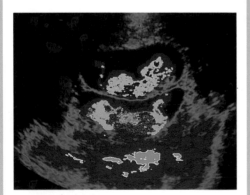

ULTRASOUND SCAN OF TWINS IN THE WOMB
Taken after the first trimester, this scan shows each twin (red and yellow) enclosed in its own amniotic sac; they are fraternal.

Q HOW MUCH LARGER WILL I BECOME WITH A MULTIPLE BIRTH?

A It is not just the weight of the babies that makes you bigger, but also the fact that you are carrying an extra or larger placenta, twice the normal amount of amniotic fluid, as well as extra body fluids. Your belly will show earlier if you are expecting more than one baby, becoming visible at 11 weeks, a week or two earlier than if you were expecting a single baby. At 20 weeks, your stomach may start to enlarge quite rapidly, and as early as 32 weeks, your womb will start to press against your ribcage. However, it is unlikely that you will reach the full 40 weeks of pregnancy; most twins or triplets are born at 36 to 37 weeks because of the womb's capacity. They are also usually smaller than single babies.

Q WILL I HAVE TO EAT MORE IF I AM EXPECTING MORE THAN ONE BABY?

A If you are expecting twins, you may not necessarily have to eat more, but you will have to pay special attention to what you do eat. You are providing nutrients for two growing babies, maintaining your own energy levels, and also coping with the extra physical demands that are being made on your body, so it is very important that you obtain the essential nutrients from your diet (see p 100). You may also feel extremely tired, sometimes to the point of exhaustion. Enlist your partner's help with the shopping and cooking so that you are able to get enough rest during the day and do not miss healthy meals.

Q CAN HAVING TWINS HARM MY BODY?

A The idea of carrying and giving birth to more than one baby can seem daunting. You may be concerned about the effect of this on your body. Some women worry that their womb, or even their abdomen, may be damaged by carrying more than one baby. This is unlikely; as your womb becomes stretched in the final part of your pregnancy, you are more likely to go into early labor. Another worry is that having twins means worse stretch marks. Stretch marks are probably linked more with the collagen and elastin content of your skin than the size of your belly – or its contents.

Q DOES HAVING TWINS MEAN I SHOULD EXPECT TWICE THE DISCOMFORT?

A With twins, you experience all the "normal" pregnancy problems, but the symptoms may be exaggerated and occur earlier in pregnancy.

■ **Morning sickness** This may be more severe with a multiple pregnancy and last beyond the first trimester.

■ **Anemia** You will be more prone to this blood condition, which is caused by a deficiency of iron, because of the extra demands on your iron supplies. Your blood will be tested for anemia. Extra iron and folic acid supplements will treat the condition.

■ **Breathlessness and abdominal pain** As your womb presses against your diaphragm, and your heart works harder pumping more blood around your body, you may find that you are short of breath and experience abdominal pain. This will be more pronounced if you are expecting twins, so you should avoid overexerting yourself. Sitting in one position for too long is inadvisable because it can further aggravate abdominal pain. Try to eat little and often rather than eat big meals that will bloat your abdomen or give you indigestion.

■ **Backache** This may be worse with twins, because of the extra weight you are carrying

■ **Varicose veins and hemorrhoids** These are more likely, because of the extra pressure on your veins. Avoid standing for too long, get regular, gentle exercise, and wear pregnancy support tights.

Q AM I MORE LIKELY TO SUFFER FROM SERIOUS CONDITIONS?

A Yes, in a multiple pregnancy, you are more vulnerable to certain complications, such as preeclampsia and edema (see p. 127), and these may occur at an earlier stage of pregnancy than is usual. The chances of premature labor are increased if you are expecting more than one baby. If your babies are born prematurely, they may need to be placed in intensive care or an incubator after the birth (see p. 214). However, because you and your babies are at a higher risk with a multiple pregnancy, you will receive extra care and attention from your doctor or midwife, and will have more checkups than women who expect only one baby. Any potential problems should, therefore, be picked up at an early stage and the relevant action taken. Your doctor or midwife will probably suggest extra rest.

Q WHERE CAN I GET HELP AND ADVICE?

A There may be an organization in your area that offers support and which can put you in touch with mothers of twins or provide useful brochures. Talk to other parents of twins who will understand your feelings and offer practical help; they may be able to offer advice on how to cope with the financial burden of having more than one child. You will also be able to see and hear how they managed with two babies after the birth, and how they manage their children now (see p. 232).

DISCUSSION POINT

DO I NEED TO REST MORE?

Resting in the hospital
Women expecting twins used to be routinely admitted to the hospital weeks before the birth because it was thought that this reduced the incidence of premature labor and meant that the babies were able to grow more. However, studies have shown that enforced bed rest does not necessarily prevent premature labor or increase the chances of the babies' survival. In some special cases, if you are expecting triplets or quadruplets, hospitalization for rest and observation is still advised, especially if you have had complications during your pregnancy. It is no longer routine medical advice.

Make sure you take it easy
Getting enough rest and relaxation is especially important with a multiple pregnancy because you will be much more tired. If you get plenty of rest you will feel better; this may also keep problems, such as varicose veins and backache, at bay. Rest and relaxation are also important because you are more likely to suffer from high blood pressure if you are having more than one child, which can lead to preeclampsia (see p. 127). Gentle exercise, such as swimming and walking, is an ideal way to relax. Swimming can also be very effective in relieving backache and any general aches and pains that you experience.

SEX DURING PREGNANCY

Q WE ENJOY OUR SEX LIFE – IS IT SAFE TO MAKE LOVE WHILE I'M PREGNANT?

A It is usually perfectly safe for couples to enjoy a sexual relationship throughout pregnancy. In fact, a healthy sex life is positively beneficial, because as well as maintaining your relationship with your partner, it helps you to unwind, reminds you that you are a sensual woman as well as a mother-to-be, and it can also be a very good form of exercise. Sexual intercourse cannot hurt your baby, safely cushioned in a bag of fluid within your womb; even deep penetration is not harmful to your baby.

Q WHEN IS SEX NOT A GOOD IDEA DURING PREGNANCY?

A You may be advised to avoid sex if you have a history of miscarriage or premature labors. It may also be sensible to avoid intercourse if there is unexplained bleeding, and if the amniotic sac has broken. Sex is also not advised in cases of placenta previa, or where the placenta has partially dislodged itself from the wall of the womb (see p. 128), because this could increase the risk of bleeding. If you have an infection, this is not a reason to stop having sex, because your baby is protected by the membranes and a mucous plug that seals the cervix.

WHICH SEXUAL POSITIONS ARE COMFORTABLE?

If you needed an incentive to be more adventurous in lovemaking, pregnancy will provide it. Most positions are feasible in the first months, but once your belly grows, you will not want your partner to rest on it.

Later, you may feel enormous and find moving difficult, so try more comfortable positions that take your belly and tender breasts into account. Not all the positions below will suit you, but it could be fun finding the ones that do.

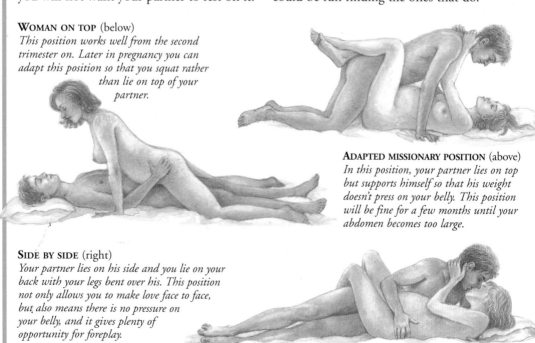

WOMAN ON TOP (below)
This position works well from the second trimester on. Later in pregnancy you can adapt this position so that you squat rather than lie on top of your partner.

ADAPTED MISSIONARY POSITION (above)
In this position, your partner lies on top but supports himself so that his weight doesn't press on your belly. This position will be fine for a few months until your abdomen becomes too large.

SIDE BY SIDE (right)
Your partner lies on his side and you lie on your back with your legs bent over his. This position not only allows you to make love face to face, but also means there is no pressure on your belly, and it gives plenty of opportunity for foreplay.

Q WHY HAS MY PARTNER LOST INTEREST IN SEX NOW THAT I'M PREGNANT?

A To some men there is nothing sexier than a woman bearing his child; to others it can all seem troubling and bring out a strong protective instinct. Some men fear that sex will hurt you or harm the baby, or bring on premature labor. Try talking to your partner about his fears and anxieties, and reassure him about how safe and natural sex is during pregnancy.

Q I'M SUDDENLY MORE INTERESTED IN SEX. AM I NORMAL?

A This is a perfectly normal way to feel during pregnancy. Some women feel at their most sensual when they are pregnant and their sex life can become more enjoyable than ever. This may be because hormonal changes have created a great sense of well-being and contentment and your body has become more sensitive to touch. An increased blood flow to the genital area can also enhance your sensitivity and sexual response.

Q WHY AM I AVOIDING SEX?

A The changes that make one woman feel more sensual can make another want to avoid sex altogether. Some women feel too sick or tired even to think of sex in the first months. Later on, their belly gets in the way. You may find the whole business too awkward. All of this is normal and reasonable. It is only a problem if your partner is not sympathetic to the physical and psychological changes you are undergoing.

Q I'VE LOST INTEREST IN SEX – WILL THIS DAMAGE OUR RELATIONSHIP?

A You must be honest with your partner about these feelings, because he may interpret your lack of interest in sex as a lack of interest in him. Also, dutiful or resentful sex is worse for your relationship than no sex at all. You could try being adventurous in your lovemaking by experimenting with different, more comfortable positions (see left). Remember too that there are other ways to express your love apart from sex; a cuddle or a massage can also provide intimate communication with your partner (see p. 114).

Q CAN SEX TRIGGER LABOR?

A If sperm comes in contact with the neck of your womb (cervix) when you are near or past your due date, it can help to trigger labor by ripening the cervix and causing it to efface. This is because sperm contains a substance called prostaglandin and artificial prostaglandins are used to ripen the cervix if labor has to be artificially started (induced). However, don't worry that having sex during pregnancy will cause you to go into premature labor. The cervix will ripen only when it is ready, at term.

Q CAN AN ORGASM CAUSE A MISCARRIAGE?

A No, there is nothing to link orgasm and miscarriage. However, in late pregnancy, orgasm can set off Braxton-Hicks' contractions (see p. 81), which can last for half an hour. These can seem like labor, but are tightenings of your womb rather than real labor contractions.

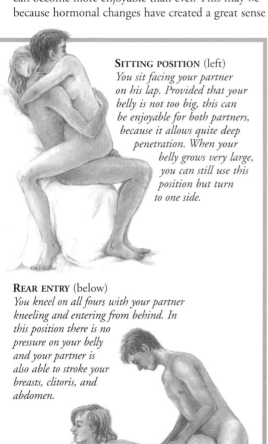

SITTING POSITION (left)
You sit facing your partner on his lap. Provided that your belly is not too big, this can be enjoyable for both partners, because it allows quite deep penetration. When your belly grows very large, you can still use this position but turn to one side.

REAR ENTRY (below)
You kneel on all fours with your partner kneeling and entering from behind. In this position there is no pressure on your belly and your partner is also able to stroke your breasts, clitoris, and abdomen.

YOUR CHANGING EMOTIONS

Q HOW AM I SUPPOSED TO FEEL NOW THAT I AM PREGNANT?

A Just as no two women are the same, there is no set emotional response to pregnancy. Pregnancy heightens the emotions – you have probably never felt so elated and yet so fearful. You may now find yourself moved at the sight of babies, even if you had little interest in them before, or weeping over bad news on the television. You may daydream about your baby or feel anxious about the future. It can feel like being on an emotional seesaw.

Q WE PLANNED THIS BABY, YET MY FIRST REACTION WAS TO CRY. WHY?

A Mixed emotions are normal, so don't feel that something is wrong if you are not happy all through pregnancy. There is a big difference between planning a baby and finding out that you are pregnant. A baby changes your lifestyle, and even women who have longed for a child will feel some pangs over the potential loss of freedom.

Q ALL I EVER THINK ABOUT NOW IS MY PREGNANCY. AM I BEING OBSESSIVE?

A As your pregnancy progresses, your thoughts may turn inward, especially if this is your first baby. It is a natural reaction to be filled with wonder at your growing body. Don't worry about being a "baby bore" – if you enjoy your pregnancy, revel in it. Share your thoughts with your partner so that he is involved in what is happening.

Q I KEEP FORGETTING THINGS. IS THIS BECAUSE I'M PREGNANT?

A Opinions differ on this. Some health professionals declare that absent-mindedness during pregnancy is largely exaggerated. Some women report that this mental vagueness is one of their most obvious symptoms, but others experience no unusual forgetfulness. Whether you feel this way or not, there is no need to feel anxious about it. Writing lists and notes to yourself may help.

DISCUSSION POINT

WHY AM I EXPERIENCING SUCH HIGHS AND LOWS?

Huge mood swings are common in pregnancy. If you feel at the mercy of your emotions, it helps to understand why this is happening to you.

Hormonal developments
Your body is flooded with hormones (see p. 73). These hormonal changes can affect your emotional as well as your physical self. The effects vary with each stage of your pregnancy and also differ from woman to woman. You will probably feel at your most erratic in the first months of your pregnancy, settle into a serene midpregnancy, then experience more ups and downs in your final trimester.

Facing change
Although your hormones may be affecting your moods, it is perhaps unfair to blame your changing emotions entirely on hormones. You are

also having to come to terms with a momentous life change. Most women with children agree that having their first baby had a far greater impact on their lives than any other event, including marriage. You can't foresee the effect that the experience of looking after and caring for a new baby will have on you and your partner. So together with pleasant daydreams and eager anticipation, you may also experience darker emotions of fear and anxiety. If you feel very depressed, however, talk to your doctor or midwife (see p. 126).

Talking to others
It will seem much worse if you keep your thoughts and emotions to yourself. Talk over with your partner any concerns you may have or discuss your fears at childbirth education classes. You may find that other pregnant women, who seem blissfully happy on the outside, are experiencing the same inner anxieties and mixed emotions.

Q **I HAVE VIVID DREAMS, ESPECIALLY OF LOSING MY BABY. IS THIS AN OMEN?**

A No, many mothers-to-be report having colorful dreams – some are happy, and others are more like nightmares. These dreams probably reflect your heightened emotions and uncertainty about the future, but you should not worry about them. It is also probable that your sleep pattern is fairly disturbed, so you are more likely to remember any dreams you have.

Q **I'M SURE SOMETHING IS WRONG WITH MY BABY. IS THIS A NORMAL FEELING?**

A Anxieties about the future often translate into fears for the health of your unborn child. Most pregnant women worry at some stage that their baby will be born with something wrong, despite having had tests that indicate there are no problems. This may be because they have had a previous miscarriage, or because there is a family history of abnormalities. Some mothers who have had one normal baby fear they will not be so lucky the next time, and others just cannot believe that they will produce a healthy child. If routine tests are all clear, it is unlikely that anything is wrong. However, no matter how many tests you have, there is no absolute guarantee that there will be no problems. If you are particularly worried or concerned, talk to your doctor or midwife.

Q **I CAN'T WAIT TO HAVE MY BABY. WHY DO I FEEL SO IMPATIENT?**

A By the time you have reached the last few weeks, you will probably feel as if you've been pregnant forever. It has been a long nine months' wait and the closer you get to your due date, the more impatient you are likely to be for labor to start and the baby to be born. Try to relax and to wait calmly (see p. 112).

Q **WHY AM I CONSUMED WITH REDECORATING THE BABY'S ROOM?**

A Toward the end of their pregnancy, many women feel an intense urge to redecorate the baby's room, shop for baby clothes, or clean closets. This is known as "nesting" and may be a sign that your baby is due soon. However, if you have recently stopped working, it may be that you simply feel the need to be active and doing something, but you should try to resist tackling any very ambitious projects because you will need to gather your energy for giving birth and the early weeks of pregnancy.

MAINTAINING A POSITIVE RELATIONSHIP

Pregnancy brings changes which can place a strain on emotional and physical relationships. Mutual understanding and a positive attitude can, however, help to enrich your life together.

Offering support
It is important that you both feel you are going through your pregnancy together. Talking about what is happening can help you to understand each other's changing needs and anxieties. Sharing the stresses as well as the joys of pregnancy can create a powerful bond between you.

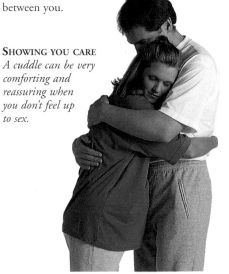

SHOWING YOU CARE
A cuddle can be very comforting and reassuring when you don't feel up to sex.

Making time for each other
Changes in your body and emotions mean that sex is not always top of your agenda in pregnancy; this can sometimes lead to tension. Try not to dwell on how often you have sex, and instead make those times you do make love very special. If you find making love uncomfortable, try new positions (see p. 90) or nonpenetrative sex, such as masturbation, oral sex, or massage. Make time to do other things you enjoy together. This can be a special time for you both as you make the transition from life as a couple to life as a family.

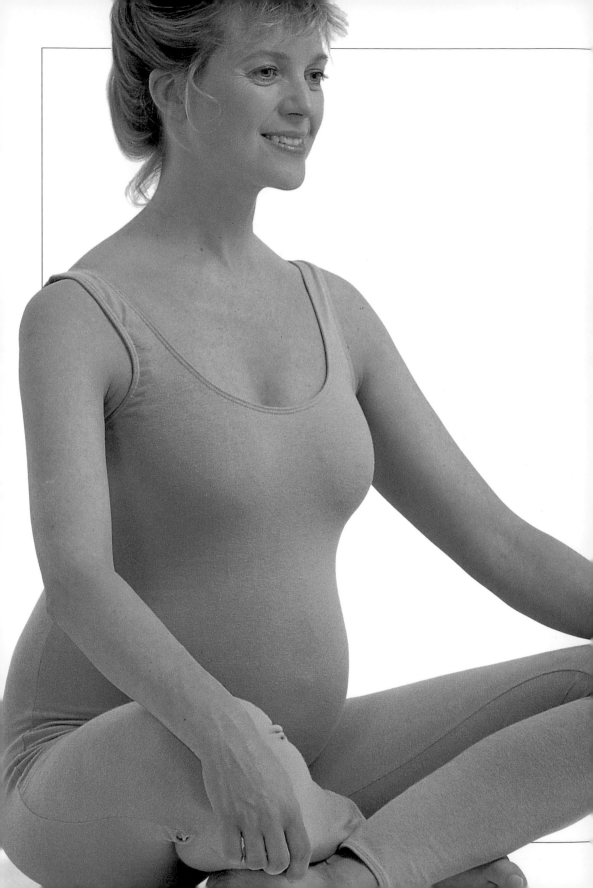

STAYING FIT AND HEALTHY

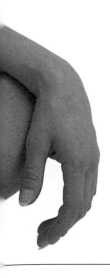

Pregnancy and childbirth place great demands on your stamina and health, so it is important to keep yourself healthy right up to and after the birth of your baby. The focus here is on giving you the knowledge, motivation, and confidence to maintain a healthy pregnancy. To prepare yourself fully for the delivery you need to eat wisely and well, keep supple, and learn how to relax to reduce tension and stress. This chapter discusses ideal pregnancy diets, exercise routines, and healthy lifestyles, which foods and drugs to avoid in pregnancy, and those complementary medicines and techniques that can benefit you and your baby.

TAKING CARE OF YOURSELF

Q SHOULD I TAKE EXTRA CARE OF MYSELF NOW THAT I'M PREGNANT?

A The more healthy and relaxed you are, the better you will be able to cope with the demands of pregnancy. A healthy lifestyle combines many factors: a balanced diet, regular exercise, and lots of rest. All of these will give you more energy and could help you avoid some of the discomforts associated with pregnancy. For instance, if you eat a balanced diet with plenty of fiber, you will be less likely to suffer from constipation, a common complaint in pregnancy.

Q WHAT CAN I DO TO STAY HEALTHY?

A Being healthy means eating the right foods (see p. 100) and getting regular exercise. This involves not only prenatal exercises (see p. 106), but also aerobic activities, such as swimming, and walking. Remember, however, that this is not a good time to begin a strenuous workout regimen.

Q WILL MY BABY BENEFIT IF I LEAD A HEALTHY LIFESTYLE?

A Yes, in general, the healthier and happier you are, the better it is for your baby's development. Many things that you eat or drink in pregnancy can affect your baby, so it is sensible to eat healthfully and avoid anything that may be harmful or toxic (see p. 98). If you make the effort to have a healthier lifestyle, your baby will ultimately benefit, and you may also feel better.

Q WHERE SHOULD I BEGIN?

A Take a long, hard look at how you treat your body and then think of ways in which you could be kinder to yourself. If you smoke cigarettes, use street drugs (even socially), or drink, seriously try to stop for the health of your pregnancy (see p. 102). You may have to make a few adjustments to your diet (see p. 100) or plan an exercise routine. Be positive about your new lifestyle – you are not only helping yourself and your baby, but you may also find that you actually enjoy being healthier. Your child needs healthy parents; look at the healthy habits you adopt now as insurance for your future good health.

Q WILL MY PREGNANCY AND DELIVERY BE EASIER IF I'M IN GOOD SHAPE?

A The stronger you are now, the more stamina you will have during the labor and the easier your recovery will be after birth. If you exercise regularly and eat healthfully, you feel more energetic and will be better able to look after a new baby. You are also more likely to regain your figure faster. Exercise is also a great stress reliever; if you feel physically fit and well, you will enjoy your pregnancy more and may be less vulnerable to feelings of anxiety.

Q I HAVE PROBLEMS RELAXING AND TAKING IT EASY. WHAT CAN I DO?

A Learning relaxation techniques can help you unwind throughout pregnancy (see p. 112). Looking after yourself also means being sure that you do not overexert yourself, which can lead to exhaustion. This is easier to say than do if you have a demanding job and/or other children, but it is important to make time to relax so that stress does not build up. Taking time out for a massage is another great way to relax (see p. 114).

Q HOW CAN I LOOK MY BEST?

A Pregnancy changes your body in ways you may not expect: as well as your growing belly, it also affects your skin, hair, teeth, and nails. You need, therefore, to take extra care of yourself during pregnancy (see opposite). Pampering yourself can give you a boost if you feel huge and ungainly during late pregnancy. Aromatherapy, massage, and other therapeutic beauty treatments are just some of the beneficial ways in which you can do this.

Q I FEEL SO HOT AND BOTHERED ALL THE TIME. WHY?

A As more blood circulates around your body, you may feel warmer and find that you perspire more. This can make you prone to rashes in your skin creases – in the groin area and under the breasts – so keep fresh by washing more frequently. Try not to put on too much weight (see p. 79); this will increase your discomfort and make you feel even hotter.

Looking good, feeling great

Hormonal changes during pregnancy can make you look healthy and radiant, but can also have the opposite effect.

Your complexion

The extra blood circulating in your body can mean that because your skin retains more moisture, it becomes more supple and less acne-prone. However, pregnancy hormones can cause certain problems: estrogen slows oil production, dries skin, and can darken freckles. Because skin texture can change, you may need a different moisturizer. Your doctor will tell you to stop taking or using acne medication in pregnancy; they can be harmful to the baby.

Oily skin

If your skin is not usually oily, don't be too concerned, as this will probably be a temporary condition during your pregnancy. Use an astringent lotion as part of your daily routine and a special moisturizer for oily skin. If you wear foundation, make sure that you use one with an oil-free base.

Dry skin

Avoid using soap, which can dry out skin; use a baby lotion or gentle facial or body wash instead. Using bath oil can help to moisturize your skin, but you should not soak for too long in the bath as this can dry your skin even more. Use moisturizer morning and evening and avoid drying astringents.

Gum infection is more likely in pregnancy, so get your teeth checked regularly

Your hair may be thicker and healthier during your pregnancy

Your nails may grow faster and break more easily than usual

Your skin will be affected by increased level of hormones and blood supply

Your hair

Hair grows in a cycle of loss and regrowth. When you are pregnant, your hair remains in the growth phase, which means it may be thicker and possibly shinier. For some women, this is good; their hair looks better than ever. For others, however, it means more unmanageable hair. If you are among the latter, you may find a shorter haircut easier to maintain. Changing your shampoo to a gentler variety may also help. For several months after the birth, you may shed a dramatic amount of hair as the growth phase of pregnancy comes to an end. Don't worry, you will not go bald; your hair should soon reestablish its normal growth-and-loss pattern.

Your teeth and gums

As soon as you are pregnant, make an appointment to see your dentist. Pregnancy makes your gums spongy and prone to infection, so it is important to have your teeth checked and cleaned regularly. You must tell the dentist you are pregnant, because you should avoid X-rays unless necessary.

Your nails

These may grow faster during pregnancy, or become brittle and break more easily than usual. If this is the case, keep them short and wear gloves when gardening or doing housework.

EATING FOR HEALTH

Q WHAT SHOULD I BE EATING?

A You do not need a special diet just because you are pregnant, but you should eat healthfully as your body has to work especially hard during pregnancy. It is now known that what you eat can have a far-reaching effect on your child's health and development. You should therefore make sure that you have a healthy, well-balanced, varied diet and that you eat regularly and often. Aim to increase your daily calorie intake by about 250 calories – the equivalent of a banana, a portion of cereal, and milk.

Q WHICH FOODS ARE BEST?

A Advice on diet often includes suggestions to eat foods that are high in nutritional content, but which you might not particularly like or enjoy, such as yeast, wheat germ, or fish oil. It is far better to be as realistic as possible in your dietary goals – eat what you actually enjoy, because it is likely that if you do restrict yourself to an artificial (and possibly quite unappealing) diet, you will probably be far more tempted to indulge in an eating binge and will consequently put on unwanted pounds. Be sure, though, to get the basic nutrients in your core diet (see opposite and p. 100).

Q WHAT FOODS SHOULD I CUT OUT?

A Try to cut out very fatty foods such as the fat on pork, fried bacon, and creamy sauces. These are likely to make you feel nauseous in the first three months as well as contribute to weight gain. Look out for the hidden fat in convenience foods such as cookies, and cakes. Avoid certain foods that carry the risk of infection and damage to your baby (see chart, p. 102).

Q DO I NEED TO TAKE EXTRA VITAMINS?

A If your diet is balanced and adequate, you should not need to supplement it unless you are a vegetarian (see below). The exception is folic acid, which is necessary before conception and in the first trimester (see p. 102).

Q SHOULD I DRINK MORE FLUIDS?

A As your blood volume increases, you need to increase your fluid intake. Drink water rather than high-calorie soft drinks or sodas, which are high in sugar and can make nausea and heartburn worse. Even if you have fluid retention, do not cut your fluid intake; try to drink up to six glasses of water each day. Drinking fluids can also prevent constipation, a common problem in pregnancy.

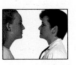

DISCUSSION POINT

HOW HEALTHY IS A VEGETARIAN DIET?

A healthy alternative
Being vegetarian does not necessarily mean that your diet is less healthy. You will, however, need to make up for the lack of meat-derived amino acids by eating a combination of incomplete vegetable proteins that are available in legumes, nuts, tofu, and grains, such as rice and whole grains. If you do this, your vegetarian diet can be healthy and should not affect your pregnancy. Indeed, you may have lower cholesterol levels than a meat eater and get more fiber from extra vegetables and fruit.

Getting the right nutrients
Your baby takes all the nutrients it needs from you. If you are not getting enough iron, this stresses your body and causes anemia (see p. 122); therefore, if you do not eat fish, eggs, nuts, and beans, you will almost certainly need iron and· calcium supplements, and probably vitamin B12. Besides making you feel very tired, anemia can affect fetal growth and your general health. Also, your body may lack the vigorous resources to counter any blood loss experienced during the birth.

Q ARE SNACKS AND JUNK FOOD BAD IN PREGNANCY?

A Snacking in itself is not a bad thing – it is much better than feeling faint from going without food for hours. If you can, you should try to snack on healthy foods. Fresh fruit, nuts, raisins, and raw vegetables are all much better for you than junk foods such as potato chips or french fries, chocolate, and doughnuts; these are high in calories, fats, sugars, and salt. Although they may produce a fast energy high, they do not contain the nutrients that will help your baby grow and develop. They are also likely to contain artificial coloring and additives. Of course, the occasional "junk" snack now and then will not do you any harm, but junk shouldn't play a large part in your diet.

Q CAN I STILL EAT FAST FOOD AND GO OUT TO RESTAURANTS?

A Although not as bad for you as junk foods, fast foods can still be high in fat and carbohydrates and, if they are kept heated for long periods of time, many of the vitamins and minerals in the food are destroyed. However, fresh pizza and restaurant meals can be nutritious for you, as long as you make sure that you maintain your basic core diet (see p. 100).

Q HOW MUCH WEIGHT SHOULD I GAIN?

A Your weight is not important during pregnancy unless you are very underweight or seriously overweight (see p. 79). What is more important is the fetal growth rate; this does not depend on your weight or how much you eat but rather on the efficiency of your placenta and the quality of your food, which supplies the appropriate nutrients. However, you will feel healthier and happier if you gain weight steadily and don't put on large amounts.

Q I HAVE BEEN TRYING TO LOSE WEIGHT. SHOULD I STAY ON A DIET?

A It is not a good idea to try to lose weight while you are pregnant. You should be eating a balanced and nutritious diet so that your baby can obtain all the nutrients he or she needs for healthy growth and development. You will also need plenty of energy to cope with the extra physical demands of pregnancy and labor. Even though you might not want to put on any weight, you will and should if your pregnancy is going well, and this is quite natural and essential.

WHAT BASIC NUTRIENTS DO I NEED?

Protein
This is an essential nutrient. After being broken down by the liver into amino acids, protein builds new tissue and is vital for the healthy fetal growth and development. On top of the normal daily requirement of 1.6 oz (45 g), you need an extra 1 oz (30 g) of protein a day during pregnancy. Protein is found in eggs, fish, meat, cheese, legumes, and dairy products.

Carbohydrates
An important food group that gives you most of your fuel or energy, carbohydrates are either sugar or starches. Eat starch-based ones, such as pasta, grains, and potatoes, rather than sugar-based ones (see p. 100), because these provide a slower release of energy over a longer period and have fewer calories.

Fats
These build cell walls and are essential for the development of the fetal nervous system, so although you should not eat too much, do not completely omit fats. Fats contain twice the calories per gram as protein and most carbohydrates, and too much fat increases your risk of heart disease and some cancers. Be moderate in your fat intake to protect your child's development and your health.

Vitamins
Necessary to maintain overall good health, some vitamins, like the B and C vitamins, aren't stored by the body, so you need to maintain a daily intake of these. All vitamins are essential, not only for the developing fetus but for your immune system, blood production, and nervous system. Folic acid is important in preventing spina bifida (see p. 12). Avoid eating liver, which is high in vitamin A, which can cause problems with fetal development (see p. 103).

Minerals
Iron facilitates many chemical processes in your body and is essential for the production of hemoglobin in red blood cells. Without iron, your body can't produce hemoglobin and you will become anemic (see p. 122). Calcium is needed for healthy bones and teeth and is also important in pregnancy. Zinc helps heal wounds and aids many digestive processes.

STAYING FIT AND HEALTHY

WHAT IS A BALANCED DIET?

You should eat sufficient protein, vitamins, carbohydrates, fats, and minerals, as well as fiber, every day to ensure a balanced diet. The food pyramid (right) shows the food groups and how much of them you should eat. You will be healthier if you limit your intake of saturated fats and sugar (top), and salt (sodium), but eat more protein for growth and carbohydrates for energy (bottom). The menu (opposite) shows a nutritious daily diet.

Fats, oils, and sweets
Use sparingly

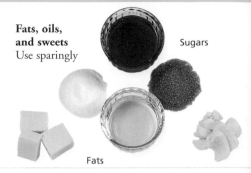

Sugars

Fats

Proteins – eggs, meat, poultry, fish, nuts, legumes, dairy products
4–6 servings of protein; 2–4 servings of dairy products a day

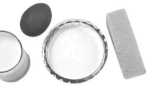
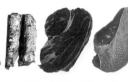

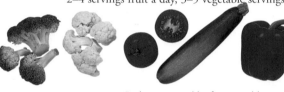

Nuts and legumes

Eggs and dairy products

Fish, meat, and poultry

Fruit and vegetables
2–4 servings fruit a day, 3–5 vegetable servings

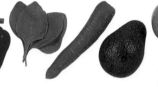
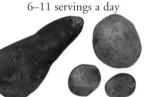

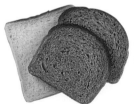

Red, green, and leafy vegetables

Carbohydrates – bread, cereal, rice, grain, pasta
6–11 servings a day

Potatoes

Grains

Rice

YOUR CORE DIET

These are the basic food groups and the quantities that you need for good health during pregnancy. These foods also contain important vitamins and minerals. Limit eating in restaurants and ordering take-outs. Make sure that your nutritional needs are met and your diet should be adequate.

Fats and sugars
Eat these in moderation. You must eat fats for your health, but they are high in calories. Of the two types of fat, saturated and unsaturated, eat less saturated fats (animal fat, cheese, cream, and butter) because they are high in cholesterol. Unsaturated fats (poly and mono) such as sunflower, olive, and safflower oils are better for your heart. Avoid sweet snacks: these are high in empty calories.

Eggs, meat, fish, nuts, legumes
4–6 servings a day of any of the following:
- 3 oz/85 g red meat or poultry
- 4–6 oz/113–170 g fish
- 1–2 oz/28–57 g cheese or 1 egg
- 4 oz/113 g legumes, grains, cereal
Eggs, meat, fish, and dairy foods are good sources of protein – essential when pregnant or breastfeeding. Vegetarian proteins include tofu, nuts, grains, and legumes.

THE FOOD PYRAMID

Eating sensibly during and after pregnancy means choosing foods from all the groups shown here. Make sure that you limit your intake of fats (top), eat adequate protein, and increase your fruits and carbohydrates (bottom).

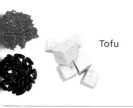

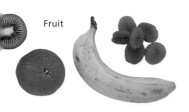

Tofu

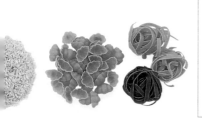

Fruit

Pasta

A SUGGESTED MENU FOR PREGNANCY

This menu gives you an idea of just how much food your daily diet should contain so that you get enough of the basic nutrients for you and your developing baby.

Breakfast

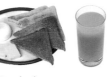

Cereal with low-fat milk

Poached egg and toast

Fruit Juice

Morning snack

A piece of fruit

Lunch

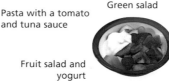

Pasta with a tomato and tuna sauce

Green salad

Glass of water

Afternoon snack

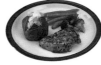

Fruit salad and yogurt

Milkshake and cookies

Evening meal

Evening drink

Chicken, baked potato, and fresh vegetables

Roll and butter

Fruit juice

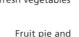

Fruit pie and ice cream

Herbal tea or warm milk

Dairy products

2–4 servings a day of any of the following:
- 1 cup low-fat milk
- 1–2 oz/28–57 g cheese
- 1 cup yogurt

Dairy products provide protein, fat, calcium (for healthy teeth and bones), and vitamins A, B, and D. Low-fat milk contains the same calcium and vitamin content but much less fat than whole milk.

Fruit and vegetables

5–9 servings a day of any of the following:
- 3 oz/85 g vegetables (at least one dark green, leafy vegetable)
- 1 mixed salad
- 1 piece of fruit/dried fruit

These are good sources of fiber and vitamins B, C, and K; some provide potassium and zinc. Dark green vegetables provide iron, magnesium, and folic acid.

Carbohydrates

6–11 servings a day of any of the following:
- 1 slice whole grain bread
- 2–4 oz/57–113 g pasta, rice, or potatoes
- 1 2oz/57g portion of cereal

Starch-based carbohydrates are a source of slow-release energy, fiber, protein, and B vitamins. You need more of these when you are pregnant or breastfeeding.

HEALTHY YOU, HEALTHY BABY

Q HOW CAN I MAKE SURE I WON'T DAMAGE MY BABY'S HEALTH?

A A lot of what you eat, drink, or inhale passes through your body to your baby. It is therefore best to cut out things known to be harmful, such as alcohol, smoking, and drugs, and avoid potentially harmful foods (see panel, below).

Q SHOULD I QUIT SMOKING?

A Yes. Smoking (and even passive smoking) reduces the oxygen and nutrients passing via the placenta to your baby. If you or your partner smoke, your baby is more likely to have a low birthweight and be vulnerable to problems in the first months of life. The risk of bleeding, miscarriage, or premature birth also increases.

Q I'M A HEAVY SMOKER. HOW CAN I QUIT SMOKING?

A You may find the decision to stop smoking easy if the queasiness of early pregnancy makes the thought of smoking sickening. If not, then giving up or cutting down can be very hard. It will help if you have support from your partner or another smoker who also wants to give up. You could join a support group, which will offer you companionship and advice. Try to quit smoking completely; it may be difficult, but the health benefits to you and your child are enormous. If you find it impossible to stop smoking altogether, then cut down to fewer than five cigarettes a day. There are other techniques to help you stop smoking, which include aversion therapy, hypnosis, and acupuncture.

FOODS THAT MAY CAUSE INFECTIONS

Although the chance of contracting one of these rare infections is limited, you can better protect your health by following these basic guidelines:

Listeriosis
Caused by the bacterium *Listeria monocytogenes*, this is a very rare infection. Its symptoms are similar to flu and gastroenteritis (see p. 122), and it can cause miscarriage or stillbirth.

Toxoplasmosis
Usually symptomless (apart from mild flu symptoms), this can cause serious fetal problems. Caused by direct contact with the organism *Toxoplasma gondii*, it is found in cat feces, raw or undercooked meat (especially pork and lamb), and unpasteurized goats' milk.

Salmonella
Contamination with salmonella bacterium can cause bacterial food poisoning. This doesn't usually harm the baby directly, but illness involving a high temperature, vomiting, diarrhea, and dehydration could cause miscarriage or preterm labor.

WHICH FOOD	RISK
Liver and liver pâtés	Listeriosis
Unpasteurized dairy products, especially soft cheeses such as camembert, brie, and blue-veined cheeses	Listeriosis
Prepared "deli" or takeout meals, like chicken and seafood	Listeriosis
Undercooked meat, especially pork	Toxoplasmosis
Undercooked eggs and poultry	Salmonella
Undercooked beef, especially ground, and rarely, unpasteurized fruit juices	Escherichia coli (may result in infection, gastrointestinal distress, or, rarely, death)
Raw fish (sushi, sashimi)	E coli (Salmonella, gastrointestinal parasites)

Q SHOULD I DRINK ALCOHOL AT ALL?

A It is impossible to say if there is a safe limit for alcohol, because its effects vary from woman to woman. What is certain, however, is that regular heavy drinking (more than two drinks a day) can lead to mental and physical problems in your baby. To be safe, avoid alcohol completely in the first three months when the baby's major organs are developing. After this, it is probably safe to have an occasional glass of wine or beer with food.

Q IS IT SAFE TO TAKE ANY DRUGS OR MEDICINES?

A The message is simple: avoid all drugs, particularly in early pregnancy, unless your doctor prescribes them (see panel, right). If you buy any medicine over the counter, you must tell the pharmacist that you are pregnant. Doctors are cautious about prescribing drugs in pregnancy, particularly in the first trimester. Some drugs must be avoided altogether (see p. 233). Others are considered safe; these include acetaminophen, and some antibiotics, such as amoxicillin and erythromycin, which may be prescribed for throat and urinary tract infections.

Q WHAT IF I HAVE TO TAKE DRUGS THAT MIGHT BE HARMFUL?

A In special situations, your doctor or midwife may prescribe a drug that could be harmful to your baby. This will occur only if the condition for which the drug is given poses a greater risk to you or your baby's health than the drug. For example, quinine, used to treat malaria, can cause miscarriage or premature labor, but the risks from the disease are far greater. If you have epilepsy or a thyroid condition, this will also need thorough treatment, or the consequences for you and your baby can be severe (see p. 124).

Q WHY IS EATING LIVER NOT RECOMMENDED IN PREGNANCY?

A Until recently, pregnant women were advised to eat liver as a source of iron. However, we now know that, in addition to iron, liver contains high levels of vitamin A, which in large doses can cause birth defects. The current advice is to avoid all liver and liver products, such as pâté, especially in the first trimester when major fetal organs are developing. A balanced diet with dairy products, vegetables (especially carrots), and fruit, provides enough vitamin A.

STREET DRUGS AND YOUR BABY

Taking street drugs is inadvisable when pregnant because it exposes you and your baby to a range of hazards. Even the relatively harmless-seeming marijuana can cause problems for the baby. Apart from the direct risks listed below, you also risk contracting the HIV virus if you inject drugs with shared needles.

Ask for advice

Consult your doctor or a help group about the potential problems of using drugs during pregnancy. If you do regularly use street drugs, you must tell your midwife or the obstetrician about this, preferably before labor, because your baby may need care after the birth.

DRUG	EFFECT
Amphetamines	Causes low birth weight
Marijuana	Causes premature labor; possible risk of chromosomal abnormality
Cocaine	Causes premature labor, serious placental bleeding, and low birth weight
Ecstasy	Apart from the possible effects on you, such as dehydration and personality changes, taking ecstasy may increase the risk of serious bleeding from the placenta
Heroin and methadone	Causes low birth weight, premature labor, higher rate of twins. After delivery: baby suffers withdrawal symptoms, higher risk of seizures, increased risk of crib death (sudden infant death syndrome: SIDS)
LSD	Causes birth defects

NATURALLY HEALTHY

Q WHAT IS COMPLEMENTARY OR ALTERNATIVE MEDICINE?

A Any treatment that lies outside traditional medicine comes under this umbrella (it includes reflexology, homeopathy, acupuncture, aromatherapy, and Chinese medicine, as well as osteopathy and chiropractic). Complementary therapy can, however, also work alongside conventional medicine. A good complementary therapist aims to treat you as a whole person and, in addition to looking at specific symptoms, will consider your lifestyle, diet, and emotional well-being before prescribing any treatment.

Q CAN COMPLEMENTARY MEDICINES HELP ME DURING PREGNANCY?

A Complementary medicines were developed after centuries of use and observation, and although it can be hard to say exactly how effective these remedies are, they do appear to be successful for many people. You can experience many extra discomforts, such as backache, nausea, and constipation, during pregnancy; you could find that natural remedies offer you gentle relief and are the ideal alternative to drugs, which you should avoid at this time.

Q WHERE DO I OBTAIN COMPLEMENTARY MEDICINES?

A You can buy homeopathic and herbal remedies from registered practitioners. Some pharmacies also sell homeopathic remedies. You can prepare your own herbal remedies, but make sure you follow the recipes carefully and use the correct quantities. If you are considering other therapies, such as reflexology, acupuncture, or aromatherapy, see a qualified practitioner for advice and treatment.

Q ARE COMPLEMENTARY MEDICINES SAFE DURING PREGNANCY?

A Most are safe, but some herbal remedies and aromatherapy oils are not recommended during pregnancy. If you are in any doubt about what you can or cannot use, always ask a qualified professional for advice. Also discuss any doubts or worries with your doctor or midwife before starting any complementary treatments.

WHICH THERAPIES CAN BE USED?

Reflexology
To relieve disorders in other parts of the body, reflexologists apply pressure to specific points on the foot to stimulate nerve endings. In pregnancy reflexology can help ease many conditions such as circulatory problems, backache, and general pains, and is used with traditional medicine for more serious problems, such as high blood pressure or gestational diabetes. Some women use reflexology in labor as a form of pain relief.

Homeopathy
Homeopathic medicines stimulate your body's own healing mechanisms. Minuscule amounts of plant, animal, and mineral extracts are used: the smaller the dose, the more potent the treatment. Minor pregnancy-related ailments, including nausea, vomiting, heartburn, and indigestion, are amenable to homeopathic treatment, but very potent doses should not be taken.

Acupuncture
This branch of Chinese medicine is based on the idea that a life force, called "chi," flows through the body, and that disorders are as a result of imbalances in this flow. Balance is restored by the insertion of fine needles into specific points on the body to unblock the "chi." Many women find acupuncture helpful in pregnancy to treat complaints such as morning sickness, headaches, allergies, indigestion, and emotional problems, such as depression, as well as more serious problems like high blood pressure. Some women also use acupuncture during labor for pain relief.

Other remedies
Aromatherapy, which involves using essential oils taken from plants and applied with massage, can help you relax in pregnancy (see p. 114). It is impossible to mention every therapy here, but there are many different possibilities.

WHICH HERBAL REMEDIES CAN I TAKE IN PREGNANCY?

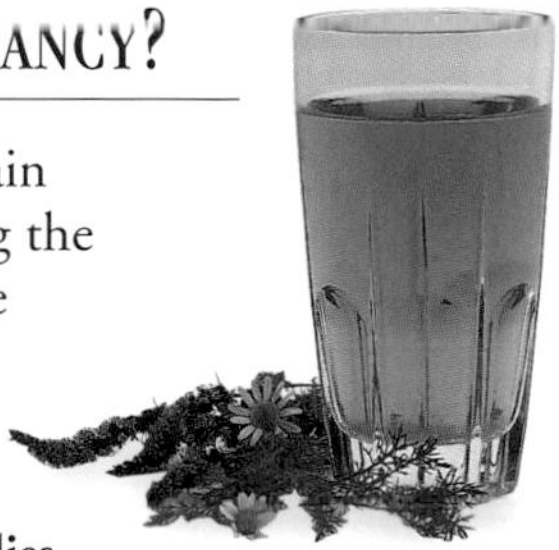

Medicinal herbs have been part of the healing traditions of certain cultures for thousands of years. Several herbal systems, including the complex Chinese system, have developed around the world. The more familiar Western herbalism, shown in the chart below, provides remedies for certain pregnancy problems.

How herbal medicine helps

Avoid all herbal remedies for the first three months of pregnancy. In later months, herbal medicines can help restore energy and to calm. In particular, herbal remedies can relieve many pregnancy ailments such as morning sickness, constipation, anemia, and heartburn. Tonic herbs can help in the preparation of the womb for childbirth. Postpartum teas, such as motherwort (*Leonurus cardiaca*), are said to help clear the uterus; do not take such teas in pregnancy.

Using herbal remedies

Herbal remedies come in several forms. Infusions are made by soaking approximately 1 oz (30 g) dried or about 2½ oz (75 g) fresh herbs in 2 cups boiling water for ten minutes. The mixture is strained and drunk hot or cold. A tincture, where herbs are preserved in alcohol and drops placed on or under the tongue, can be bought from a health food store or herbalist. Always check with your herbalist that the herbs you buy are safe for use in pregnancy.

AILMENT	HERBAL REMEDY	WHAT TO DO	EFFECT
Nausea	Ginger *Zinziber officinale*	Drink as an infusion or take 2–5 drops of tincture with water when needed	Has a soothing effect on the digestive system and helps prevent vomiting
	Peppermint *Mentha x piperita*	Drink as an infusion after meals or take in a tincture	Aids digestion, increasing the flow of digestive juices, and reduces nausea
Tension/anxiety	Lemon balm *Melissa officinalis*	Use in aromatherapy or as an infusion or take in a tincture with water	Acts as a relaxant and has a calming effect, relieving tension and mild depression
Depression	St. John's Wort *Hypericum perforatum*	Drink as an infusion or take in a tincture with water three times a day	Traditionally used to treat nervous complaints, this helps ease stress
Constipation	Dandelion *Taraxacum officinale* Crampbark *Viburnum opulus*	Drink as an infusion Take in a tincture with hot water twice a day	This can help stimulate the liver; acts as a gentle laxative
Heartburn	Cardamom *Eletteria cardamomum*	Drink as an infusion or take in a tincture three times a day	Has a soothing effect on most digestive problems; relieves gas and indigestion
Fatigue	Ginseng *Panax quinquefolius*	Take as a powder in a capsule	Acts as a stimulant and tonic; avoid high doses in pregnancy

STAYING FIT AND HEALTHY

EXERCISE IN PREGNANCY

Q HOW ACTIVE SHOULD I BE DURING MY PREGNANCY?

A Unless your lifestyle already keeps you very active with normal occupations such as housework, walking, or gardening, you will probably feel better if you keep up some form of regular, gentle exercise during your pregnancy. With a fairly inactive daily routine, exercise such as walking or swimming, will increase your fitness and stamina and will help you cope with the workload of pregnancy and the demands of labor. Listen to your body and stop exercising when it tells you to. It will probably not be until the final stages of your pregnancy that you feel too uncomfortable to exercise.

Q ARE THERE ANY SPECIAL EXERCISES FOR PREGNANCY?

A Yes, the pelvic floor exercises (see opposite). The weight of your womb and fetus place a great strain on the muscles of your pelvic floor. It is important to strengthen these muscles during your pregnancy to prevent tearing in labor, and also to aid recovery after birth. Exercising your pelvic floor muscles will help to support the weight of the womb, and can also help control the need to urinate. There are also specific exercises that help tone up your muscles and improve the suppleness of your joints that can make your pregnancy more comfortable (see p. 108) and relieve specific problems, like backache (see p. 110).

WHICH KIND OF EXERCISE IS BEST?

Swimming is an excellent exercise because the water supports your body weight and allows you to tone your muscles without strain. It can also improve your stamina. Some swimming pools or health clubs now offer water exercise classes designed for pregnant women. These are ideal for less confident swimmers because they are done while standing in shallow water. Brisk walking, yoga, and dancing are also good ways to keep fit and supple.

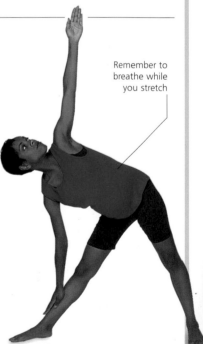

Remember to breathe while you stretch

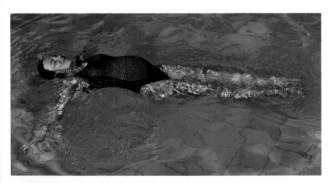

SWIMMING
This can be particularly enjoyable in late pregnancy because you will feel much lighter and the water will cool you. Avoid the breaststroke if you have pain in the symphysis pubis area or sacroiliac joints (see p. 83).

YOGA OR GENTLE STRETCHING
Gentle yoga or stretch exercises are excellent for releasing tension, increasing the mobility of joints, and improving circulation and breathing.

Q HOW OFTEN SHOULD I EXERCISE?

A Several times a week is ideal, but it's fine to vary the activity – swim one day, walk on another, and perhaps do an exercise class or yoga on a third. If you are used to this type of regular exercise, you can continue with it for as long as you feel comfortable, but always listen to your body and slow down if necessary. However, if you are new to exercise, you should start slowly, gradually building up stamina. A little stretching every other day is better than a long hard workout once a week.

Q ARE THERE SPECIAL EXERCISE CLASSES?

A There are now many classes organized specially for pregnant women. Some offer prenatal exercises, some are for yoga, others are childbirth education classes. Some gyms, pools, and health clubs also offer exercise classes in water run by qualified professionals.

Q WHAT SHOULD I WEAR?

A Make sure you wear supporting exercise footwear to prevent jarring and damage to the joints. Choose loose, comfortable clothes that won't make you overheat. It is a good idea to wear a support bra during any exercise.

Q WHEN SHOULD I AVOID VIGOROUS EXERCISE?

A There are certain times when vigorous exercise is not recommended in pregnancy: if you have previously had problems in pregnancy or your doctor or midwife has advised against it; if you have a temperature or feel unwell; in very hot weather. Most importantly, make sure that you do not exhaust or overexert yourself doing any exercise that you are not used to.

Q ARE THERE ANY PARTICULAR ACTIVITIES THAT I SHOULD AVOID?

A This is not the time to participate in violent or hazardous activities where there is a chance of injury to you or the baby. Activities or sports to avoid include strenuous athletics such as high jumping or sprinting, and any that require intense training; also, any high-risk activities, such as horseback riding and downhill skiing, that could result in physical injury. As always, if you are contemplating doing something you don't normally do, check with your midwife or doctor first.

THE PELVIC FLOOR

The pelvic floor supports the pelvic organs (the bladder, the womb, and part of the bowels). Pelvic muscles also help control your bladder and bowels. These muscles can be stretched by the weight of the womb; this causes discomfort and can result in stress incontinence (see p. 120).

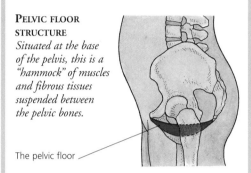

PELVIC FLOOR STRUCTURE
Situated at the base of the pelvis, this is a "hammock" of muscles and fibrous tissues suspended between the pelvic bones.

The pelvic floor

PELVIC FLOOR EXERCISES

Strengthen your pelvic floor muscles by pulling and squeezing in your anus, vagina, and urethra as if holding back the flow of urine. Hold and release.

Slow pull-ups
Pull up and hold the squeeze as hard as you can, and count up to ten. Let go and relax for a few seconds before repeating.

Fast pull-ups
Squeeze tight and let go several times.

How often
Practice several times daily, especially near the end of pregnancy, and as soon as possible after birth. As your muscles strengthen, increase the number of squeezes and length of holding time.

Checking yourself
To check that you are doing the exercise properly, try any of the following tests:
■ When you are urinating, see if you can stop or slow down in midflow.
■ Hold a mirror between your legs to see if there is a lift in the perineal area.
■ Put a finger into your vagina and feel it tighten when you practice.

STAYING FIT AND HEALTHY

A BASIC STRETCH ROUTINE

Giving birth tests your physical resources to the limit, and taking care of a baby can be hard work, so it makes sense to prepare yourself. These nonstrenuous stretching and toning exercises can increase your strength and suppleness. They also help reduce aches and tiredness.

EXERCISE HINTS

- Try to exercise as part of your daily routine.
- Exercise with a friend or partner if possible.
- Warm up and cool down when exercising.
- If you are unused to exercise, start gently to build your strength and stamina gradually.
- If you are a beginner in a class, don't try to keep up with more experienced students.
- Make sure that your exercise teacher knows you are pregnant.
- Exercise should never be painful or make you feel sick, dizzy, or breathless. If an activity causes pain or discomfort, stop immediately.
- Make sure you do not become overheated with vigorous exercise: overheating may be linked with problems in early pregnancy.
- Drink plenty of fluids (preferably water) to avoid becoming dehydrated.

PELVIC TILT

These pelvic tilt exercises help to strengthen your lower back and abdominal muscles, preventing bad posture.

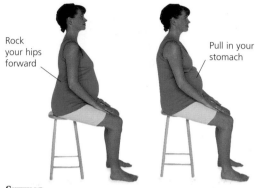

Rock your hips forward

Pull in your stomach

SITTING
Sit on a chair or stool, making sure your feet can rest flat on the floor. Rock your pelvis forward. Then pull in your stomach and rock back on your hips. Repeat.

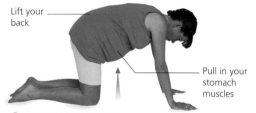

Lift your back

Pull in your stomach muscles

ON HANDS AND KNEES
On all fours, lift your back and pull in your stomach muscles. Imagine your spine stretching. Return your back to a level position, holding stomach muscles firm.

HIPS AND TORSO

Mobility can be increased by twisting and circling exercises that loosen the trunk area. You may also find these exercises a comforting movement in the first stage of labor.

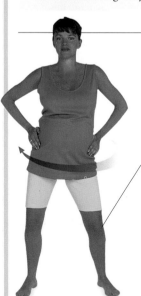

Bend your knees slightly

HIP CIRCLING
With your feet apart and knees slightly bent, place hands on hips. Slowly circle your hips from the waist in one direction five to ten times; then repeat the other way.

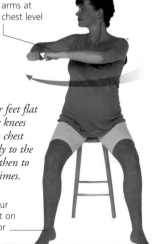

Hold your arms at chest level

TWISTING
Sit on a chair with your feet flat on the ground and your knees apart. Lift your arms to chest level and twist your body to the right as far as you can, then to the left. Repeat several times.

Rest your feet flat on the floor

LEG STRETCHES

The legs carry a lot of extra weight during pregnancy, so stretching and strengthening your leg muscles will be beneficial. The exercises will also improve the circulation in your legs, which could make you more comfortable later in pregnancy.

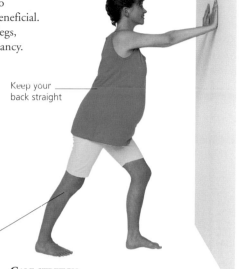

Keep your back straight

LEG STRENGTHENING
Stand with your back against a wall and your feet apart. Slowly bend your legs until you feel some pull on your thigh muscles but before you feel uncomfortable. Hold for a count of 20, then return to standing. Repeat five times.

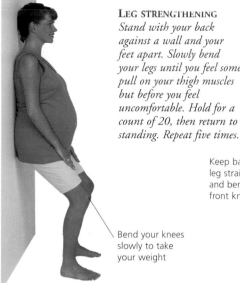

Keep back leg straight and bend front knee

Bend your knees slowly to take your weight

CALF STRETCH
Stand facing the wall, bend your elbows, and lean against the wall, resting your weight on your forearms. Now, with both feet facing the wall, place one foot behind the other. Feel the stretch in the calf muscles. Hold the stretch for a few seconds, then repeat with the other leg. Repeat five times.

FEET AND ANKLES

Pregnancy hormones relax the walls of veins; this slows the blood to the heart and can cause varicose veins and swollen ankles and legs. Do these exercises regularly during the day to stimulate the circulation in the legs and help relieve the discomfort of swollen ankles. This is important for women who sit at a desk all day or stand for long periods.

You can either sit on the floor or on a chair for this exercise

UP AND DOWN
Move one foot up and down from the ankle, without pointing the toes. Repeat with the other foot. Perform ten to 20 times per foot twice a day.

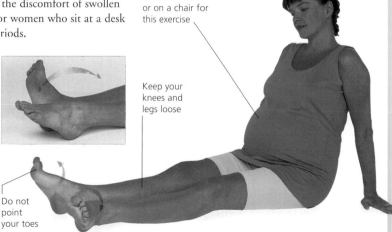

Keep your knees and legs loose

ROTATIONS
Make circling movements with each foot ten times one way and again the other way. Keep the toes relaxed.

Do not point your toes

TAKE CARE OF YOUR BACK

Backache in pregnancy can have several causes. Early in pregnancy, hormones cause the ligaments and joints of the spine to stretch more easily, which makes backache more likely. Added to this, the weight of the womb pulls the spine forward. While prevention is always better than cure with backache, if you are in pain, here are some ways to alleviate the severity (see also panel, below).

YOUR POSTURE

Be conscious of how you sit or stand: your back should always be in a straight line, not arched, and your shoulders should be held back. Try to relax your back a few times every day.

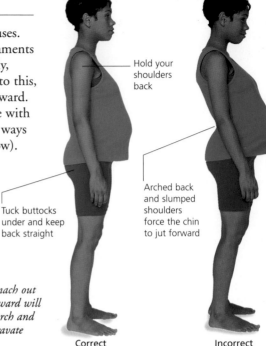

Hold your shoulders back

Tuck buttocks under and keep back straight

Arched back and slumped shoulders force the chin to jut forward

Correct

Incorrect

CORRECT
As your belly grows, it is tempting to lean back and stick your stomach out, but this puts pressure on the ligaments and joints of the spine.

INCORRECT
Sticking your stomach out and slumping forward will make your back arch and may cause or aggravate lower backache.

SITTING WELL

It is also important to sit well, especially if you spend a lot of time working at a desk or sitting watching television.

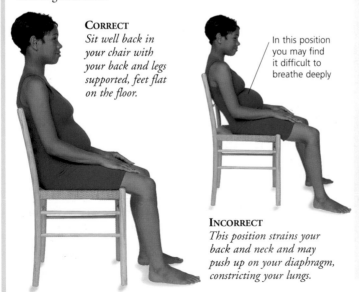

CORRECT
Sit well back in your chair with your back and legs supported, feet flat on the floor.

In this position you may find it difficult to breathe deeply

INCORRECT
This position strains your back and neck and may push up on your diaphragm, constricting your lungs.

ALLEVIATING YOUR BACKACHE

Backache can sometimes be the worst aspect of an otherwise problem-free pregnancy, but there are ways you can help reduce its severity:

■ Improve your posture.
■ A good back massage can ease some backache (see p. 114).
■ Apply local heat; use a hot water bottle on the aching areas.
■ Gentle stretching exercises (see opposite, above) can keep your muscles and joints supple and may relieve low back pain.
■ Take acetaminophen for pain relief, if your doctor approves.
■ Consult your doctor, physical therapist, or osteopath if symptoms are severe.

STRETCHING YOUR LOWER BACK

A few simple stretches will help you reduce low back pain. The pelvic tilt exercise (see p. 108) also helps strengthen the lower back.

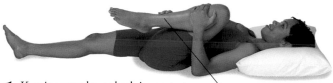

1 Keeping your lower back in contact with the floor, and one leg straight, bring the other knee up to your chest and hug it. Hold for a few moments. Repeat with the other leg.

Clasp your ankle with your other hand for support

2 Bring both knees up to your chest and hug them with both arms. Hold for a few moments. Release slowly. If your belly is too large, bring your legs up on either side of it.

Lying in this position is good for the lower back

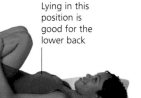

HOW TO GET UP

It is important to protect your back when you are pregnant. As your stomach muscles are separating to allow your belly to grow, they cannot be used in the same way as before.

Rest one leg over the other

1 First, turn on your side so that you are ready to pivot yourself up.

2 Support yourself with your hands, and let your arms take your weight.

3 Move into a kneeling position. Stand up, one leg at a time, keeping your back straight.

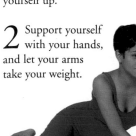

Push up from the floor

LIFTING YOUR CHILD SAFELY

If you lift a small child correctly, it is safe. As your stomach grows, however, you may find your child difficult to hold. Instead, give your child lots of attention while sitting down.

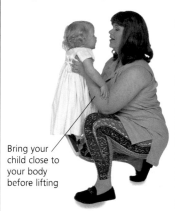

Bring your child close to your body before lifting

1 To lift your child (or a heavy object) bend your knees and lower yourself to his or her level.

Keep your back straight

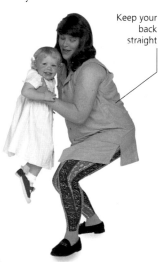

2 When you lift your child, keep your back straight and use your legs, making sure that you hold your child as close to your body as possible.

REST AND RELAXATION

Q WHY IS IT IMPORTANT TO LEARN TO RELAX IN PREGNANCY?

A The more relaxed you are, the more comfortable your pregnancy will be and the more you will enjoy it. Your mind and body will work better, you will feel healthier, and your baby will thrive. You will have more energy with less tension and stress, because these are physically draining. You will also sleep better.

Q WHAT IS THE DIFFERENCE BETWEEN RESTING AND RELAXATION?

A During the day when you stretch out, or when you sit in a chair watching television, for example, you may be physically resting, but not necessarily relaxed: your mind may be active and your body could feel stiff and tense. Reaching a state of complete relaxation allows you to switch off from worries and achieve a calm, positive frame of mind; this will allow your body and muscles to unwind and any tension to ebb away.

Q WHAT IS THE BEST WAY TO RELAX COMPLETELY?

A You don't have to be sitting still or lying down to relax. Taking regular walks or going for a quiet swim can relieve physical tension and clear your mind. Massage and aromatherapy (see p. 114) are luxurious ways to unwind. However, one of the most effective ways to release stress is by learning relaxation techniques (see opposite).

Q HOW WILL LEARNING RELAXATION TECHNIQUES HELP ME?

A If you practice relaxation techniques regularly, you will find that they provide a short break from physical and mental stress and make it easier to deal with day-to-day pressures. You will be more aware of how your body feels when it is tense, and learn how to relieve the tension. This is particularly useful during pregnancy, when sleep may be difficult; relaxation techniques can also help relieve anxiety and therefore help with pain during labor.

WHAT IS THE BEST POSITION FOR SLEEPING?

A good night's rest can seem an impossible quest, especially in late pregnancy when your baby may kick and turn in the night. Sleeping on your stomach or your back no longer feels comfortable. Sleeping on your side is the answer; it takes the weight off your back and thus your circulation, which allows an unrestricted flow of blood to the placenta. This position also allows you to try the relaxation technique opposite.

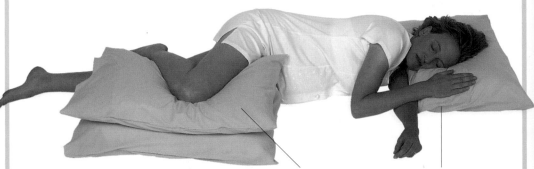

GETTING COMFORTABLE
Lie on your preferred side, put one or two pillows between your legs, and rest your upper leg on the pillows. You may also need a pillow under your belly.

Use one or two pillows to lift your upper leg

One pillow under your head is usually adequate

TAKING TIME OUT TO RELAX

The main difference in the busy, active life of a pregnant and a nonpregnant woman is that the pregnant woman has the added physical weight and discomfort of pregnancy. As the pregnancy progresses, you may find it helpful to take time out to relax mentally and physically. Relaxation helps relieve tension, anxiety, and tiredness.

GET COMFORTABLE

Make sure you are sitting or lying comfortably. If you prefer to sit in a chair, make sure that your back is supported with a pillow and that your feet are flat on the floor or resting on a cushion or similar support. Alternatively, you could lay your head on your folded arms on top of several pillows placed on a table (see below). You can either close your eyes or leave them open, whichever seems least distracting.

CALM YOUR BREATHING

Begin by slowly exhaling through your mouth to empty your lungs completely. Then close your mouth, and slowly breathe in through your nose. You will find that this makes you take a deeper breath than you normally might and you should find that this is calming. Breathing in this way will also help clear stale air from the bottom of your lungs. Repeat this several times. Your body will begin to relax on the exhale. Continue in this way until you are breathing in a slow, comfortable rhythm.

CALM YOUR MIND

Calming your mind is as important as relaxing your body, but it takes practice and patience. As much as possible, try to eliminate any distractions from your environment: turn off the TV and any music and take the phone off the hook. Close your eyes and concentrate on steadying your breathing and the way your body feels as you begin to relax. If your mind starts to wander off to familiar nagging worries, gently call it back. Picture a pleasant scene where you feel happy and relaxed. Explore this scene and conjure up all the details, imagining that you are actually there. Try to do this for at least 20 minutes, and then open your eyes and stretch gently to finish the exercise.

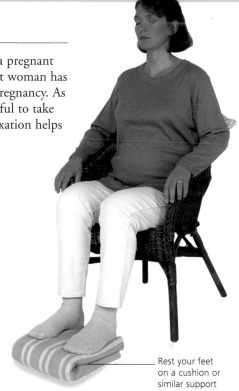

Rest your feet on a cushion or similar support

SITTING IN A CHAIR
If you don't want to lie down, you can practice while sitting in a chair. Support your lower back with a cushion, and rest your feet on a cushion or folded blanket.

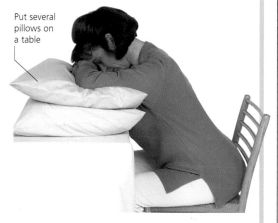

Put several pillows on a table

AT A TABLE
This position, which allows you to stretch out and relaxes your lower back and neck, is comfortable in late pregnancy, when your baby is high under your diaphragm and it is difficult to breathe.

STAYING FIT AND HEALTHY

MASSAGE IN PREGNANCY

Q WHAT ARE THE BENEFITS OF MASSAGE?

A Recognized for centuries as a comfort and a tonic, massage is an aid to relieving muscle pain and stiffness. Most importantly, it gives you a great feeling of well-being as it releases tension and restores and boosts vitality. Your circulation is stimulated by a massage, which can have either a calming or an invigorating effect. Regular massages during pregnancy will help you to relax and will reduce tiredness as well as relieve any aches and pains, particularly backache.

Q HOW IS IT DONE?

A The muscles and soft tissue are stroked, rubbed, and kneaded gently and rhythmically, usually with the hands, sometimes with specialist tools, which is soothing and restorative.

Q IS MASSAGE IN PREGNANCY SAFE?

A It is safe to stroke most of your body but vigorous rubbing or kneading of the abdomen is not advised. You may find that, except in the first trimester, you are not comfortable lying on your stomach. Certain essential oils should not be used because they are too astringent (see below).

Q WHAT ABOUT BEAUTY PARLOR MASSAGES?

A These are fine, but tell the masseur or masseuse that you are pregnant, because some restrictions should be observed. However, a chiropractor, professional masseur, or qualified aromatherapist will probably give you a better massage.

Q WHAT IS AROMATHERAPY?

A Aromatherapy is the treatment of the whole body with essential oils or essences from plants and flowers to regulate the body and relax the mind and spirit. The oils can be absorbed through the skin either in massage, when they are added to creams or oils, or during bathing; they can also be inhaled from vaporizers. Aromatherapists also use herbs and teas as a means of detoxifying the body.

Q WHAT PROBLEMS CAN AROMATHERAPY HELP ALLEVIATE?

A In pregnancy, aromatherapy can be used to help alleviate nausea, painful Braxton-Hicks' contractions, edema, and heartburn. It can also be of benefit in cases of tiredness, insomnia, depression, and anxiety. When used in conjunction with massage in the first stage of labor, it can be helpful for its relaxing and calming effects, and for pain relief.

WHICH ESSENTIAL OILS CAN I USE?

Oils used in massage are the "essence" of plants or flowers. Each oil has a different action, fragrance, and sometimes color. Oils can be antiseptic or antibiotic, astringent and stimulating, or calming and aphrodisiac.

The essential oils recommended in pregnancy
Chamomile, citrus oils, geranium, lavender, neroli, rose, sandalwood.

The essential oils to be avoided in pregnancy
Basil, clary sage, hyssop, juniper berry, marjoram, myrrh, pine, rosemary, sage, thyme, bay.

Recipes for massage treatments
Mix the following oils in a small jar or bottle and apply with warm hands.

For relaxation 50 ml grapeseed oil, 5 ml wheatgerm oil, 8 drops neroli, 8 drops sandalwood.

To moisturize the skin 25 ml avocado oil, 25 ml almond oil, 5 ml wheatgerm oil, 10 drops chamomile, 5 drops sandalwood, 5 drops frankincense.

During pregnancy 50 ml almond oil, 5 ml wheatgerm oil, 4 drops lavender, 4 drops sandalwood, 2 drops tangerine, 2 drops geranium.

RELAX WITH A MASSAGE

Massage can release tension and restore the body's natural energy levels. During pregnancy and labor, a comforting massage can help you relax and sleep better. Lie down or sit comfortably in a warm room. It is best, but not essential, to remove your clothes, keeping the areas not being massaged covered with warm towels.

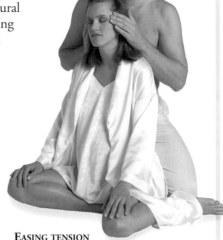

WHERE TO START

Your partner should begin the massage with stroking movements, using the balls of the fingers softly but rhythmically, then using the hands to work more firmly on tense muscles. The palms can be used to apply pressure, or the knuckles for really tense spots.

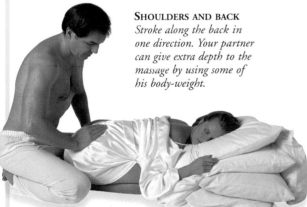

SHOULDERS AND BACK
Stroke along the back in one direction. Your partner can give extra depth to the massage by using some of his body-weight.

EASING TENSION
Rubbing in small, circular movements on the face and around the forehead and temples can relieve tension headaches.

MASSAGE TIPS

■ Warm the hands; remove jewelery.
■ Scented oils, powder, or creams will allow the hands or massage tool to slide easily over the skin.
■ Never pummel the belly or breasts.

MASSAGE FOR BACKACHE

The best position for back massage in early pregnancy, when you can lie on your stomach, is face down on a bed or the floor. Later on, sit on the edge of a sofa or chair and support your arms on the back of a chair, or lie on your side on a firm bed or comfortable floor surface.

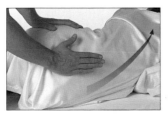

STROKING
Start the back massage with firm, stroking movements from the base of the spine up to the neck, using one or both hands.

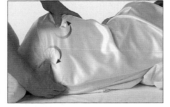

CIRCULAR MOVEMENTS
Gentle pressure applied in circular movements at the base of the spine with the thumbs relieves muscle tension and relaxes the whole back.

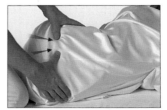

DEEP PRESSURE
Steady, direct pressure applied to either side of the spine is especially good for easing lower back pain in pregnancy and labor.

WORK AND TRAVEL

Q CAN I CONTINUE TO WORK?

A It is good to work for some, if not most, of your pregnancy. This may be a physical strain, especially in later months, but there are benefits: you will have company during the day; you will be leading a normal life, even if your body is changing; working and continuing with normal routines will confirm that you are not abnormal or ill.

Q IS THERE ANY WORK I SHOULD NOT DO IN MY CONDITION?

A If you are pregnant (or are breastfeeding) you should work with your employer to ensure that the work you do is not likely to put your or your baby's health at risk. This may mean that your working conditions have to be changed, or that a suitable alternative must be found. You can't be fired or laid off just because you are pregnant (see p. 230).

Q WHEN SHOULD I TELL MY EMPLOYER?

A Every work situation has its own nuances and expectations. Women who work with supportive peers may be comfortable sharing news of their pregnancy early on, but for women in competitive or demanding professions, later may be better. It's often wise to wait until after the first trimester or until you have had amniocentesis results (see p. 36), if you have had a test, before you tell your colleagues.

Q DOES MY EMPLOYER NEED TO BE INFORMED IN WRITING?

A While there are federal regulations governing maternity leave, each province also has its own requirements. Written notice is required, but the length of advance notice may vary. Check with your local government service office. Give your employer a written note after you discuss your plans, outlining what you have agreed, to avoid misunderstandings.

DISCUSSION POINT

MATERNITY LEAVE

When to give up work
This depends on how you feel, how far you have to travel, and how stressful your work is, and the benefits available to you. Many women work until the last week or two before their due date. You will have to stop earlier if you have a pregnancy-related illness or medical problem; your doctor will give you a medical certificate for disability coverage. Otherwise you can continue for as long as you want. Remember that if you are expecting twins or another multiple birth, you may well need to stop working earlier (see p. 88).

Once you've left work
Your priorities may change as you prepare for your new life. This can be a creative period with lots of time to think, but you may also be at a loss as to how to fill the hours. Try to make the most of this time to yourself. As you get bigger you will probably wish to be less active and get more rest.

Returning to work – it's your decision
Many women enjoy their work and wish to pursue their careers after the baby arrives. You may also have to return to work for financial reasons, or you may return because you feel more fulfilled doing a job and having a family to take care of. You must decide what is best for you and try not to let other peoples' opinions influence your decision. Even if you ultimately change your mind after your baby arrives you can still do so, although you should make sure that you know your legal obligations to your employer.

Worry about leaving your baby
Before the birth you cannot know how you will feel about leaving your baby. Inevitably, you will find it a wrench after being with your baby every day for a few weeks or months. Whatever you decide, be prepared to feel guilty. However, what is good for you is also usually good for your baby.

Q WHAT ARE MY RIGHTS AND BENEFITS IN PREGNANCY?

A It is important to get help and advice as soon as soon as you become pregnant because the situation for rights and benefits is constantly changing, both at the federal government level and within companies. Be sure to familiarize yourself with your company's maternity policies and practices before you get pregnant (see p. 230).

Q CAN I TAKE TIME OFF FOR MY VISITS TO THE DOCTOR OR MIDWIFE?

A Employers are not required to give you time off for prenatal care. Many employers, especially in white-collar industries, will do so. If you make appointments during nonworking hours, this may impress your employer and work in your favor when you negotiate maternity leave and pay.

Q I FEEL SICK AND TIRED – SHOULD I GIVE UP OR TRY TO WORK THROUGH IT?

A The first trimester is usually the hardest to get through, but this phase of nausea and tiredness will pass. Many women find that the middle trimester and later weeks are a good period for work because they do not feel as tired.

Tips for working through pregnancy

■ If possible, avoid standing for too long. Do not work for prolonged periods without breaks, and make sure you eat at lunchtime rather than go shopping.

■ Try to find a few minutes during the day to do some light exercises for your neck, legs, ankles, and shoulders (see p. 108).

■ If your job is particularly stressful or you are having medical problems, it may be a good idea to suggest working shorter hours or even from home.

■ Ease up on your daily workload, perhaps by being less fastidious about the housework or perhaps by asking your partner to help out more around the home.

■ Be sure that any business travel you undertake is cleared by your doctor or midwife.

QUESTIONS TO ASK

If I continue to work, will I find it more difficult to cope with my pregnancy?

What maternity benefits am I entitled to?

Can I collect disability insurance during my pregnancy?

GETTING OUT

Is it safe to continue to drive?
It is as safe for the baby as it is for you. However, after 37 weeks it is advisable, particularly on long journeys, to have someone with you to share the driving chores. Being driven will also help reduce your fatigue level; also, having someone with you, in the event of you going into labor, is prudent. Some women report that getting behind the wheel is difficult in the last few weeks.

Should I wear a seat belt when I'm in a car?
It is now a legal requirement for drivers and front seat passengers to wear seat belts. Being pregnant does not exclude you from this legislation. Seat belts may be uncomfortable, but wearing a properly fitted belt best protects the mother and baby in an accident. If you are in an accident, even if you do not feel you have been hurt, you must be checked by your obstetrician or midwife: in rare cases, the belt can cause injury to the placenta or the womb.

When is it safe to travel by air?
If you are having a normal pregnancy, there should not be any problems. Some airlines, however, will not allow pregnant women on board after week 34. It is best to avoid air travel in the last four to six weeks of your pregnancy because you could go into labor at any time. Check with your doctor or midwife to be sure.

Can I have vaccinations before traveling?
Doctors tend to avoid giving live vaccines to pregnant women, although it is unlikely that they will harm your baby. If you absolutely must visit an area where polio, yellow fever, or malaria are common, you should be vaccinated, as these diseases pose a greater danger to you and your baby than a vaccination. Consult your obstetrician or midwife before traveling.

Should I pack medicines for my vacation?
Unless you have prescription medications, only pack acetaminophen. Motion-sickness medications should be avoided. If you are likely to be traveling in areas where pharmacies are not easily found, you should take rehydration medication if you get diarrhea.

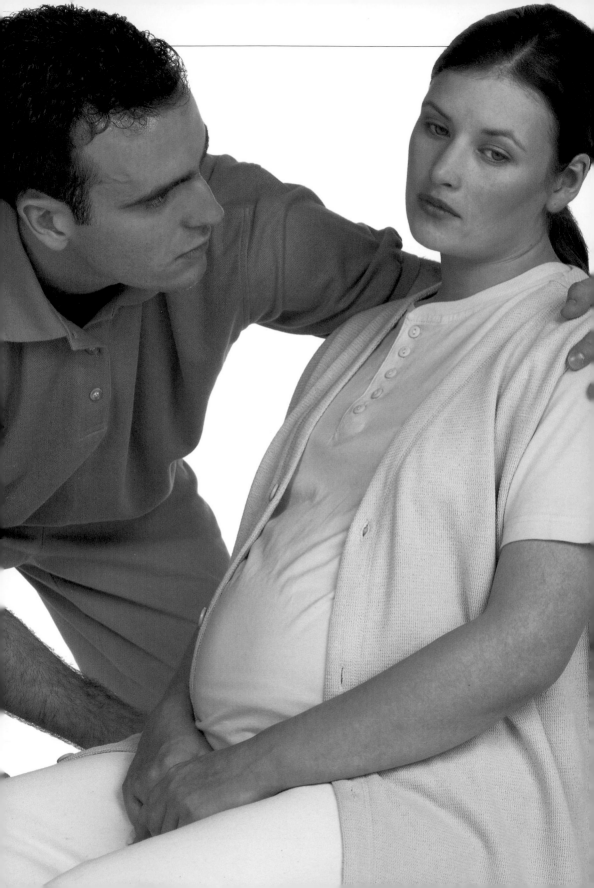

ISSUES IN PREGNANCY

Few pregnancies run their course without some problem occurring – most are minor, but a few are more significant. Like many couples, you and your partner may find even minor complaints worrisome; however, most can usually be dealt with relatively quickly. Only very rarely are there indications of a serious condition. This chapter shows you what to watch for during pregnancy, which problems are common and need no additional treatment, and which need to be brought to the attention of your doctor or midwife. By understanding what is happening, you will be able to cope more easily with any unexpected developments.

COMMON DISORDERS

Q WHICH PROBLEMS DO I NEED TO CONSULT MY DOCTOR ABOUT?

A The numerous changes your body undergoes throughout pregnancy can cause many problems. Most of these are normal and will not need special medical attention. However, there are sometimes more serious developments in pregnancy, such as infections (see opposite) or gestational diabetes (see p. 125), which need particular attention from your obstetrician or midwife. Always mention anything that is troubling you to your doctor or midwife so that they can reassure you or take further action as necessary.

Q WHAT IS CAUSING MY ABDOMINAL ACHES AND PAINS?

A Pregnancy will invariably cause various twinges in your abdomen. The main offenders are the ligaments of your womb, which are stretching, those of your pelvis, and those supporting the sacroiliac joints, which are loosening. These pains often lessen if you change position, for instance, or lie down for a while. You may find that gentle exercises or swimming will help.

Q MY LOWER ABDOMEN ACHES AND I FEEL SICK. WHAT IS WRONG?

A Not every pain is simply due to your pregnancy. If you have stomach pain with other symptoms, such as nausea or vomiting, then it may be caused by indigestion, food poisoning (gastroenteritis), cystitis (a urinary tract infection, see opposite), or even appendicitis, all of which can occur in pregnancy. Pregnancy can mask symptoms and exaggerate others; some, cystitis for example, have slightly different symptoms during pregnancy. Seek help if you suspect that anything is wrong.

Q I SUFFER FROM MIGRAINES. WILL THESE GET WORSE IN PREGNANCY?

A Some women suffer more, others find that their migraines completely disappear. Migraines may be linked to blood flow to the brain, which is affected by high estrogen levels. Some of the symptoms of migraine are similar to those of preeclampsia; should you experience a headache with blurred vision or spots in front of your eyes, you should see a doctor.

Q WHAT IS A FIBROID AND CAN IT AFFECT MY PREGNANCY?

A A fibroid is a benign lump of muscle inside your womb, and is normally noticed when you have an ultrasound or an internal examination. Fibroids rarely develop during pregnancy, but if you already have one, the high levels of estrogen produced by your body in pregnancy can cause it to grow larger. If a fibroid degenerates, it may cause pain in your abdomen. Although unpleasant, this is not usually serious. It is unusual for a fibroid to affect your baby or your labor unless it grows very large or obstructs your cervix. A fibroid may also increase the risk of heavy bleeding after the birth (see p. 178).

Q IS URINE LEAKAGE A COMMON PROBLEM DURING PREGNANCY?

A Leaking urine when you cough, sneeze, laugh, or run is exceptionally common from midpregnancy onward. This is known as stress incontinence, and you may wish to wear a sanitary pad if it happens fairly frequently. You can help alleviate the problem by practicing pelvic floor exercises (see p. 107), and by cutting down your intake of diuretics like tea, coffee, and alcohol. Cystitis is often a cause of stress incontinence, or it makes the problem worse if you already have it (see opposite). If you were suffering from incontinence before you became pregnant, and it gets much worse during your pregnancy, you may need to have your bladder examined to evaluate these chronic problems.

Q WHY, WHEN I STAND UP, DO I FEEL PAIN AND WEAKNESS IN MY PELVIS AND LEGS?

A As you approach 37 weeks, your baby's head moves down toward your pelvis and presses against the pelvic bones, causing the ligaments to stretch and making your pelvic area feel really uncomfortable. The baby's head may also press against your sciatic nerves, which influence movement, pain, and sensation in your legs, and this can cause numbness, tingling, and weakness down one or both legs. Known as sciatica, this is fairly common. If it is severe, however, you should see your doctor to eliminate other possible causes, such as a slipped disc (see p. 83).

INFECTIONS IN PREGNANCY

Infections are caused by viruses or bacteria. Chickenpox, rubella (German measles), and herpes are caused by viruses. Viruses contain types of DNA that are incorporated into your cells and then infect your body. They cannot be treated by antibiotics. Bacteria are live organisms that can infect your body by multiplying rapidly in tissue and in the bloodstream. These include organisms that cause urinary tract infections, food poisoning, and diarrhea. More serious bacterial infections include toxoplasmosis and listeriosis. Unlike viruses, these can be treated with antibiotics. Pregnancy was believed to increase the risk of infection, but there is no strong evidence for this.

Can infections affect my baby?

It is unusual for bacteria or viruses to cross the placenta, but there are some exceptions to this rule. The baby may be indirectly affected by an infection (like a kidney infection) that causes premature labor.

Urinary tract infections (UTIs)

A urinary tract infection can affect any part of the urinary tract, including the bladder and kidneys. Symptoms include a constant need to urinate, irritation, or a burning sensation when urinating, and low abdominal pain and, if untreated, blood in the urine, and fever. If you have any of these symptoms, you need antibiotics. Delay in treatment may cause kidney infection, which can make you ill and can cause miscarriage or premature labor.

Yeast infections

Yeast infections are common and usually harmless vaginal infections caused by the fungus *Candida albicans*. About 40 percent of pregnant women develop yeast infections; they are even more usual in women who have diabetes or are on antibiotics. Its main symptoms are vaginal soreness and itching, and a white discharge. Treatment involves a course of medicated cream and vaginal suppositories. Natural remedies, such as applying yogurt, are also used, but their effectiveness is not known.

Toxoplasmosis

If you think you have been in contact with this infection (see p. 102), your blood will be tested for antibodies that your body produces to fight it. If present, you will be referred to an expert to see if your baby is affected. The fetus may need treatment, and fetal growth will be checked by regular scans. If the infection were missed, there would be a risk of miscarriage or stillbirth, or your baby might be born mentally disabled or blind. This infection is rare.

Listeriosis, Salmonella

These food-borne bacteria are found in soft cheeses, pâtés, some meat, eggs, unpasteurized juices, and some precooked foods (see p. 102). If infection is suspected, your blood will be tested and, if the results are positive, you will need antibiotics and your baby may need to be delivered early. Listeriosis can cause premature labor, miscarriage, or stillbirth. If your baby has to be delivered, he or she may be very ill and need antibiotics to prevent septicemia (blood poisoning) and meningitis.

Rubella (German measles)

This virus is no longer common in pregnancy because most young adults have been vaccinated against rubella as children. Rubella can cause your baby to have heart and brain defects, deafness, and cataracts. If you are infected in the first three months of pregnancy, there is a more than 50 percent chance of your baby being affected; after the first three months, the risk is reduced.

Chickenpox (varicella zoster)

This can cause a severe lung infection or pneumonia if contracted in pregnancy, but there is only a small chance that this will harm your baby. If you have been in contact with anyone with chickenpox and are not immune, you will be injected with immunoglobulins to reduce any risk.

Herpes

This virus can cause painful blisters in and around the perineal area. The risk of passing this on to your baby at birth, even with recurrent herpes, is low. However, if your first attack is in pregnancy and you have ulcers at the time of delivery, you may be offered a cesarean section because there is a risk of your baby being infected, which may cause brain damage.

How do I know when a complaint needs treatment?

Most of the complaints you will experience during your pregnancy are common and nothing for you to worry about; in fact, they are probably a sign that your pregnancy is progressing normally. However, if any discomfort persists or keeps coming back,

SYMPTOMS	POSSIBLE CAUSES	COMMON/MILD CASES
Headaches with blurred vision	Migraines; preeclampsia	May be linked to high levels of the hormone estrogen in pregnancy. Just as some women get headaches with the Pill, which contains estrogen, pregnancy can have the same effect.
Severe tiredness, lethargy, inability to carry out simple tasks, palllor	Anemia	Anemia is usually caused by insufficient iron, either in your diet or from the demands of pregnancy. This reduces the hemoglobin in the red blood cells.
Severe vomiting, inability to keep food or even fluids down, thirst	Severe morning sickness	Morning sickness is common, although its severity varies. If you are expecting more than one baby, this can worsen and prolong morning sickness.
Aching under ribs, shortness of breath	Baby's position	In late pregnancy, your womb presses on internal organs, which press on your ribs.
Abdominal aches	Baby's size	Muscles stretch to accommodate the womb, and ligaments become loose.
Abdominal pain – with vomiting and/or diarrhea	Food poisoning; cystitis; appendicitis	Cause unrelated to pregnancy.
Low backache	Baby's weight and position	Hormones cause the joints and ligaments of your pelvic area and spine to soften, which places strain on your back; this is made worse by bad posture.
Intense itchiness, usually on stomach and back or in folds of skin (under breasts)	Dry skin; liver problems	May be due to dryness from lack of vitamin B; varicose veins cause itchiness; a skin rash can occur due to excess weight and extra sweating.
Leaking urine when you cough, sneeze, laugh, or run	Baby's weight; cystitis	Your bladder is being squashed by your womb, causing it to leak; this is common from midpregnancy onward.
Numbness, tingling, and weakness in fingers, difficulty in gripping objects, may have shooting pain in wrist and arm	Fluid retention	Swollen tissues in the wrist compress nerves, causing pain and weakness. This is called carpal tunnel syndrome.
Pain in pelvic area, numbness, tingling, or weakness down one or both legs	Sciatica; slipped disc	In late pregnancy, your baby's head fills your pelvis, stretching ligaments, and may also press against sciatic nerves.
Swollen ankles, toes, and puffy fingers	Fluid retention (edema); preeclampsia	May be caused by increased blood volume. This condition tends to be worse in hot weather or if you are expecting more than one baby.

mention it to your doctor or midwife, because it may be symptomatic of another underlying and possibly more serious condition. The chart below lists common pregnancy complaints, their symptoms, whether they need treatment, and whether they might be signs of a more serious condition. If you have any of the symptoms below, don't try to diagnose yourself. Talk to your doctor or midwife.

IN SEVERE CASES	TREATMENT
If you have a severe headache, blurred vision, and/or spots in front of your eyes after 20 weeks of pregnancy, this may indicate preeclampsia (see p. 127), and you should contact your doctor immediately.	Prevention is the best option because, apart from acetaminophen, most treatments are not safe in pregnancy. Avoid migraines by not getting dehydrated or hungry, and avoid triggers like bright light, stress, loud noise, cheese, chocolate, and red wine. If a severe headache is diagnosed as preeclampsia, you will be hospitalized.
When severe, this reduces your immunity and your ability to cope with the demands of pregnancy.	Eat a balanced, nutritious diet containing iron, folic acid, and vitamins (see p. 100). Take your vitamins. Your doctor may prescribe iron supplements; you can improve their absorption by taking them with an acidic drink, such as orange juice.
You may be dehydrated and lacking in energy, especially if it continues past the first trimester. You may also have a urinary tract infection (see p. 121).	Drink plenty of fluids; very severe morning sickness may need hospital treatment to replace the nutrients and fluids you have lost. You may be given injections, or suppositories, of antiemetic drugs, that are considered safe in pregnancy. If you suspect a UTI, consult your doctor.
The baby may be in the breech position or you are expecting more than one baby.	Pain and pressure may be relieved by lying on your side rather than your back; or by resting your head on your raised arms (see p. 113).
This does not usually become a serious problem.	Aches may improve if you change position, or lie down; swimming can help by taking the weight of the womb off the rest of your body.
Indicates food poisoning (gastroenteritis), cystitis, or appendicitis.	If you are vomiting and/or have pain and diarrhea, see your doctor.
If pain is very severe, this may be caused by strain on your sacroiliac joint, which can make it difficult to walk (see p. 83).	Be aware of your posture (see p. 110), avoid any twisting movements, don't lift heavy objects, and have a massage (see p. 114). If severe, you may need to be treated by an osteopath experienced in treating pregnant women. Ask your doctor or midwife to recommend one.
In rare cases this may indicate a liver problem (cholestasis), but this will be accompanied by other symptoms (see p. 126).	Aloe vera cream or calamine lotion, bought over the counter at a pharmacy store, can relieve rashes. Your doctor may prescribe antihistamines; you could also use talcum powder to keep your skin dry. If a liver problem (cholestasis) is suspected, you will be referred to a specialist immediately.
If this occurs with other symptoms, such as abdominal pain, or blood in the urine, it may be a sign of cystitis (see p. 121).	Practice pelvic floor exercises (see p. 107) and cut down on tea, alcohol, and coffee; wear a sanitary pad if needed. If this persists after pregnancy, you may be referred to a urinary specialist.
This usually does not become a serious problem.	Try not to lift heavy objects. If you must use a keyboard, try to rest your hands in your lap every 15 or 20 minutes. If the pain is severe, acetaminophen may help. If symptoms persist, your doctor may refer you to a physical therapist.
The sciatic nerves may be trapped. Or if very severe, this may indicate a slipped disc.	Pain should cease or lessen before giving birth, when the baby's head has fully engaged (see p. 65).
If severe, may be a sign of excess fluid retention, called edema. Blood pressure should be monitored to check for preeclampsia (see p. 127).	Avoid salty foods, which make you retain water, and avoid standing too much; wear support hose. Don't drink less fluid, as this won't relieve the problem and may cause you to become dehydrated.

HIGH-RISK PREGNANCIES

Q WHAT ARE HIGH-RISK PREGNANCIES – IS MY BABY AT RISK?

A These are pregnancies that warrant close attention because you have an existing medical condition such as asthma, diabetes, or epilepsy, or because you develop a serious condition caused by your pregnancy (see p. 126). You will be closely monitored by your doctor or midwife, and may have more frequent checkups and ultrasounds. With careful management, there is usually no reason why your pregnancy should not proceed normally.

Q I AM ASTHMATIC. HOW WILL THIS AFFECT MY PREGNANCY OR MY BABY?

A Mild asthma should not cause problems during your pregnancy if you normally control the asthma with a bronchodilator or a steroid inhaler. Severe asthma, such as an attack that required hospitalization and oral medications, will be a problem for you and your baby only if your asthma increases and the oxygen supply to your baby becomes dangerously low. Whatever you do, don't stop taking your asthma medication unless your doctor or midwife has advised you to.

Q I AM EPILEPTIC. WILL I HAVE A NORMAL PREGNANCY?

A While there is a slightly increased risk of epilepsy in children of a parent with epilepsy, the risk is low. Epilepsy should not prevent a normal pregnancy. Your doctor may change or increase your medication before or during pregnancy to be sure that your epilepsy is controlled.

Q SHOULD I STOP TAKING MY EPILEPSY MEDICATION DURING MY PREGNANCY?

A No. Epilepsy may worsen in pregnancy, so you must take the medication that controls it. If you do have a seizure, the fetus may be harmed if you fall on your belly or if the oxygen getting to it is reduced during the seizure.

Q I HAVE THYROID PROBLEMS. WILL THIS AFFECT MY BABY?

A If you have an existing thyroid condition, your thyroid function will be regularly checked by blood tests. Your medication should not affect your baby's development, but your baby's thyroid function may be affected and will be checked after birth.

CAN HIV AFFECT MY PREGNANCY?

If you know you are HIV-positive, but otherwise healthy, your pregnancy should not be affected. There is no evidence to suggest that pregnancy increases your chances of developing full-blown AIDS sooner. You will need to take extra care of yourself as your ability to fight infections is reduced during pregnancy. You should take iron and folic acid supplements to prevent anemia, and to help fight any infections.

Will I receive special care?

Most large hospitals have special arrangements for caring for pregnant women with HIV. You may have several specialists caring for you during your pregnancy, including a midwife, an obstetrician, and/or a doctor who specializes in genitourinary medicine. Although these people will know that you are HIV-positive, if you prefer, they may be able to keep this information completely confidential by not recording it on your chart or hospital notes.

What is the risk to the baby?

The risk of passing HIV on to a fetus while it is in your womb is about 1 in 5. This risk is probably higher if you contract HIV when pregnant, because your body hasn't had a chance to fight the virus. You may be advised to opt for a cesarean delivery rather than a vaginal delivery. The risks of transmission are also reduced by the antiviral drug azidothymidine (AZT), given during the birth. Breastfeeding is thought to increase the chances of passing HIV to your baby, and should be avoided.

Q CAN SICKLE CELL ANEMIA HARM THE FETUS OR ME DURING PREGNANCY?

A Sickle cell anemia is a condition that affects red blood cells and can cause chronic anemia; it is most likely to affect black African people and people of Mediterranean origin (see p. 30). If you carry the trait for this condition, but do not suffer from it, you may already be anemic, which can worsen in pregnancy. You may need supplements of iron and folic acid; if you have severe anemia you may require a blood transfusion. You will have specialist prenatal care with frequent checkups. Sickle cell anemia can cause premature birth and a low birthweight baby. If the fetus has sickle cell anemia, he or she will not be affected while in your womb because symptoms only develop in the first months of life. Your baby will be tested for the disease after the birth.

Q I HAVE THALASSEMIA. HOW WILL IT AFFECT MY BABY?

A Thalassemia is an inherited blood disorder that affects the red blood cells and causes anemia. It appears in two forms. The minor variety of thalassemia often goes unnoticed and does little harm. Major thalassemia, however, can seriously restrict growth and damage major organs. Affected children only start to show symptoms of thalassemia within three or four months of birth, so prenatal screening is used to detect the disease (see p. 30). A baby born with the more serious variety of thalassemia may need to receive a blood transfusion after the birth. In extremely serious cases, where an affected fetus is considered unlikely to live, the parents may be offered the choice of a termination.

HOW WILL DIABETES AFFECT MY PREGNANCY?

There are two types of diabetes in pregnancy: preexisting diabetes mellitus and gestational diabetes. Diabetes can be controlled to minimize any dangers.

Preexisting diabetes mellitus

You and the fetus will be monitored closely throughout your pregnancy, usually by an obstetrician. Pregnancy doesn't necessarily make diabetes worse, but your insulin requirements and your blood sugar regulation will change; you will also be more susceptible to developing high blood pressure (preeclampsia) or having a premature labor.

Gestational diabetes

If you develop diabetes in pregnancy, this is known as gestational diabetes and tends to be less serious than normal diabetes. Your blood sugar levels can either be controlled through your diet, or insulin may be required. This type of diabetes improves after you have had your baby.

How gestational diabetes is diagnosed

Normally, the signs of diabetes are thirst, passing urine frequently, feeling weak, and losing weight. However, in pregnancy, these classic symptoms may not occur because of other metabolic changes; diabetes is often diagnosed only through routine testing of your blood and urine.

Controlling your diabetes

To be sure that your pregnancy progresses smoothly, your diet must be strictly controlled and normal blood sugar levels maintained. Your doctor will discuss your diet with you but, in essence, you need lots of carbohydrates such as pasta and potatoes, plenty of fiber, and a limited intake of fats and sugar. Eat little and often and do not miss meals. You may be given insulin injections if you are unable to control your blood sugar through your diet. Contact your doctor if you suddenly feel unwell, drowsy, or feverish, or if you cannot feel significant fetal movement.

Diabetes and your baby

Good blood sugar control during the first few weeks of a pregnancy reduces the fetus' chances of developing a congenital abnormality, such as a cleft palate. Babies of diabetic mothers can grow very large or have restricted growth. With the care you will receive and careful control of your diet, your baby should develop well and be healthy at birth.

Prenatal care with diabetes mellitus

Your doctor can monitor your blood sugar control, and your insulin dose may have to be increased. Your blood pressure and urine will also be checked. You will be offered scans every two to four weeks after 20 weeks to monitor fetal growth. If your baby seems to be too large, your obstetrician may want to deliver you earlier, around 37 to 38 weeks.

CAUSES FOR CONCERN

Q CAN I DEVELOP SERIOUS CONDITIONS BECAUSE OF MY PREGNANCY?

A Yes, there are conditions that may arise because of your pregnancy and, if they develop, you will require special treatment. These conditions include preeclampsia (see opposite), thrombosis (see p. 129), and, more rarely, liver diseases (see right). The purpose of prenatal care is to detect these conditions, and to monitor and deal with them before they become serious. However, without becoming unnecessarily anxious, if you are aware of some of the potential problems that can occur during pregnancy, you can alert your doctor or midwife if you suspect that something may be wrong.

Q I HAVE EXTREMELY ITCHY SKIN. WHAT CAN I DO?

A This is common in pregnancy, usually caused by dryness or a rash. It can be controlled with special moisturizing creams. Occasionally, your doctor may prescribe antihistamine tablets.

Q CAN ITCHY SKIN BE SERIOUS?

A Yes. There is a rare condition affecting the liver called obstetric cholestasis, which may cause premature delivery or stillbirth; the symptoms are: very itchy and yellowish skin, dark urine, and feeling generally unwell. If you have these symptoms, seek help immediately.

IS IT COMMON TO FEEL VERY DEPRESSED DURING PREGNANCY?

Many women become significantly depressed during pregnancy. This is thought to be caused by hormonal changes during the first trimester, and often eases without needing treatment. Depression is also more likely if you felt low at the start of your pregnancy, or if you have suffered from depression before becoming pregnant. You are likely to experience depression if you are having problems with your partner, if the pregnancy was unplanned, or if you are not sure if you really want to have a child now.

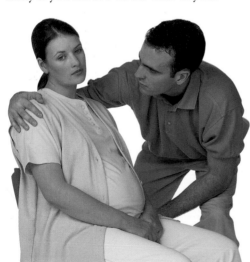

PROLONGED DEPRESSION
The hormonal changes that accompany the onset of pregnancy (see p. 73) can cause depression; if it continues after the first trimester, consult your doctor.

Symptoms of depression
Early signs of depression are: you feel irritable and anxious, especially about your baby; you feel continually tired; you have no energy, and find it difficult to enjoy yourself; it is difficult to get to sleep because you feel so anxious about things, or you wake up in the early hours of the morning feeling stressed or despondent.

Relieving depression
Mild depression in pregnancy is often easily helped by reassurance and support from your partner, family, or friends. If your depression is severe and you feel desperate, do not keep it to yourself; consult your midwife or doctor immediately. You may benefit from professional help, or your doctor may recommend some medication. There are drugs that are very effective in treating depression and are safe for you and your baby during pregnancy, although ideally these should be avoided in the first trimester.

What is preeclampsia?

Preeclampsia is a condition that can only develop in pregnancy, and its symptoms include: high blood pressure (hypertension); protein in the urine; swollen legs, ankles, and fingers (edema); headaches; nausea, and vomiting; blurred or disturbed vision; abdominal pain; and excessive weight gain. It very rarely occurs before week 24, but can strike quickly. Its severity ranges from slightly swollen ankles and a small rise in blood pressure to the "full blown" condition of dangerously high blood pressure and seizures, known as eclampsia (see below).

How common is preeclampsia?

Around seven percent of women develop preeclampsia with their first pregnancy. It is much less common in subsequent pregnancies; if you suffer from high blood pressure, diabetes mellitus, or a kidney disease, then preeclampsia is more likely. The risks of developing preeclampsia are also increased if you are over 35, have already had preeclampsia, or are having a multiple pregnancy. However, if you have any of these conditions, you will be closely monitored by your doctor or midwife throughout your pregnancy.

I had preeclampsia in my first pregnancy. Does this mean I will have it in future pregnancies?

Your chances of developing preeclampsia are lower in your second pregnancy, as long as you did not suffer from it in your first pregnancy. However, there is a very small minority of women who have severe preeclampsia in their first pregnancy and may, for an unknown reason, develop it in subsequent pregnancies.

Am I more likely to develop preeclampsia if my mother had toxemia?

Toxemia, gestosis, proteinuric pregnancy-induced hypertension, hypertension of pregnancy, and preeclamptic toxemia (PET) are all terms for preeclampsia. If close relatives of yours have suffered from this, you should not worry too much, as it is only slightly more common in women whose mothers or sisters have suffered from the condition; you still have more than a 90 percent chance of *not* developing preeclampsia.

Can preeclampsia be prevented?

As the cause of preeclampsia is not known, prevention is not guaranteed. But doctors and midwives are familiar with the symptoms. As you attend all your prenatal checkups, your blood pressure is monitored and early signs of the condition may be noticed. If you had high blood pressure before pregnancy, you may need to change your medication during pregnancy. Your blood pressure will be checked every week or two. Low doses of aspirin may be given to pregnant women who are at high risk after 12 to 14 weeks, because aspirin may reduce the severity of preeclampsia if it occurs.

How is preeclampsia treated?

Mild preeclampsia shouldn't warrant a hospital stay, but your blood pressure will be more frequently monitored, and your urine checked. Relaxation, rest, gentle exercise, and a nutritious diet are recommended. If you have a severe headache, blurred vision, or the baby isn't moving as usual, you will need close hospital supervision. If your blood pressure continues to rise, drugs may be used to control it. Severe preeclampsia means that your baby may be delivered early, often by a cesarean, because of the risk of your having a seizure.

How is the fetus affected by preeclampsia?

A fetus can be seriously damaged by a poorly functioning placenta: "placental insufficiency". This can cause fetal growth in the womb to be restricted, which may require early delivery.

When does preeclampsia turn into eclampsia?

This can happen if preeclampsia is not carefully supervised and treated. If eclampsia develops, the mother may have seizures and become unconscious. This occurs in the later stages of preeclampsia, before, during, or after delivery, and may be fatal for the baby and/or the mother. Thankfully, eclampsia is now extremely rare because doctors have learned to treat preeclampsia before it becomes eclampsia.

Is the immediate delivery of my baby the only cure for severe preeclampsia?

If your blood pressure, kidney function, or baby's health becomes critical, there is no time to wait, irrespective of prematurity. Preeclampsia is dangerous for you and your baby if uncontrolled.

BLEEDING IN PREGNANCY

Q IS VAGINAL BLEEDING A SERIOUS PROBLEM IN PREGNANCY?

A Vaginal bleeding at any stage of pregnancy should be taken seriously. Even if you think the bleeding is harmless, it should be brought to the attention of your doctor or midwife so that the cause can be identified and treatment given. Severe bleeding in the early weeks may be a sign of miscarriage or, after 24 weeks, of premature labor. Seek medical advice at once.

Q WHERE IS THE BLEEDING COMING FROM – ME OR THE FETUS?

A Your doctor will ascertain where the bleeding is coming from. Apart from a threatened miscarriage, the most common sources of bleeding are the cervix (the neck of the womb) and the placenta (see below and panel, right). It is very unusual for blood to come from the fetus.

Q SHOULD I BE WORRIED ABOUT BLEEDING FROM MY CERVIX?

A During pregnancy, the rise in estrogen can cause the cervix to become slightly reddened, causing an "erosion." This is quite common and usually clears up after the birth. Occasionally, there may be light bleeding from your cervix, especially after intercourse. If you have had abnormal Pap smears, bleeding from your cervix may be more important and you should see your doctor.

Q HOW SERIOUS IS BLEEDING FROM THE PLACENTA?

A Bleeding from the placenta occurs for two reasons; you may have a low-lying placenta, known as placenta previa; or the placenta may have come away from the side of the womb, known as placental abruption (see right). With placenta previa, the placenta is low, covering, or partially over the cervix, and this may prevent a normal vaginal delivery. Placental abruption is serious and may necessitate immediate delivery.

Q CAN A YEAST INFECTION CAUSE BLEEDING?

A Yeast infection can make your vagina sore and itchy, which may mean that you might have a raw area that bleeds, especially after intercourse. It can be treated with vaginal suppositories and cream, although it commonly recurs during pregnancy.

WHAT HAPPENS IF I HAVE BLEEDING FROM THE PLACENTA?

Bleeding in pregnancy is often one of the first signs of placenta previa. If it is suspected that the placenta is situated low in your womb, you will be given ultrasound to establish its location.

What a low placenta means

Early in your pregnancy, ultrasound shows the placenta's position. If the placenta is low, you will have regular scans to see if it has moved. Sometimes, as the womb expands, it moves up away from the cervix. If it does, you may be able to have a normal delivery. Also, if the placenta is very near the cervix, but not actually in the way of the baby's head, a vaginal delivery may be possible. However, if the placenta completely obstructs the cervix, the baby will have to be delivered by cesarean.

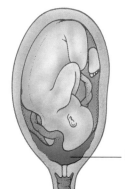

PLACENTA PREVIA
When the placenta is positioned directly over the cervix, it is called a major previa. You will need a cesarean delivery if the placenta is in this position.

Placenta

Placental abruption

If the bleeding is fresh (bright red) and you have abdominal pain, the baby is not moving normally, and your womb feels tense and tight, contact your doctor or go to the hospital at once. You may have placental abruption – the placenta has partially come away from the womb wall. This is serious because it means that your baby may have to be delivered as soon as possible, even if you are not at term.

BLOOD CONDITIONS

Q AM I LIKELY TO GET A BLOOD CLOT DURING PREGNANCY?

A A blood clot, or thrombosis, is more likely to happen in pregnancy because of the changes in the way your blood clots. When a thrombosis occurs, it is likely to occur in the veins in the calves of your legs. It is not a common condition, but there are certain risk factors that increase the likelihood, including smoking; being overweight or inactive for long periods of time; if you or members of your family have previously had a deep vein thrombosis or pulmonary embolus.

Q HOW DO I KNOW IF I'VE GOT A BLOOD CLOT?

A If you have a pain in your calf or thigh, sometimes with slight swelling and redness, this is a sign of a blood clot. Your leg may also be painful to walk on and the area tender to touch. This can occur at any stage in pregnancy, but more commonly in later months or just after the birth.

Q IS A BLOOD CLOT A SERIOUS CONDITION?

A A blood clot is painful and may make your leg swell, but its real significance is that part of the clot may break off and pass to your lungs. If this happens it is called a pulmonary embolus; although not common, it is potentially very serious, if not fatal.

Q HOW WOULD I KNOW IF I HAVE A PULMONARY EMBOLUS?

A A pulmonary embolus makes you short of breath and gives you chest pain, especially when breathing in. If you develop either of these symptoms, especially if you know you have any of the risk factors mentioned above, you must inform your doctor as soon as possible. You will need to have a special lung scan and an X-ray test called a venogram or a Doppler scan (see p. 34), to visualize the veins in your legs. Blood-thinning injections of heparin or warfarin tablets may also be prescribed.

WHAT IS RHESUS DISEASE?

Each person's blood has a Rhesus (Rh) factor, which is either positive (85 percent of the population) or negative (15 percent). This is a problem only when an Rh-negative woman has a partner who is Rh-positive – this may result in an Rh-positive baby. If the mother's and the baby's blood come into contact during the birth, her body produces antibodies against the baby's blood.

How does this affect my baby?
Your blood is tested every few weeks to check if you are making antibodies. If you do, the present baby won't be affected, but a subsequent fetus may become severely anemic because the mother's antibodies will cross the placenta and destroy the fetal red blood cells. This is now rare as pregnant women and women who have had a miscarriage or termination are injected with Rh_o immuneglobulin to prevent the manufacture of maternal antibodies.

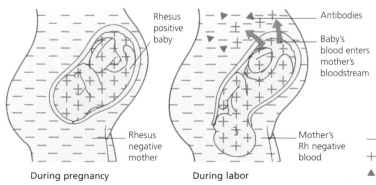

RHESUS DISEASE
Antibodies produced against Rhesus positive blood by the mother during delivery (left), cross the placenta in later pregnancies and cause severe anemia in the baby, or even miscarriage.

— Rhesus negative blood
+ Rhesus positive blood
▲ Mother's antibodies

During pregnancy   During labor

ISSUES IN A MULTIPLE PREGNANCY

Q HOW WILL MY PREGNANCY BE AFFECTED IF THERE IS MORE THAN ONE BABY?

A If you are pregnant with more than one baby your pregnancy is automatically classed as high-risk. Besides all the normal symptoms of pregnancy, you have a greater chance of developing a potentially serious condition, such as preeclampsia (see p. 127). Your pregnancy will be more closely monitored by your doctor or midwife, and you will have experienced staff to supervise the birth. It is also unlikely that you will carry your babies to 40 weeks.

Q AM I MORE LIKELY TO GET PREECLAMPSIA IF I'M HAVING TWINS?

A Multiple pregnancies place extra strain on your body's resources at an earlier stage in the pregnancy, so you are slightly more likely to suffer from high blood pressure and excessive weight gain, two of the possible symptoms of preeclampsia.

Q WILL I HAVE MORE FREQUENT CHECKUPS IF I'M EXPECTING TWINS?

A Yes, you will have more frequent checkups to monitor the fetal growth rates, and your blood pressure and urine will be tested more frequently. You may be offered more frequent ultrasound scans.

Q ONE OF MY TWINS IS LARGER THAN THE OTHER. IS THIS A PROBLEM?

A It is relatively common for twins to grow at a different rate in the womb. If there is a big size difference, your babies may be delivered early. Size difference also needs to be investigated to eliminate a rare condition called twin-to-twin transfusion syndrome (see opposite). This only occurs if your twins are identical and share a placenta.

Q AM I LIKELY TO HAVE A PREMATURE LABOR?

A Yes, it is very likely that your babies will be born early. With twins, you can probably expect to go into labor between 34 and 38 weeks, and with triplets between 32 and 36 weeks. This is partly because of the increased weight that you are carrying, and because the extra amniotic fluid stretches your womb and puts extra pressure on your cervix. If your babies are born before term, they will probably be smaller than full-term babies and may need to spend time in a neonatal intensive-care unit (see p. 214).

Q MY TWINS ARE IDENTICAL, WILL THIS AFFECT THE DELIVERY?

A It is very important, not least for the delivery, to determine whether the twins are identical or not and, if they are identical, whether they are in separate placental sacs. Identical twins are more likely to be born by cesarean delivery, as they usually share a placenta and are occasionally in the same amniotic sac. These factors can make a vaginal delivery difficult and dangerous. Provided that at least one of them is head down (cephalic), fraternal twins can often be delivered vaginally.

Q AM I MORE LIKELY TO HAVE A CESAREAN DELIVERY?

A Yes, twin or multiple deliveries are more likely to be by cesarean delivery, especially if the first baby is not head down in the womb, or if there are any other complicating factors. The cesarean delivery will usually be a planned procedure involving a team of professionals, with an obstetrician, an anesthesiologist, and a pediatrician on hand for each baby.

Q CAN I INSIST ON A TRIAL VAGINAL DELIVERY?

A For the reasons given above, twin vaginal deliveries are considered to be higher risk than the delivery of one baby. Ask your doctors exactly why they are suggesting a cesarean. It is unlikely that they are proposing this simply as a standard procedure; there is probably a specific reason for avoiding vaginal delivery. However, you do have the right to refuse their advice if you feel strongly, but you may put your health at risk.

Q IF ONE FETUS DIES IN THE WOMB, CAN THE OTHER CONTINUE TO DEVELOP?

A Yes, if one fetus miscarries early in the pregnancy, the healthy fetus may continue to develop in the womb. This does not usually cause serious problems for the surviving baby and the lost fetus may even be absorbed into the placenta. However, if one fetus dies during or after the second trimester, its placenta can remain in the womb and may act as a focus for infection. During the third trimester, the death of one baby is more likely to cause premature labor; or the dead twin may simply remain in the womb while the other twin continues to grow.

Q WILL I BE ABLE TO TELL IF ONE TWIN IS NOT MOVING?

A Usually, after about 24 weeks, the babies stay on one side and you can tell what position they are in. Most women can feel their babies moving separately and are even able to tell when one is sleeping. If you notice that one twin's movements have signficantly changed, or a twin has stopped moving, inform your doctor or midwife immediately.

Q WHY DO I FEEL GUILTY ABOUT LOVING MY SURVIVING TWIN?

A It will obviously be distressing for you and your partner if a twin dies. Even though you still have one baby to cherish, you will feel the loss of your other baby. However, it is important to realize that you can be overjoyed by the arrival of your healthy baby, and at the same time grieve deeply for the one who died.

Q WILL THE LOSS OF ONE TWIN AFFECT THE SURVIVING BABY?

A You may worry that the death of one twin will affect the emotional well-being of the surviving one, but there is no evidence of this. The living twin has every chance of being healthy and happy.

QUESTIONS TO ASK

Are my twins identical or fraternal?

Will I have regular ultrasound to check the babies' growth?

Will I be seen by a professional experienced in dealing with multiple pregnancies?

Do I need to change my diet to support more than one pregnancy?

TWIN-TO-TWIN TRANSFUSION SYNDROME

This is a rare condition that occurs only in identical twins with a shared placenta. It is caused by an abnormal blood vessel in the placenta that connects one fetus directly to the other. As a result, one fetus (the donor) uses most of its energy pumping blood not only around its own body but around the other fetus' body (the recipient). This means that the donor twin does not grow properly, and its amniotic fluid is reduced. The recipient twin grows much bigger and an excessive amount of amniotic fluid accumulates rapidly over hours or days.

What are the symptoms?
The rapid increase in amniotic fluid may cause swelling and pain in the abdomen, and premature labor may begin.

What is the outlook for the babies?
This depends on how severe the condition is and how early it is discovered. There have been attempts to treat this condition using lasers to destroy the abnormal blood vessel and by draining the amniotic fluid from the sac around the larger twin. Neither technique is ideal and the risk of premature labor and stillbirth in severe cases is high.

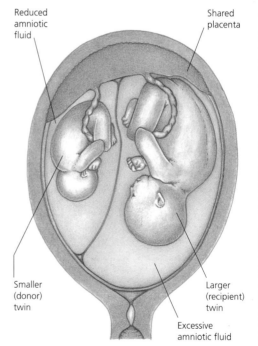

Reduced amniotic fluid

Shared placenta

Smaller (donor) twin

Larger (recipient) twin

Excessive amniotic fluid

WHY THE WOMB SWELLS
The larger "recipient" twin receives more blood than the smaller one and therefore excretes more fluid into the surrounding amniotic fluid. This swells the womb and causes the mother to experience increasing pain.

IF SOMETHING IS WRONG

Q WHAT ABNORMALITIES CAN OCCUR IN MY BABY?

A Different types of abnormalities can occur: congenital abnormalities, that is, physical defects that are present at birth for no reason, such as cleft palate or club foot; these do not endanger the baby's life. Chromosomal abnormalities occur when there is a problem in the baby's genetic makeup; these include conditions such as Down syndrome (see opposite). Genetic defects, such as cystic fibrosis, can be inherited from the parents (see p. 35).

Q ARE FETAL ABNORMALITIES COMMON?

A Up to two percent of babies are born with what is called a congenital abnormality, but often this is something relatively minor, such as an extra digit, or a heart murmur. More rarely, a baby is born with a serious abnormality, such as a heart defect, or spina bifida. Chromosomal abnormalities, such as Down syndrome, are relatively rare.

Q WHEN ARE ABNORMALITIES USUALLY DISCOVERED?

A Since the widespread introduction of ultrasound, many major abnormalities are picked up at an early stage in pregnancies (around 18 to 22 weeks). Some of the less obvious abnormalities may sometimes be missed, even by experienced technicians, and in this situation you may not find out about a problem until your baby is given a postpartum check after the birth.

Q WHAT SUPPORT WILL I BE GIVEN IF MY BABY IS FOUND TO HAVE A PROBLEM?

A If an abnormality is discovered or suspected during a prenatal scan, you will usually be referred to a neonatalogist who specializes in fetal medicine. Ask the doctor or radiologist (or both) to explain everything on the scan; ask what the outlook is (see opposite), and whether you will need further ultrasounds or invasive tests (see p. 36). You will be given time to think about the situation, obtain further information, talk to your family or your own doctor, and be invited to come back with questions.

Q WHAT IS THE NEXT STEP ONCE AN ABNORMALITY IS DISCOVERED?

A With major abnormalities, such as cardiac defects, where an operation is needed that may endanger your baby's life or where your baby may have a permanent disability, ask to see the pediatric surgeon and obstetrician to discuss this. Only then can you make an informed choice. With minor abnormalities that won't endanger your baby's life, or need only a small operation, the situation is less serious but should still be discussed with the pediatric surgeon.

Q COULD I HAVE DONE ANYTHING TO PREVENT MY BABY'S ABNORMALITY?

A No reason can be found for the majority of abnormalities. Only rarely are abnormalities caused by factors such as diabetes, infections, anti-epilepsy drugs, or alcohol. It will be difficult, but it is most important that you do not feel guilty about what has happened.

Q WHAT IS THE DIFFERENCE BETWEEN A MAJOR AND A MINOR DEFECT?

A Parents are invariably shocked and upset if a defect is found in their baby, no matter how small, but doctors divide abnormalities into minor and major ones. Minor defects such as cleft palate or blemishes will not endanger your baby's life. They require no treatment or just a small operation, or physical therapy, to correct. Major abnormalities, such as serious heart defects, can endanger the baby's life and may require major surgery. The baby may also have a permanent disability.

QUESTIONS TO ASK

What does the ultrasound show?

Would you advise a second opinion?

How serious is the condition?

Will my baby need surgery after birth?

Is it likely that my baby will have a normal life?

What are the options in continuing with the pregnancy?

WHAT IS THE OUTLOOK IF MY BABY HAS AN ABNORMALITY?

The outlook for your baby depends on how severe the abnormality is. It also depends on whether you have access to pediatric surgeons who can carry out corrective surgery. It is usually very hard for the parents to come to terms with their baby's abnormality, no matter how minor, even though many conditions can be treated successfully in the first few months of life.

Disfiguring blemishes
Marks on the baby's face from labor, bruising from forceps, and even acne, are fairly common at birth; most are not serious or permanent and usually disappear within days.

Cleft palate
Babies with this defect have a palate and/or lips that do not join properly in the middle, leaving a gap. Once the baby is born, depending on the severity, plastic surgery can be carried out (often successfully); sometimes several operations may be required over a number of years.

Club foot
A baby born with a club foot usually has one foot twisted at the ankle so that it doesn't point in the normal direction. Physical therapy or corrective surgery (involving several operations for severe cases) can correct the problem after the birth.

Extra or absent fingers and toes
Often a hereditary defect, extra digits are quite easily removed by surgery after the birth. Absent digits are very rare and usually not correctable.

Water on the kidney (hydronephrosis)
This is a swollen kidney as a result of a blockage lower down in the urinary tract that stops the flow of urine. Minor cases often get better spontaneously at or before delivery. More severe cases, however, can eventually cause kidney damage, and surgery will be needed after the birth to remove the obstruction, or even the damaged kidney itself.

Heart (cardiac) defects
These are relatively common, varying from a small hole in the heart that often closes naturally, to more serious conditions of the heart and arteries, which may need major surgery once the baby is born.

Diaphragmatic hernia
This is a condition where the baby's abdominal contents (bowels and sometimes liver) push up through a hole in the diaphragm into the chest cavity, compressing the lungs and stopping them from developing fully. Major diaphragmatic hernias can also compress the heart, pushing it to one side. This condition must be operated on within a few days of birth. The outlook depends on how big the hernia is and whether and how severely the lungs and heart have been damaged.

Spina bifida
This defect occurs when the bones, usually at the bottom of the spine, don't join properly so that the spinal cord, which contains vital nerves supplying the lower part of the body, is exposed. It is only after the birth that the true extent of the nerve damage becomes obvious. Severely affected babies can suffer from disabilities including paralysis of the legs and bladder problems. Spina bifida often occurs in conjunction with hydrocephalus (water on the brain), which can cause mental retardation. Minor degrees of spina bifida, in which the spinal defect can only be detected by an X-ray, can also occur; successful corrective surgery after the birth is possible. With the advent of diagnostic testing, this condition is more easily identified. The condition is becoming rare; the incidence of spina bifida is known to decrease if mothers take supplements of folic acid in early pregnancy.

Down syndrome
Although universally dreaded, Down syndrome is quite rare, affecting about one in every 650 fetuses. Caused by the presence of an extra chromosome, Down syndrome may be detected on a nuchal scan at 11 to 14 weeks (see p. 34), by AFP test screening, or by ultrasound scanning at 18 to 22 weeks (see p. 32); but diagnosis can only be confirmed by an invasive test (see p. 36). Most Down syndrome children have some physical abnormalities; the face and features tend to be small, while the hands are short and broad; there are also varying degrees of mental disability. Medical and surgical advances, together with enhanced long-term care facilities, have greatly improved the outlook of Down children, who can make the most of their capabilities with constant educational and environmental stimulation.

IF YOU LOSE YOUR PREGNANCY

Q WHAT IS A MISCARRIAGE?

A A miscarriage occurs if your pregnancy ends before the fetus is capable of sustaining life – normally considered to be before about 24 weeks. Most miscarriages happen in the first ten weeks of pregnancy; in fact, at least 30 percent of all conceptions end this way.

Q WHY DO MISCARRIAGES HAPPEN?

A There are several reasons why every pregnancy does not lead to a successful birth. It may be because your pregnancy was ectopic (see below); the fetus may not have developed normally; or the placenta, the egg, or the sperm was defective. There may also have been a chromosomal problem.

Q ARE ALL MISCARRIAGES THE SAME?

A Not all miscarriages happen in the same way – there are several terms to define what takes place: "threatened," "missed," and "inevitable." In the first trimester, if there is bleeding but no pain, and the fetus stays alive and healthy so that the pregnancy continues to term, this is called a threatened miscarriage. You may have what is called a missed miscarriage if the fetus dies, but stays in the womb and is either expelled later or is removed by an operation. An inevitable miscarriage is the term used when there is bleeding and pain, the cervix opens and the fetus is expelled from the womb. If the miscarriage leaves small fragments of the placenta or blood clots in the womb, this is known as an "incomplete" miscarriage (see opposite).

WHAT IS AN ECTOPIC PREGNANCY?

When a fertilized egg develops and implants outside the womb, either in a fallopian tube or, more rarely, in the abdominal cavity, the developing egg outgrows its blood supply and dies, causing severe bleeding. This condition is rare.

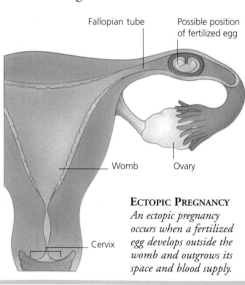

Fallopian tube   Possible position of fertilized egg

Womb   Ovary

Cervix

ECTOPIC PREGNANCY
An ectopic pregnancy occurs when a fertilized egg develops outside the womb and outgrows its space and blood supply.

Symptoms and treatment
If you are experiencing severe pain in your abdomen (usually on one side), heavy vaginal bleeding, and you feel faint (particularly if you have already had a positive pregnancy test), go to an emergency room at once. Ectopic pregnancies can't be saved. The situation may be life-threatening to you because it can cause severe internal bleeding and will need prompt surgery. In serious cases, the affected fallopian tube may need to be removed. Sometimes, an early ectopic pregnancy can "miscarry" itself, known as a tubal abortion, without your knowledge.

How likely is an ectopic pregnancy?
You are at risk if you have previously had an infection in your fallopian tubes or pelvic inflammatory disease, or if your fallopian tubes have been otherwise damaged. The chances also increase if you become pregnant while wearing an IUD or while taking the minipill.

Can I still have a normal pregnancy?
You can still have a healthy pregnancy after an ectopic pregnancy, although your chances of conception may be slightly reduced.

Q HOW DO I KNOW IF I AM HAVING A MISCARRIAGE?

A Vaginal bleeding with periodlike cramps are frequently a sign that you are about to have a miscarriage. Bleeding at any stage of pregnancy, with or without pain, should always be taken seriously; seek immediate medical advice.

Q WILL I NEED TREATMENT AFTER A MISCARRIAGE?

A Yes, you will probably have an ultrasound scan to see what has happened. You will not need treatment if the scan shows that your womb is clear. If the womb is not entirely empty, known as an incomplete miscarriage, you may need a procedure called a D & C (dilation and curettage) to clear your womb. If your womb is not cleared in this way, an infection could develop which could affect your chances of a future pregnancy. You will have a general anesthetic for this procedure.

Q I HAVE HAD SEVERAL MISCARRIAGES. DO I NEED TO SEE A SPECIALIST?

A One or two miscarriages are unlikely to have a long-term effect on your ability to carry a pregnancy to term. Early miscarriages are very common, and investigations are unlikely to help unless you have had more than three in succession. Even then, further investigations will prove useful only if you have a treatable condition.

Q CAN ANYTHING BE DONE TO PREVENT A LATE MISCARRIAGE?

A When a threatened miscarriage occurs in the second trimester and the cause is identified – if, for example, there is a weakness in the cervix or an infection – this can be treated and miscarriage can often be avoided. If, however, no cause is found, nothing can be done to prevent it.

Q WILL I SEE AND HOLD THE FETUS AFTER HAVING A MISCARRIAGE?

A If you miscarry in the second trimester of your pregnancy, you can see the fetus if you wish. However, not everyone wants to do this, and you should not feel you have to. Most hospitals have a trained professional, usually a doctor or midwife, to guide you and your partner through this difficult time. If your baby is born and dies after 24 weeks, this is legally not a miscarriage but a premature birth, and the birth and death have to be recorded and, if you wish, funeral arrangements made (see p. 231).

DISCUSSION POINT

HOW WILL LOSING MY PREGNANCY AFFECT ME?

Feelings of guilt and anger
You will almost certainly feel guilty and also possibly angry after a miscarriage, even though it is unlikely that you or your partner were in any way responsible for the loss. These feelings are very understandable. Ask your caregivers to explain exactly what may have happened and to answer your questions.

The need to grieve
Whether you miscarried early in pregnancy or very late, and particularly if you had already felt your baby move, you may think of your pregnancy as a person and grieve for your loss. Grieving is important, just as it is when you lose any loved one. It may take some time to come to terms with your loss.

Healing
If you lose your baby late in pregnancy, it may help you both to see and hold him or her and spend some time alone together. You may want to give your baby a name, either informally, or with a religious ceremony, and to keep a memento such as a photograph, a lock of hair, or a handprint. Holding a funeral can also help the healing process. There are support groups, usually run by people who have experienced miscarriage or the death of a baby, that can help with the grieving process (see p. 232).

The future
It is a good idea to see the obstetrician about six weeks or so afterward to talk about what happened and why. You may want to ask for advice about future pregnancies. However, it may be wise to wait awhile before planning another pregnancy so that you can recover mentally and physically. The time will come when you feel ready. Remember, many women lose pregnancies, and most women who have had a loss go on to have a healthy baby.

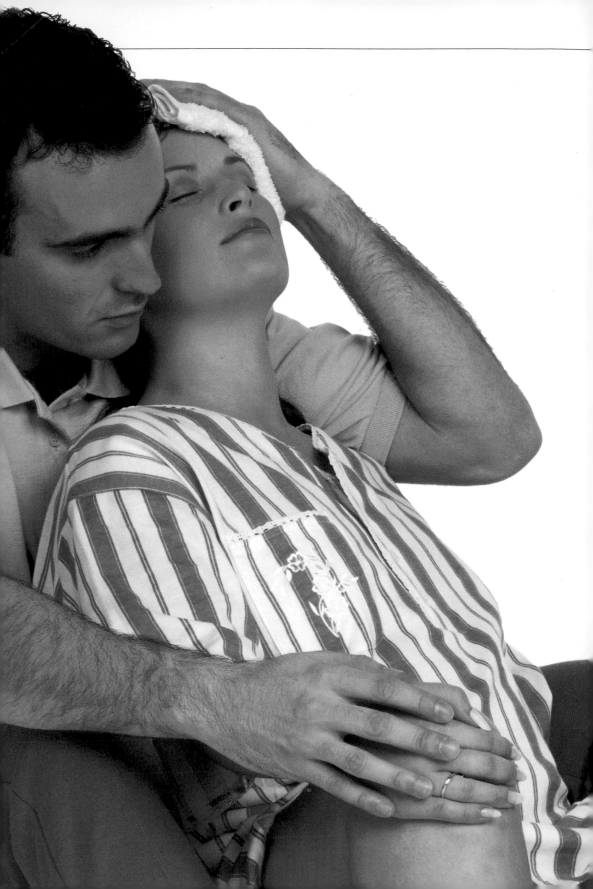

LABOR
AND
BIRTH

Few other events in life can compare with the anticipation and excitement of the birth of a baby; soon you will meet the tiny human being you have carried and nurtured for so long – and you will treasure the moment forever. You may have fears about what will happen during the delivery, and you may be concerned about how you will react to the physical exertion of labor. This chapter explains the types of delivery, your choices in pain relief and their relative effectiveness, and what happens during the three stages of labor. With this information, you can feel truly positive about what is to come.

PREPARING FOR LABOR

Q **HOW WILL MY LABOR BE INFLUENCED BY HOSPITAL POLICIES?**

A Hospitals have policies on all aspects of labor, birth, and postpartum care, so it's worth discussing these with your midwife or doctor. However, these are usually only guidelines and, if you have a request that conflicts with hospital procedure, you can often negotiate.

Q **WHAT ASPECTS OF MY LABOR CAN I NOT DECIDE ON?**

A You can be involved in all aspects of the planning of your labor, but when it comes to the actual delivery, it's important to listen to the professionals. They will guide you in the choices available to you, based on the immediate needs of you and your baby. If any medical intervention is necessary, there is usually a good reason for it.

Q **HOW CAN I LET THE HOSPITAL KNOW WHAT KIND OF LABOR I WANT?**

A One way is to outline your ideas in a birth plan (see opposite). A birth plan is a document that tells hospital staff how you would like your labor and delivery to progress. It can cover the type of delivery you want, who you would like with you, and your preferences for pain relief. However, certain requests depend on the facilities available, such as whether or not there is a labor pool.

Q **WHY IS WRITING A BIRTH PLAN A GOOD IDEA?**

A Even jotting down a few lines is an excellent way to focus your mind on the choices that are available to you during labor; it can also make you feel more confident and more in control. Also, there will probably be periods during your labor when you won't feel like answering lots of questions: if you have prepared a birth plan, the staff will look at this when you start your labor and will be aware of your preferences.

Q **WHO SHOULD I TALK TO ABOUT MY BIRTH PLAN?**

A Discuss your birth plan with your midwife or doctor at around 32 to 36 weeks. They will be familiar with the hospital's policies and facilities, and will know whether your plan is feasible.

Q **HOW LIKELY AM I TO GET WHAT I REQUEST IN MY BIRTH PLAN?**

A Most doctors and hospitals will try to accommodate your wishes, but be flexible and open-minded: your labor may not go as expected, so try not to be disappointed if something happens that means that you have to abandon all or part of your birth plan. Be positive and emphasize the things you are looking forward to, such as breastfeeding your baby afterward, or your partner cutting the cord.

Q **CAN I SAY THAT I DON'T WANT STUDENTS PRESENT DURING LABOR?**

A Yes, you can, but the students are not only there to learn about birth, they can also provide useful support to the main medical team and to you, and are always closely supervised.

Q **DO I HAVE TO WRITE A BIRTH PLAN?**

A You don't have to. In fact, many women choose not to, especially if they have had a baby before. However, if you have particular likes or dislikes, fears and requests, a birth plan is the place to state these. However, during labor, the medical team will always consult you before carrying out any treatment.

Q **CAN I CHANGE MY BIRTH PLAN?**

A What you put in your birth plan is not written in stone; keep a copy of it with your packed hospital bag so that you can change it at any time if, on further reflection, your original thoughts don't seem like such a good idea.

QUESTIONS TO ASK

Is it this hospital's policy to follow birth plans as closely as possible?

Shall I bring an extra copy of my birth plan to the hospital?

Does the hospital have the facilities to comply with my requests?

Are all the medical staff open to discussion about procedures?

WRITING A BIRTH PLAN

There is no set format for a birth plan; it can consist of a few simple instructions, or detailed notes. It is important to include those issues that most concern you, and to list your preferences, but try not to sound too confrontational. Discuss the plan with your doctor or midwife, and ask him or her to sign and date it. You need at least two copies, one for yourself and one to add to your hospital records.

WHAT IT MIGHT COVER	WHAT YOU SHOULD CONSIDER
Who you want to have present as a birth partner	■ Who will be your birth partner: your partner, a friend, or a relative? Can you have more than one person with you? If you need to have a cesarean section or stitches, would you prefer your birth partner to leave?
THE FIRST STAGE	■ How do you feel about being induced if you go past your due date? ■ Do you want to be as active as possible during labor? ■ How do you feel about fetal monitoring, which could confine your movements? ■ How do you feel about your labor being artificially speeded up, either by having your water broken or by a hormone drip (see p. 159)? ■ Have you practiced certain breathing or relaxation techniques, and would you like to be coached in these during labor to relieve the pain? ■ If you are giving birth in a teaching hospital, do you object to medical students or student midwives and nurses being present?
Pain relief	■ Do you want to be offered pain relief or do you want the medical team to wait until you ask for it? ■ Do you have preferences for certain kinds of pain relief – and at what stage of labor would you like to receive them (see p. 154)? ■ If you have an epidural, would you prefer it to be timed so that it wears off when you are ready to push?
THE SECOND STAGE	■ In what position would you prefer to deliver your baby (see p. 166)? ■ Would you prefer to be allowed to tear naturally or would you prefer a cut made to the perineum (an episiotomy) to make room for your baby's head on delivery? ■ Would you like to see your baby's head being delivered? ■ Would you like your birth partner to cut the umbilical cord?
When your baby is born	■ Would you like your baby to be delivered straight onto your abdomen? ■ Does the hospital routinely suction the baby's air passages after birth? ■ Do you want a midwife or nurse to help you breastfeed? ■ Would you and your partner prefer to be left alone with your baby in the delivery room?
THE THIRD STAGE	■ Does the hospital routinely use drugs to speed up the delivery of the placenta? Would you prefer to deliver it naturally? ■ If you need stitches to your perineum, would you prefer an experienced doctor or midwife to do them rather than a student? Would you object to having a local anesthetic for this? ■ Providing all goes well, how soon would you like to leave the hospital?

LABOR AND BIRTH

GIVING BIRTH IN A HOSPITAL

Q WHAT PLANS SHOULD I MAKE BEFORE MY LABOR IN A HOSPITAL?

A There are a number of arrangements that need to be made well in advance of your labor so that everything runs smoothly when you need to go into the hospital. Make a list of relevant contact numbers, keep them by the telephone, and tell another person where they are in case of an emergency. You should include your doctor or midwife's contact number, or the number of the maternity department, and your labor partner's daytime telephone number. Keep your hospital notes handy.

Q WHAT OTHER ARRANGEMENTS MUST I MAKE?

A Work out your travel arrangements in advance, because once your contractions start, you should not attempt to drive yourself to the hospital. If no one else is available to drive you to the hospital, call a taxi or, in an emergency, call an ambulance. If you have children, you should make arrangements for someone to come over at short notice to look after them. They should be prepared to come even if you go into labor in the middle of the night.

GETTING READY FOR YOUR HOSPITAL BIRTH

Plan what you will need to pack in your hospital bag, and make sure that it is ready at least three weeks before your baby is due. If you leave the packing until you go into labor, you are more than likely to forget something in the excitement.

WHAT YOU NEED

In most hospitals you will need the basic essentials shown here, but you can take other things for relaxation and massage.

Socks

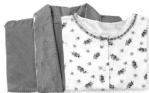

A big T-shirt or nightgown for labor

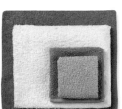

Washcloths and towels

Slippers

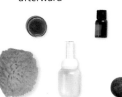

A robe and nightgown for afterward

Extra items

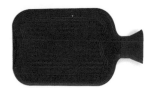

A hot water bottle for backache

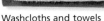

A sponge, lip salve, water spray, massage oil, and equipment

Essentials for your labor
- A nightgown or big T-shirt
- Socks
- Washcloths and towels
- Slippers
- Robe and several nightgowns
- Shower bag with toiletries

Extra items
- Hot water bottle
- Sponge and lip salve
- Water spray bottle
- Massage equipment and oils
- Music for relaxation
- A small hand mirror

After delivery for you
- Nursing bras and breast pads
- Disposable briefs
- Sanitary pads
- Personal stereo and books

Q WHAT DO I NEED TO TAKE TO THE HOSPITAL FOR MY LABOR?

A You will need to pack a bag of basic essentials. Before you begin to pack, ask your midwife for a list of basics you need to bring as well as what the hospital provides in the way of toiletries. Assemble the things you'll want for your comfort during the delivery, such as a cooling face spray and a natural sponge to suck when your mouth feels dry, as well as your usual toiletries for washing and freshening up. Usually you can wear your own clothes for labor such as a large T-shirt or short-sleeved nightgown. For later on the maternity ward, you will need a robe as well as fresh nightgowns (front-opening if you intend to breastfeed). Don't forget to pack your sanitary towels, maternity bras, and breast pads.

Q APART FROM ESSENTIALS, SHOULD WE BRING ANYTHING ELSE?

A You may both be glad to have something to distract you during a prolonged early labor, so your partner could arrange to bring in tapes and a cassette player, games, or playing cards. Remember to bring your favorite massage oils and equipment if you are using them. If you want to record the birth of your baby, pack a camera or video camera. Change or a phone card for the hospital telephone is essential, as cellular phones – which can interfere with equipment – are not allowed. You might consider refreshments for your partner during a long labor, because few hospitals provide food during the night, or vending machines that contain food. A change of clothes for your partner is also useful.

WHAT YOUR BABY NEEDS

You need to provide a set of clothing for when your baby is born. The following list is very basic, but should cover your baby's immediate needs after the birth. You will undoubtedly buy much more clothing than this over the coming months (see p. 196).

Essentials
- Two to three sleepers or nightgowns, and undershirts
- Scratch mittens
- A shawl or baby blanket
- Cream, such as vitamins A & D cream, or petroleum jelly, for baby's bottom
- Disposable diapers
- Cotton balls

Afterward for taking your baby home
- An extra layer of outdoor clothes and blankets
- A car seat
- A hat

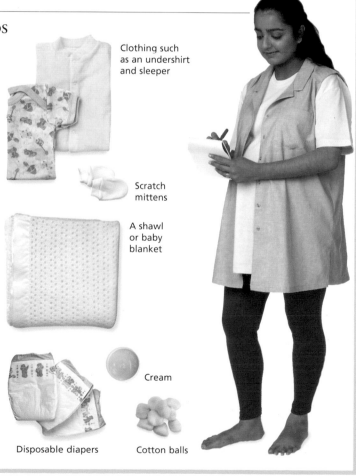

Clothing such as an undershirt and sleeper

Scratch mittens

A shawl or baby blanket

Cream

Disposable diapers

Cotton balls

THE DELIVERY ROOM

A hospital environment can seem frightening to an outsider, but if you understand exactly what is going on when you have your baby, you can be more relaxed. Your hospital will invite you to tour its obstetric's department as part of your prenatal preparations. It is a good idea to go to see the delivery rooms and maternity wards, and to ask any questions you might have about the hospital's procedures and equipment.

WHAT IS THE EQUIPMENT FOR?

The labor room is full of equipment, some of which can seem intimidating to prospective parents. Below is a guide to the most important items you will see:

■ **Bassinet** This is where your baby is laid when being checked over by the midwife or doctor.

■ **Delivery bed** Although high, the delivery bed is practical: for delivery, the bed can be raised and lowered, and the end of the bed can be removed to facilitate the delivery and any stitching that needs to be done.

■ **Resuscitation cart** This cart is equipped with oxygen for your baby and suction apparatus to extract any mucus from your baby's lungs. There is also a heater in the cart for the newborn baby. This equipment is always prepared and available in the event of a problem arising during delivery.

■ **Sphygmomanometer** This instrument measures your blood pressure.

■ **Gas and air** Available in some hospitals, gas and air is a mixture of oxygen and nitrous oxide that you can inhale through a mask during your labor to help take the edge off your pain.

■ **External fetal monitor** This records your contractions and your baby's heartbeat, and shows them on a continuous printout.

■ **Extra comforts** Some hospitals supply aids, such as a bean bag, birthing chair or stool, or a rocking chair, for a more active birth.

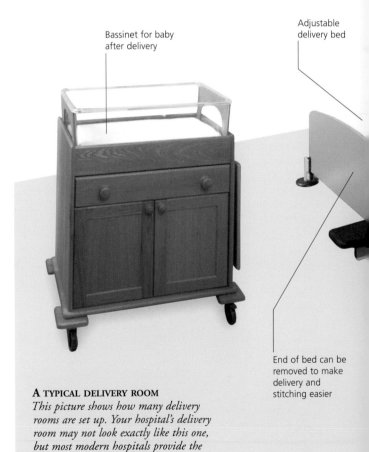

Bassinet for baby after delivery

Adjustable delivery bed

End of bed can be removed to make delivery and stitching easier

A TYPICAL DELIVERY ROOM
This picture shows how many delivery rooms are set up. Your hospital's delivery room may not look exactly like this one, but most modern hospitals provide the equipment shown here. Some also offer private bathroom facilities, and there may be a shower or tub.

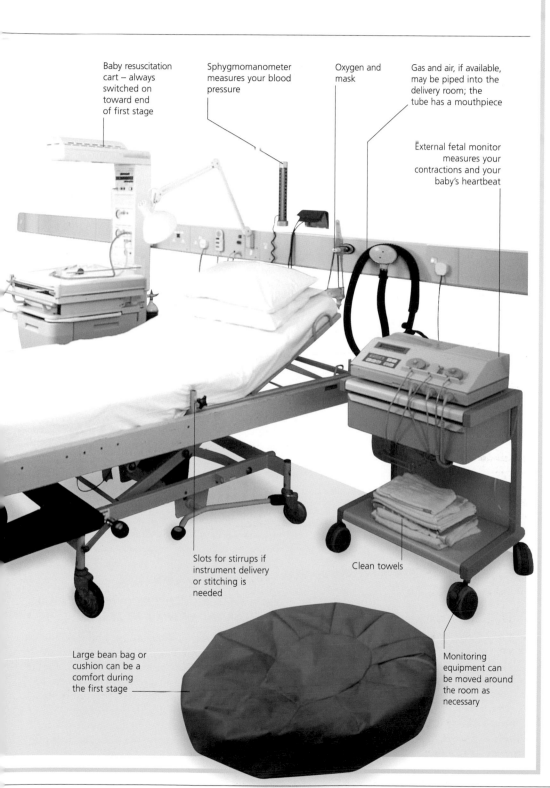

Baby resuscitation cart – always switched on toward end of first stage

Sphygmomanometer measures your blood pressure

Oxygen and mask

Gas and air, if available, may be piped into the delivery room; the tube has a mouthpiece

External fetal monitor measures your contractions and your baby's heartbeat

Slots for stirrups if instrument delivery or stitching is needed

Clean towels

Large bean bag or cushion can be a comfort during the first stage

Monitoring equipment can be moved around the room as necessary

LABOR AND BIRTH

PREPARING FOR A HOME BIRTH

Q **WHAT ARE THE ADVANTAGES OF HAVING MY BABY AT HOME?**

A There are many positive aspects, the most important being familiarity with your surroundings; you and your partner will not have to travel anywhere when you go into labor, and you may both feel more relaxed about participating fully in the event. You will also have more freedom to move around, and to give birth in whatever position feels natural and comfortable. You can create a soothing atmosphere with music and candles, and your labor can be as private – or as social – an event as you wish, yet you will have the reassurance of a professional presence in your midwife. If you have other children, they can come in immediately afterward.

Q **IS A HOME BIRTH AS SAFE AS A HOSPITAL BIRTH?**

A If your pregnancy and labor are considered to be straightforward, there is no evidence to suggest that a home birth is less safe than a hospital one. You may feel more reassured if you talk to your midwife to find out exactly which situations she can deal with.

Q **WHAT DO I NEED TO DO IN PREPARATION?**

A When your midwife visits you, ask her about what equipment you should provide for her in preparation for labor; she will probably supply a list of essential and optional items. You also need to prepare the room or areas in which you intend to give birth (see p. 146).

QUESTIONS TO ASK

Are there any medical reasons why I should not consider having a home birth?

What are my options if labor does not proceed normally?

How can I find a midwife who will be sympathetic to my ideas about home birth?

What kind of pain relief can the midwife offer me during a home birth?

Q **WHAT KIND OF ROOM IS BEST FOR A HOME BIRTH?**

A It can be anywhere in your home, but it should be warm (with extra warmth available for the baby when he or she arrives), quiet (where you are not likely to be interrupted by other members of the household), and ideally near a bathroom. If you intend to have an active or water birth, the room must be spacious enough for you to clear a birthing area and cover it with plastic sheets for protection, with space for pillows or bean bags if you wish. You'll also need a clear tabletop that can be used as a work area for the midwife's equipment, as well as somewhere to put all your comfort aids. Your midwife will inspect your room beforehand to check that there are no problems.

Q **CAN I ASK MY FAVORITE MIDWIFE TO ATTEND MY LABOR?**

A Midwives usually work with a small team, and you should have the chance to meet most of your team during the prenatal period. If you have a favorite midwife, ask her if she minds putting herself on "extra" call to look after you, but there is a chance that she might not be able to.

Q **WHAT HAPPENS WHEN LABOR STARTS?**

A Call your midwife and your birth partner as soon as you feel that your labor has begun (see p. 156). Your midwife will give you her beeper number, or a cellular phone number if she has one. Keep the relevant numbers on hand as your estimated date of delivery approaches.

Q **WHAT SHOULD WE DO WHILE WE WAIT FOR THE MIDWIFE TO ARRIVE?**

A You will be relaxing and breathing through your contractions. If you have not already done so, your birth partner can prepare the room by moving away furniture, laying out plastic sheets, bringing in pillows and cushions from other rooms, and creating a comfortable atmosphere with heating, lighting, and relaxing music. He or she can also organize care for your other children, and prepare drinks and snacks for everyone to have later.

Q WHAT WILL MY MIDWIFE DO DURING MY HOME BIRTH?

A When your midwife arrives, she will ask questions about your progress. She will probably give you an internal examination to confirm the stage of labor and the position of your baby, and she will record the strength and frequency of your contractions. She will check your blood pressure, temperature, and pulse to ensure that there are no problems, and will regularly monitor your baby's heartbeat (usually with a handheld Doppler sonicaid device), to check that your baby is not in distress. Your midwife will deliver your baby and the placenta and, if necessary, stitch any tears or cuts after the birth.

Q WHAT IF PROBLEMS DEVELOP DURING THE BIRTH?

A Your midwife is trained to spot potential problems, and if any develop, she will call an ambulance to take you to hospital. She will then accompany you to the hospital, stay with you, and deliver the baby with the appropriate medical back-up. This may be disappointing if you've had your heart set on a home birth, but it is important to keep an open mind about transferring to hospital. Remember that the safe delivery of your baby will always be your midwife's priority, whether you are giving birth at home or in a hospital.

Q IS IT REALLY NECESSARY TO BOIL WATER FOR A BIRTH – OR IS THIS A MYTH?

A Midwives used to have to sterilize their equipment in boiled water, but this is no longer necessary. Some warm water will be needed to clean your baby after he or she is born.

Q CAN MY CHILDREN WATCH THE BIRTH?

A Only you can gauge how your child or children will react, but if he or she is likely to be frightened by seeing you in pain, it may not be a good idea. Also, you may lose your partner's support while he or she tends the child or children elsewhere in the home. The child or children could perhaps be there to meet the new arrival immediately after the birth.

Q WHAT WILL HAPPEN IN THE FIRST FEW HOURS AFTER MY BABY IS BORN?

A Once delivered, you will be able t hold your new baby; he or she will then be cleaned, examined, and weighed (see p. 175). The midwife will need warm water, cotton balls, and a diaper ready. This is a time for you and your partner to bond with your baby; the home is ideal for undisturbed contact. The midwife stays long enough to be sure that all is well. She will usually return to check you both later in the day.

DISCUSSION POINT

DECIDING ON A HOME BIRTH

Some women feel more secure if their labor is managed by doctors in a hospital; others relish the chance to have their babies without medical intervention. If you are self-confident enough to ask, you can usually get the kind of birth you want.

The medical reaction
Because they cannot predict how your labor may progress, doctors generally are not enthusiastic about first babies being delivered at home, so you may find that your doctor prefers you to have had at least one normal delivery in a hospital before agreeing to a home birth. However, if you are set on a home birth, and there are no medical objections (see p. 22), talk to your midwife.

Pain relief
You may choose a home birth because your goal is a more natural approach, and you particularly want to avoid medical intervention such as an epidural anesthesia and electronic fetal monitoring. This is fine, but however determined you are to keep the birth as natural as possible, you may change your mind and ask for pain relief once the labor begins. Your midwife may be able to offer you an injection of meperidine (Demerol); she cannot give you an epidural.

Organization
Organizing a home birth is perhaps not as easy as simply going into a hospital, but most women who do manage it find that having their baby at home is a very satisfying experience.

LABOR AND BIRTH

What do I need for a home birth?

Because you have chosen to give birth in your own home, you and your partner are in control of your birth environment and can provide the atmosphere you prefer. There are, however, certain essentials you should provide; ask your midwife for a list.

What you will need

The midwife attending your delivery will bring with her all the necessary medical equipment (see panel, right). Decide where you would like to have your baby; the only requirements are warmth and cleanliness. In addition to some items of equipment you will be required to provide, consider the optional items shown below.

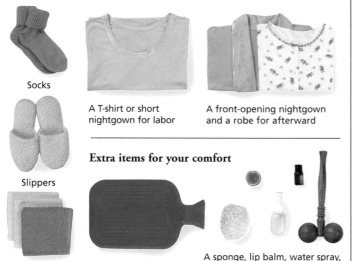

Socks

A T-shirt or short nightgown for labor

A front-opening nightgown and a robe for afterward

Slippers

Extra items for your comfort

Washcloths

Hot water bottle

A sponge, lip balm, water spray, massage oil, and equipment

Essentials for you
- Something comfortable to wear (a large T-shirt or short nightgown)
- Socks, washcloth

Extra items for your comfort
- Small natural sponge to suck on
- Ice chips or cubes
- Hot water bottle
- Water spray bottle
- Lip balm; massager, oil

Items you will need afterward
- A fresh nightdress
- Slippers and dressing gown
- Nursing bra and breast pads
- Disposable briefs
- Sanitary pads
- Towels

Equipment you will need to provide

Your house probably already contains most of the things you need, but you may want to provide extra cushions so that you have several alternatives for changing positions as you cope with contractions. Dim lights may help you relax during labor, but your midwife will need a bright light for stitching.

Extra pillows or large cushions

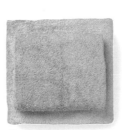

Clean towels

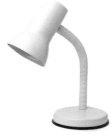

Lamp

FOR YOUR BABY

About three weeks before your baby is due, start assembling all the basic items that will be necessary for your new baby. The main requirements are diapers, warm clothing, and somewhere to sleep.

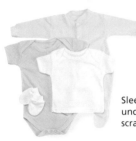

Sleepers, undershirts, and scratch mittens

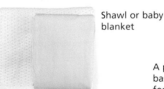

Plenty of diapers, diaper cream, and cotton balls

Shawl or baby blanket

Essentials

- Soft, clean towels and sheets
- Diapers (disposable or cloth as preferred)
- Clothing such as two to three sleepers, undershirts, or nightgowns
- Scratch mittens
- Shawl or baby blanket
- Cotton balls
- Vitamins A & D cream or petroleum jelly
- Bassinet or crib
- Changing pad (optional)

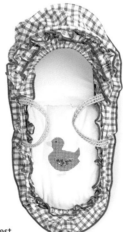

A portable bassinet is best for a newborn baby

THE MIDWIFE'S PACK

Your midwife arrives with a delivery pack containing essential medicines and sterile instruments for the safe delivery of your baby.

Basic labor kit

- Antiseptic solutions
- Blood pressure monitor
- Thermometer; stethoscope
- Doppler sonicaid
- Syringes
- Urine testing sticks
- Oxygen
- Equipment for stitching
- Gloves, scissors

For pain relief

- Narcotic drugs such as meperidine (Demerol). (Your midwife may ask you to get this with a prescription from your doctor beforehand)
- Local anesthetic

In case of emergency

- Resuscitation equipment for your baby
- An intravenous drip in case of hemorrhage

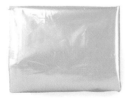

Plastic sheeting

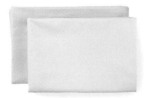

Clean sheets

Checklist for the labor

- Clean sheets for your bed in case you use it, and/or waterproof cover for the mattress
- Plastic sheeting for the floor
- Lamp or bright flashlight for stitching, if necessary
- Pillows or cushions
- Hot water, soap, and clean towels
- Energy snacks and drinks for you, your partner, and the midwife

For afterward

- Bags for trash disposal
- Clean sheets for your bed

Optional extras

- Bean bag(s) or large floor cushions
- Handheld or portable fan
- Portable electric heater if the room needs extra warmth
- Music, candles, and/or scented oils to create a relaxed atmosphere
- Camera or videocamera loaded with film
- A low stool
- Handheld mirror
- Birthing pool – you rent this in advance, if wanted

LABOR AND BIRTH

YOUR CHOICES IN CHILDBIRTH

Q WHAT ARE MY CHOICES IN TYPES OF CHILDBIRTH?

A You can choose between a natural, or alternative birth, an active birth, or an actively (medically) managed birth – or even a combination of these.

Q WHAT DOES A NATURAL BIRTH INVOLVE?

A A natural birth avoids the use of drugs for pain relief, encourages active labor positions; it also favors the use of natural or complementary types of pain relief (see below).

Q WHAT ARE THE BENEFITS OF NATURAL OR COMPLEMENTARY PAIN RELIEF?

A Stress in labor increases tension and reduces your capacity to deal with pain. Natural methods of pain relief (see below) or distractional stimuli, such as massage, stimulate your body to release endorphins, its own natural "painkillers"; these help you cope with the pain, which reduces stress and enables you to feel more in control of your labor. Whether you go for a completely natural childbirth, or combine natural with medical pain relief, be prepared for your plans to alter.

WHAT NATURAL PAIN RELIEF METHODS ARE AVAILABLE TO ME?

Natural pain-relieving methods soothe and relax you, but will not entirely stop all pain; however, by easing tension, they increase your capacity to deal with pain. You will need to organize, practice, and familiarize yourself with these methods before the birth. Most methods can be used with medical types of pain relief (see p. 154). Most midwives and doctors accept these approaches and are open to their use during labor, but if you decide to have a natural birth, discuss this before labor.

ALONE OR WITH YOUR PARTNER

■ **Heat and cold** Applying heat or cold is soothing in labor and can ease tension; in itself it will not get rid of pain but it can make pain easier to cope with. A hot water bottle alternated with a washcloth soaked in cold water can reduce backache or cramping. Some women find that a cold washcloth on the face can ease tension.

■ **Movement** Keeping mobile improves your circulation and can help to reduce backache, as well as acting as a distraction to the pain. Try different positions in labor, using cushions, bean bags, or chairs for support, until you find a position that suits you best.

■ **Massage** This relieves tension in your shoulders, neck, face, and back, as well as relaxing you and improving circulation, thereby reducing the intensity of labor pains. You and your partner can practice this together before labor (see p. 114).

■ **Aromatherapy** This technique involves essential oils combined with massage, which helps reduce tension, and can relieve, but not eliminate, pain, particularly in early labor. You can also place oils in vaporizers in the room to help soothe you.

WITH AN EXPERT

If you are considering using any of the following methods you will need to arrange for a qualified practitioner to be with you throughout labor to ensure that everything is done correctly.

■ **Acupuncture** Fine needles inserted into specific body points (see p. 104) relieve pain by releasing the body's own painkillers, endorphins.

■ **Reflexology** Applying pressure to specific points on your feet can relieve pain and muscular problems in other parts of the body (see p. 104). Gentle foot massage can also be very relaxing.

■ **Hypnosis** This works by suggestion: if you believe that you can control the pain, you may be less disturbed by it. Try hypnosis only if you have tested it before labor.

Q WHAT DOES AN ACTIVE CHILDBIRTH MEAN?

A An active childbirth means that you move around during the early part of labor, and give birth in any position other than the traditional one of lying on a bed on your back. Many women find it easier and less painful to give birth in this way. You can sit, stand, squat or kneel on all fours; you will, however, need assistance from your birth partner, midwife, or hospital staff. An active childbirth should not be confused with the "active management of labor." This is a medical phrase that originated in the 1960s and was based on the close supervision of labor and, if necessary, providing early intervention in the labor process with labor-inducing drugs or by artificially rupturing the membranes (see p. 159).

Q WHAT ARE THE BENEFITS OF AN ACTIVE BIRTH?

A Active positions may help your labor to progress through the use of gravity; they can make your contractions more effective in the first stage of labor, increase your stamina, and help your cervix to open more easily. In the second stage of labor, an upright rather than a supine position means that you won't feel as if you are pushing uphill, which can help progress.

Q HOW DO I PREPARE FOR AN ACTIVE CHILDBIRTH?

A The principles of this type of birth are usually covered in independent prenatal classes; you will be taught to trust your body and your instincts, as well as to strengthen your breathing techniques.

WATER FOR PAIN RELIEF

Immersion in water was originally used just for pain relief during the first stage of labor, and it was not intended that the actual birth take place under water. Births taking place in water are not generally considered safe.

The benefits of water
Sitting in water is often used as a form of pain relief in labor and can be very pleasant. Water supports the body and might also speed up a slow labor. Laboring in water may reduce your chances of tearing during labor because it helps you relax.

Arranging for a labor pool
Some hospitals now have labor pools or large bathtubs available. If your hospital does not offer this option, ask about a birthing room with a private shower. Discuss these options with your doctor or midwife.

Assistance
Not all midwives and doctors are experienced in the use of water and labor pools during labor. If you would like to use a water pool at any time during your labor, check with the doctor or midwife beforehand to ensure that you will have the assistance of a professional experienced in the supervision of this type of birth.

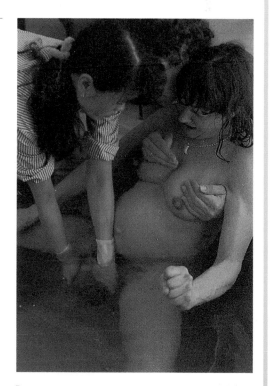

LABORING IN WATER
While the mother and her partner watch, a midwife guides the head of the baby out into the water during this water birth. Many women stay in the water only for the first stage of labor, and get out to deliver their babies; this is much safer for the baby.

COPING WITH PAIN IN LABOR

Q DO MOST WOMEN USE SOME TYPE OF PAIN RELIEF DURING LABOR?

A Although many women think that they would like to go without pain relief in labor, it is very common to have some kind of help, whether it is self-administered or given by a midwife or doctor. A minority of women need no assistance, while some women use every method of pain relief available. The majority of women, however, falls between these two extremes. Remember, giving birth isn't a race or an endurance test, and you shouldn't feel that you are a failure if you ask for a pain-relieving drug.

Q WHAT IS THE PAIN OF LABOR GOING TO BE LIKE?

A As you will probably have experienced degrees of pain before in your life, you will have some idea of your particular pain threshold. The pain of labor is, however, unlike any other, inasmuch as it is not a warning that something is wrong. Also, unlike most other pains, labor contractions come and go, giving you intervals of respite. Some women say they are like strong menstrual cramps; others say that they seem to overwhelm the whole body and are so excruciating that they are hard to bear.

WHAT ARE THE MAIN METHODS OF PAIN RELIEF?

The main medical types of pain relief used in childbirth are meperidine, or a similar drug, and epidural anesthesia (see p. 152). Nonmedical methods include breathing techniques, such as Lamaze, and the TENS machine which, although they may not completely eradicate the pain, can take the edge off it. Some women combine other nonmedical pain relief methods (see p. 148) with drugs and anesthesia.

MEPERIDINE (OR OTHER NARCOTIC)

Meperidine (Demerol) is a synthetic analgesic drug that is similar to morphine. This type of pain relief is administered by an injection into the muscle of your buttock or thigh every three to four hours.

How does it work?
Meperidine relieves pain by stimulating specific "opiate" receptors in your brain and spinal cord that are also the target of endorphins, your body's own painkillers.

Why choose this method?
Meperidine can be an effective pain reliever; it is useful when you can't have, or don't want, other forms of pain relief, such as epidural anesthesia.

What are the drawbacks?
Reactions to this drug include nausea, vomiting, blurred vision, sleepiness, and mood changes. If you are given meperidine within the two hours prior to the birth, it can make your baby sleepy and affect his or her ability to breathe and move spontaneously or to respond to stimuli. For these reasons, meperidine is not given too late in labor.

NITROUS OXIDE (GAS AND AIR)

Nitrous oxide is offered in some hospitals and other forms of anesthesia may also be available. Nitrous oxide is a mixture of gas and oxygen; this has been used in labor since the middle of the last century and is considered a safe form of pain relief.

How does it work?
You inhale it, slowly and deeply, through a special mask or mouthpiece. It helps ease your perception of pain but does not remove the pain entirely. Its effect is not immediate; if inhaled at the start of a contraction, it takes effect by the time the contraction is at its peak.

Why choose this method?
Nitrous oxide is particularly useful during early labor, but can be used at any time, and in combination with other methods of pain relief. It is unlikely that you will overdose on gas and air during your labor.

What are the drawbacks?
Some women find that it is not really strong enough if contractions are very severe. It can also make you feel "out of it" and nauseous.

Q WHAT IF I CAN'T COPE WITH THE PAIN OF LABOR?

A Remember that labor pains are simply a sign that your body is working hard to open up your cervix and move the baby down the birth canal. No one can predict how you will cope with the pain of your first labor; and subsequent labors often do not follow the same pattern, so try not to panic or feel disappointed if you need help.

Q WHAT FACTORS MIGHT AFFECT HOW I DEAL WITH PAIN DURING LABOR?

A How you cope during labor will depend primarily on the intensity of the pain. Certain factors can also affect your capacity to deal with the pain, such as when you last ate and slept, how long your labor lasts, how your baby is lying, and how comfortable and relaxed you are. A birth partner can really help make you feel relaxed by being supportive, talking you through the contractions, and distracting you.

Q HOW CAN I PLAN MY PAIN RELIEF BEFORE I START LABOR?

A It is a good idea to think about the method of pain relief you might prefer and to find out which methods are available, their benefits, and possible side effects. It is also important to find out whether or not you have to practice or organize them before the onset of labor. Keep an open mind about this, however, because labors do not always go according to plan.

USING A TENS MACHINE

TENS (Transcutaneous Electrical Nerve Stimulation) is a battery-operated device with wires that are attached to your body by adhesive pads.

How does it work?
A tiny electrical current passes through your skin, reducing pain messages to your brain and at the same time stimulating the production of endorphins, the body's natural painkillers.

Why choose this method?
By using a handset, you are in control of the machine and the intensity of the current. You can walk around and stay upright; it can also be used with relaxation and other self-help methods.

What are the drawbacks?
Most hospitals do not supply the machine; if you decide to try it, you will have to rent your own set beforehand and take it with you when you first go into labor (see p. 232).

USING TENS
Press a button on the handset at the start of a contraction. Electric impulses give a mild tingling sensation that blocks the pain.

BREATHING TECHNIQUES

Special breathing methods, such as Lamaze, help you relax and cope with the pain; they can be used with other types of pain relief (see p. 154).

How do they work?
Known as psychoprophylaxis, this method involves the use of practiced levels of breathing during contractions. Concentration on breathing distracts you from the pain and also relaxes your muscles so that tension, which heightens pain, is eased. To be effective, these techniques should be learned and practiced in a prenatal class. Take your partner so that he or she can help you during labor.

Why choose this method?
It is a natural method that does not involve drugs or medical supervision; you are in control.

What are the drawbacks?
This method is not always successful because it depends on your reaction to your labor pains, which cannot be predicted, and on your ability to concentrate on something other than the pain.

Two pairs of pads are taped to your lower back

HAVING AN EPIDURAL

Q WHY SHOULD I CONSIDER AN EPIDURAL?

A An epidural should be considered when you, or your obstetrician or midwife feel that the pain is more than you can cope with. You are more likely to need epidural pain relief if your baby is in the posterior position and intensive contractions result in little progress (see p. 160). You might have an epidural if you need a cesarean delivery, or with a forceps or vacuum extraction delivery. An epidural may also be necessary with a multiple birth or if your baby is in the breech position. Your doctor or midwife will tell you if he or she thinks you need an epidural, but the final decision will be yours.

Q HOW WILL AN EPIDURAL AFFECT ME?

A An epidural should act as a total pain block, numbing all sensation in your abdomen. However, it can also affect the nerves that control the movement in your legs and bladder, which means that your legs may feel quite heavy and difficult to move, and you may not be able to feel when you need to urinate. When an epidural is inserted, you may be encouraged to lie down, and a small plastic tube (catheter) may be passed into your bladder to keep it from becoming too full; an overly full bladder could impede the progress of your baby or cause bladder problems.

HOW DOES AN EPIDURAL WORK?

An epidural anesthetic works by numbing the nerves in your spine that lead to your abdomen. A small amount of local anesthetic is injected into the lower part of your back to numb the area before the main anesthetic is injected. This procedure usually takes around 20 to 40 minutes, and the effect should last for several hours. The anesthetic can then be "topped off" every few hours through the end of the catheter where a filter valve is attached in order to prevent bacteria from entering your body.

THE PROCEDURE

■ To stop your blood pressure from dropping suddenly, you will be connected to an intravenous drip. You will be asked to lie still on your side or to sit up, and your lower back is washed with soap.

■ The anesthetist will give you a local anesthetic.

■ The anesthetist will carefully place a fine, hollow needle between two vertebrae in the lumbar region of your lower back.

■ To check that the needle is in the right place, a small amount of anesthetic is given through the needle. If this numbs your abdomen satisfactorily, a catheter is inserted through the needle, and a full dose of anesthetic is delivered.

CONNECTING THE CATHETER
The catheter or tube is taped into position along your back so that you will then be able to move around if you wish and be "topped off" later, if necessary.

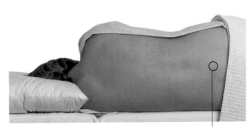

Position for an epidural   Insertion point

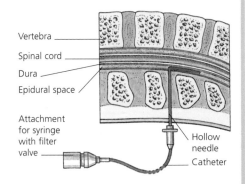

Vertebra
Spinal cord
Dura
Epidural space
Attachment for syringe with filter valve
Hollow needle
Catheter

Q WHO WILL GIVE ME AN EPIDURAL – AND WHEN SHOULD I ASK FOR ONE?

A Epidurals are normally given by a trained anesthesiologist. The majority of hospitals do have such anesthesiologists available around the clock; however, check on this with your local hospital before labor to avoid disappointment or misunderstanding. When you are in labor it might be a good idea to request an epidural sooner rather than later, just in case the anesthetist is not available immediately. If you wait too long, you may find that your labor is too advanced to have an epidural because the baby is descending into the birth canal and you need to push.

Q WILL I STILL BE ABLE TO PUSH MY BABY OUT IF I HAVE AN EPIDURAL?

A It is commonly believed that you cannot push if you have had an epidural because you can no longer feel your contractions. You can push, but your midwife or obstetrician will have to tell you when to push, either by watching a tracing on an external fetal monitor or by feeling your abdomen. It is not as easy to push without the strong urge that comes with normal second stage contractions, but it is possible. Alternatively, your midwife or doctor may wait for the epidural to wear off slightly so that you are able to feel the contractions again and push for yourself.

Q WILL I BE CONFINED TO BED WITH AN EPIDURAL?

A You will have to remain in a bed because it will probably be difficult for you to move your legs. Some hospitals offer "mobile epidurals," which use a type of anesthetic drug that blocks the pain and still allows you to walk around and empty your bladder. However, these are not available everywhere, and not all anesthesiologists are familiar with them.

Q CAN I HAVE A CESAREAN DELIVERY UNDER AN EPIDURAL?

A With the improvements in cesarean procedures, an epidural anesthetic is preferable to a general anesthetic; it will also enable you to see and to hold your baby as soon as he or she is born (see p. 182). More importantly, an epidural anesthetic is safer for you than a general anesthetic. Having an epidural anesthetic also means that you won't be sleepy or have to spend as much time recovering after the operation as you would under a general anesthetic.

Q WHAT IS THE DIFFERENCE BETWEEN AN EPIDURAL AND A SPINAL ANESTHETIC?

A An epidural anesthetic, where a catheter is attached to your back, allows the anesthetic to be maintained over time, freeing you from pain for many hours. With a spinal anesthetic, the needle is inserted into your spinal canal, a small dose of anesthetic is given, and the needle is removed. This takes effect more rapidly than an epidural anesthetic, but it only lasts one to two hours, and cannot be "topped off."

Q IS THERE A RISK OF BACKACHE WITH AN EPIDURAL?

A There has been a lot of research in recent years into whether women who have had an epidural experience more backache after delivery than those who haven't. However, there is no evidence to link chronic postpartum backache with epidural anesthetics. Many women experience backache for some time after giving birth, but this could be due to a long, difficult labor rather than the epidural. An epidural can sometimes cause a headache that may last for a few hours or days; this is not dangerous and is also very rare, occurring in less than one percent of epidurals.

Q CAN AN EPIDURAL GO WRONG?

A It is virtually impossible for an epidural to injure or paralyze you. The only problem that can arise is if the epidural anesthetizes only half your abdomen (called an incomplete block). In this event, the anesthesiologist will be called back to get the epidural working properly. The anesthesiologist does this by gently moving the tube in your back to allow the anesthetic to reach all the relevant nerves. It should not hurt. Occasionally, the epidural needle needs to be completely repositioned, which takes a few minutes.

QUESTIONS TO ASK

Is there an obstetric anesthesiologist available at the obstetrics department at all times?

If I have an epidural, will I have to be catheterized?

Do my previous back problems mean that I won't be able to have an epidural?

WHICH TYPE OF PAIN RELIEF IS BEST FOR ME?

	BREATHING	AROMATHERAPY	REFLEXOLOGY/ HYPNOTHERAPY/ ACUPUNCTURE	MASSAGE
Do I need to organize or practice this in advance, or is it supplied?	You need to learn how breathing techniques work, and to practice them, before going into labor.	You need the oils and vaporizer or burner and, if combined with massage, to have a person present who can massage you.	You should have contacted a therapist and tried these prior to labor, then arranged for the therapist to be with you during labor.	Your partner should practice massaging you before labor (see p. 114), or your midwife may be happy to do this if she is free.
How will it affect me?	Deep, controlled, slow breathing distracts you from pain by making you focus on something else; it also reduces nausea and dizziness.	It relaxes you and can reduce stress and tension; only use oils that are suitable during pregnancy (see p. 114).	These all help relax you and reduce pain, or distract you from pain during labor (see p. 104).	It will help you relax by relieving stress and tension, and by helping to soothe aching and tense muscles.
How will it affect my baby?	It will not affect your baby. This helps you relax, so your labor should progress better.	It will not affect your baby and, if you are relaxed, your labor may progress better.	These will not affect your baby.	It will not affect your baby.
How quickly does it work if I decide to use it?	Immediately	If you have the essential and base oils with you in labor, aromatherapy can begin to work immediately.	Once the therapist begins using the treatment, you should feel the benefits within 15–30 minutes.	Immediately, but make sure someone is present who knows how to massage you.
How long will it last?	As long as you control your breathing.	Whether used intermittently or continuously, you should feel the benefits throughout the labor.	The effects vary, depending on which therapy is used and for which symptom; all can be made to last the entire labor.	If done properly, the effects of massage can last for a considerable time.
Can I combine it with other methods of pain relief?	Yes, you can use this technique in conjunction with any other types of pain relief.	Yes, it is commonly combined with massage (see p. 114) and other types of pain relief.	Yes, you may find that these do not provide adequate pain relief on their own.	Yes, you can combine this with any other method of pain relief.
Can I use it in a home birth?	Yes	Yes	Yes	Yes
Can I use it before I come to the hospital?	Yes	Yes	Yes	Yes

WATER	TENS	GAS AND AIR (nitrous oxide and oxygen mixture)	NARCOTIC DRUG, SUCH AS DEMEROL	EPIDURAL ANESTHETIC
The labor room may have a bath that you can use in early labor, or a birthing pool; you may have to reserve the pool in advance.	You may be able to rent a TENS machine from the hospital. If not, you can rent or buy one from a hospital supply company.	This may be supplied in the hospital.	This is supplied in all hospitals, and brought to a home delivery by your midwife (see below).	It will be supplied by the hospital and is not something you can arrange or reserve in advance.
This relieves tension by supporting you, but you may have to get out of the water for your baby to be monitored (see p. 158).	It makes pain less intense by reducing pain stimuli from reaching the brain, and by stimulating the body's natural painkillers, endorphins.	This takes the edge off contraction pains, but may make you feel light-headed, sleepy, and sometimes nauseous (see p. 150).	This relieves pain, but can cause light-headedness and nausea; you may need an antiemetic injection with it (see p. 150).	This should numb your stomach, rectum/anus, and vagina, stopping all feeling; your blood pressure may drop slightly (see p. 152).
It will not affect your baby as long as careful attention is paid to the water temperature.	It will not affect your baby.	It will not affect your baby.	If given late in labor, it can make your baby sleepy and affect his or her breathing; some oxygen may be given to wake your baby.	It won't affect your baby unless your blood pressure drops and the blood flow to the placenta is reduced.
It will begin to work as soon as you get into the water.	After switching on the machine and adjusting the output to the correct strength, the effects can be felt immediately.	The effect should be immediate.	This can take 10–20 minutes; an internal exam will be carried out to be sure that you are not about to give birth imminently.	This can take 30–45 minutes; an internal exam ensures that you aren't about to deliver, and an anesthesiologist is called.
The effect will last if you stay in the water, but you may find it less effective as labor progresses.	The stimulus affects a contraction, but the overall effect should last longer; it may be less effective in more painful labor.	The effect wears off in a few seconds, but you can use it consistently throughout the first stage of labor.	It takes 20 minutes to take effect and should last for about three hours.	This depends on the type of epidural (see p. 153), but it can be "topped off," giving pain relief throughout labor.
Yes, within limits. You can have meperidine, but it is impossible to have an epidural while lying in water.	Yes, except in water.	Yes, you can use this with all other methods of pain relief.	Yes, you could try gas and air, or even an epidural with it.	This should totally block the pain and you shouldn't need anything else.
Yes	TENS is ideal for use in a home birth.	Your midwife may be able to bring it with her.	Yes, your midwife can bring this; it may have to be prescribed and obtained from a pharmacy in advance.	No, because it must be administered by an anesthesiologist; you and your baby will need monitoring.
Yes NB. If your doctor agrees, you can labor in water after your water breaks.	Yes, practice using it prior to labor; the start of labor is the most effective time to use it.	No, it can only be used under medical supervision.	No, these drugs require a prescription.	No, this must be administered in hospital by an anesthesiologist.

LABOR AND BIRTH

THE FIRST SIGNS OF LABOR

Q WHAT ARE THE SIGNS THAT LABOR HAS BEGUN?

A Several signs can indicate whether or not you may be starting the first of three stages of labor. These signs can be divided into two groups: those that are possible indicators and those that are absolute signs (see chart, opposite). Certain signs, such as a "show" (see below) days or even weeks before you actually start labor, can lead you to think that labor has begun. In fact, the only true sign that labor is underway is the occurrence of frequent and regular contractions that are causing your cervix to dilate (open).

Q WHAT DOES A "BLOODY SHOW" MEAN?

A During pregnancy, a plug of jellylike mucus seals the lower end of your cervix to keep infections out of your womb. This plug comes out toward the end of your pregnancy, and although it may mean that labor is going to start soon, it can dislodge (with no harm to the baby) up to six weeks before your labor starts. Some women have a show after an internal exam, especially when they are at or near term.

Q WHAT SHOULD I DO IF I HAVE A SHOW?

A Try not to panic. It's normal for a show to contain either fresh red blood or old dark blood (like at the end of your period) as part of the clear or cloudy mucus of the plug. Unless you have other symptoms, such as strong, regular contractions, a show is not an absolute sign that labor is starting, but it is best to call your midwife or doctor for advice.

Q HOW DO I KNOW IF I'M JUST IN FALSE LABOR?

A You will be experiencing regular Braxton-Hicks' contractions (see p. 81), which – particularly if they are strong and if this is your first baby – can be mistaken for the real thing. The difference between these "practice contractions" and real labor pains, however, is that they occur irregularly, perhaps one or two an hour, then fade away, whereas true labor pains usually begin slowly and build in intensity and frequency.

Q I'M HAVING REGULAR, UNCOMFORTABLE CONTRACTIONS. WHAT SHOULD I DO?

A Time your contractions from the beginning of one to the beginning of the next, and also record how often they occur. There are no hard-and-fast rules, but as a rough guide: if they are regular (less than 30 minutes apart), and painful (you have to stop what you are doing until they pass), you should contact your midwife or doctor.

Q WHAT DOES "BREAKING WATER" MEAN, AND WHEN SHOULD MINE BREAK?

A The "water" is the amniotic fluid (contained in membranes) that surround and protect your baby in the womb. The membranes usually break (see p. 164) as your cervix opens, once labor is actually in progress. The contractions that are opening your cervix may cause the baby to press down, creating pressure that bursts the membranes. If they don't break spontaneously, they may be broken artificially by your midwife or doctor to speed up your progress (see p. 164).

Q HOW DO I KNOW IF MY WATER HAS BROKEN, AND WHAT DO I DO?

A This question can be worrying, especially as any slight leakage could be urine. If there is a large amount of fluid, you will be in no doubt about what has happened. But if your water breaks and produces a trickle, and you are still in doubt, put on a sanitary pad and then examine the pad. Urine looks and smells different than amniotic fluid. Amniotic water is normally clear or a light straw color, with little odor, and trickles beyond your control. If you think your water has broken, contact your midwife or doctor. What happens next depends on whether you are actually in labor.

Q WHAT IF MY WATER BREAKS BEFORE I AM IN LABOR?

A If you are between 37 and 42 weeks pregnant and your water breaks without your contractions having begun (see opposite), it is quite likely that you will spontaneously go into labor within 24 hours; within 48 hours, over 90 percent of women will have gone into labor. In certain situations, you may be induced to help your labor get started (see p. 159).

Q HOW WILL I KNOW IF THERE'S ANYTHING TO BE CONCERNED ABOUT?

A If you see a dark green fluid when your water breaks, it means your water contains meconium, the substance in your baby's digestive system (see p. 62) that is usually passed in the first bowel movements after birth; if passed earlier, it can mean fetal distress, and you should contact your midwife or doctor immediately. If you have a lot of blood mixed with the fluid, or bright, fresh bleeding that continues after your water has broken, this also needs to be checked out at once.

Q WHAT SHOULD I DO IF I THINK I AM IN LABOR?

A True labor contractions occur very regularly, and grow stronger and more frequent. If you think you are in labor, contact your midwife or doctor for advice. Your midwife will probably come to see you, or you will be asked to go to your hospital to check if labor has indeed started. Remember to take your hospital notes and your labor bag with you. It is important to try not to panic; you have prepared for this moment, and should have plenty of time.

HOW CAN I TELL IF I AM IN LABOR?

The only true sign that you are in the early first stage of labor is regular contractions that are causing your cervix to soften and open. Whether or not this is happening, however, needs to be confirmed by an internal examination. However, if you are in any doubt about whether you are in labor, check your symptoms on the chart below and contact your midwife or doctor for information and reassurance.

YOU ARE HAVING	IF...	WHAT TO DO	BUT IF...	WHAT TO DO
Contractions	1 or 2 contractions per hour	Wait; labor has not begun	Contractions 5–10 minutes apart	Call your midwife or doctor
Baby's movements have become less frequent	With or without contractions	Contact your midwife or doctor for advice	All movements have stopped	Go to the hospital immediately
Strong contractions	Less than 5 minutes apart	Contact your caregiver and get to the hospital at once	Some contractions are weak and irregular	Contact your caregiver or hospital
Water breaks	⟶	Contact your midwife or doctor for advice	With dark green stains (meconium)	Call your caregiver; go to the hospital immediately
Had a show	⟶	Contact your midwife or doctor for advice	With lots of blood	Call your caregiver; go to the hospital immediately
Constant backache	It can be eased by changing position, or by massage	Wait and see	It does not ease and with other signs (see above)	Contact your midwife or doctor for advice
Diarrhea	Without other signs (see above)	Wait and see	With other signs (see above)	Contact your midwife or doctor for advice
Strong urge to push	⟶	Labor is in progress	⟶	Contact your midwife or doctor immediately

LABOR AND BIRTH

IN THE HOSPITAL

Q DO I HAVE TO ARRANGE MY MEDICAL INSURANCE BEFORE I GO TO HOSPITAL?

A Yes, it is usually a good idea to establish insurance information with the hospital before your due date. Your doctor or midwife will be able to give you a hospital preadmission form. Fill this out, and then return the form to the doctor or midwife or directly to the hospital. You may wish to call the hospital billing department after two weeks to make sure they have received the form and that everything is in order.

Q WHAT HAPPENS WHEN I ARRIVE AT THE HOSPITAL?

A After the inevitable paperwork, you will be welcomed to the obstetrics department, and meet your midwife or doctor. You can then change into a nightgown or a T-shirt (hospital gowns are ideal) and familiarize yourself with the staff. Your caregiver will discuss your symptoms and check the notes and any birth plan you have brought with you.

Q WILL I BE GIVEN MEDICAL CHECKS AT THE HOSPITAL?

A Your temperature, blood pressure, and pulse will be checked, and your urine will be tested for the presence of protein, sugar, and blood. Your abdomen will be examined to check your baby's position and the strength and frequency of your contractions. Your baby's heartbeat will also be checked by an external fetal monitor to be sure that he or she is not in distress (see below). Continuous fetal monitoring may be needed if there are any complications, such as a breech baby, twins or triplets, a very small or a very large baby, or the presence of meconium.

Q HOW WILL MY CAREGIVER CONFIRM THAT I AM IN LABOR?

A Your caregiver will confirm that you are in labor by timing your contractions and by giving you an internal examination to see if your cervix is dilating and has softened (see p. 161).

HOW IS MY BABY'S HEARTBEAT MONITORED?

An external fetal monitor records your baby's heart rate and your contractions. If your baby's heartbeat is normal and there is nothing else of concern in your labor, you can be disconnected from the monitor so that you can move around. Your caregiver will listen to your baby's heartbeat intermittently during the labor.

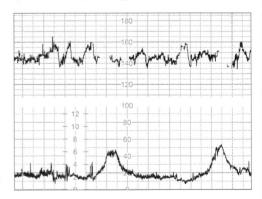

HOW THE MONITOR WORKS
The external fetal monitor is securely attached to your abdomen by a belt. Your baby's heartbeat is detected by ultrasound.

WHAT THE PRINTOUT SHOWS
The top line of the printout (above) shows your baby's heartbeat, the lower shows your contractions. These can be interpreted to discover if your baby is distressed.

WHAT IS AN INDUCED LABOR?

It is sometimes necessary to start labor artificially. This is known as induction of labor or, if your water has already broken, stimulation of labor. Induction of labor is usually easier if you have had one or more babies before by vaginal delivery, and if your cervix (neck of the womb) is ripe.

Why labor might be induced

■ When you are beyond 41, or in some cases, 42 weeks pregnant (known as "postdates" pregnancy).

■ If your doctors are concerned that your baby's growth has slowed down or stopped, your baby is not moving well, there is a reduced amount of amniotic fluid, or the placenta is no longer nourishing your baby (placental insufficiency).

■ If you have reached 40 weeks and you have a medical condition that means that an early delivery would be in your best interest.

■ If you are at 40 weeks, and you have a vital personal reason to have your baby delivered.

■ If your baby has a condition, such as a hole in the heart, that needs surgery, it is in your baby's interests to be delivered during working hours when the necessary staff are on call and available.

■ If you develop preeclampsia, your doctors may decide, for your own and for your baby's safety, that your labor should be induced; this may be as much as a few weeks before your baby is due. Your blood pressure will be controlled during the labor.

The procedure for inducing labor

First, your obstetrician will check that your baby is "head down" in your womb, and has engaged low in your pelvis, then will ascertain if your cervix is ripe. You will be asked to return to the hospital at a certain time on a certain day to have your labor induced. When you come in, your baby's heartbeat will be monitored for about half an hour on an external fetal monitor (see left) to check that he or she is not in distress. You will then be induced by one of the following methods:

■ **Prostaglandin (vaginal gel or tablets)** This substance is found naturally in your womb lining and one of its functions is to stimulate uterine contractions so that labor can begin. If your cervix is firmly closed, your midwife or doctor may put a gel or a tablet containing synthetic prostaglandin into your vagina, which helps to ripen your cervix. This procedure may be repeated several times in one day, or even continued the next day, until you go into labor or your cervix has opened sufficiently for your water to be broken. The advantage of this method of induction is that it allows you to remain mobile and to eat.

■ **Artificial rupture of the membranes** If your cervix is sufficiently ripe, this can be an effective way of inducing labor. Your doctor or midwife will give you an internal examination, then use a long, thin plastic hook to brush against the delicate membranes, which is usually enough to break them (see p. 164).

■ **Oxytocin** This is a synthetic substance fed into your arm via intravenous drip to increase the strength and regularity of your contractions; it is similar to natural oxytocin, the hormone produced by the pituitary gland, which causes the womb to contract, stimulating labor. This method is often combined with the artificial rupture of your membranes (see above). It is very safe, but too much oxytocin can cause your womb to contract too much; it can also make your contractions very painful (and sometimes causes double contractions).

Why inductions are not more common

Although inductions are usually successful, labor is not induced more frequently or on demand because there is a risk that you will not go into labor. If the induction fails, you may then need to have a cesarean. If your labor is induced you are also more likely to need an assisted delivery with forceps or a vacuum cup (see p. 180). An induced labor is less likely to be successful if your cervix is completely closed and your baby's head has not fully engaged in your pelvis.

What to consider

An induced labor may be more painful and take longer than one that starts naturally. You may need to have an epidural; this means that you will be prepared if you later have to have a cesarean, or even an assisted delivery with forceps or with a vacuum extraction cup.

THE FIRST STAGE OF LABOR

Q WHAT ARE THE MAIN STAGES OF LABOR?

A Labor has three distinct stages: the first starts with regular contractions that open up your cervix, and lasts until the cervix is fully open (about 10 cm). The second stage of labor begins when your cervix is fully open and concludes with the birth of your baby. The third stage is from the birth of your baby until the delivery of the placenta.

Q HOW LONG DOES EACH STAGE OF LABOR LAST?

A Every birth is different and the timing varies, but as a rough guide, doctors expect the first stage of labor to last eight to 14 hours, the second stage one to two hours, and the third stage ten to 60 minutes. If this is your first baby or your labor is induced, it can take longer; if this is not your first baby, labor may be quicker.

Q WHEN SHOULD I DISCUSS MY BIRTH PLAN OR PREFERENCES FOR THE BIRTH?

A Once it is confirmed that you are in labor, you should discuss your birth plan if you haven't done so (see p. 138). Remember, this is to make your feelings clear. If you feel unable to converse because of the contractions, ask your partner to discuss your birth plan with the caregivers and staff.

Q WHAT WILL HAPPEN ONCE IT IS ESTABLISHED THAT I AM IN LABOR?

A Once you are having between two and four contractions every ten minutes, you, your baby, and the progress of your labor will be closely monitored. Many hospitals use a system whereby the progress of labor is recorded on a graph called a partogram that shows the rate at which your cervix is dilating and acts as a visual guide so that problems can be spotted immediately.

THE POSITION OF YOUR BABY

Your baby's position in the womb will affect your labor. For an easy passage through the birth canal, the best position for your baby is head-down (cephalic) with the back facing your abdomen (anterior position). If your baby's back has turned toward your back (posterior position), your baby presents the widest part of the head (occiput) into the birth canal; this can give you back pain, and also a prolonged labor that may have to be assisted (see p. 180). A breech presentation means that the feet or buttocks are delivered first; this also requires the assistance of an experienced doctor or midwife.

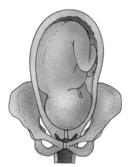

OCCIPUT ANTERIOR
Your baby's head is down with his or her back turned toward your abdomen.

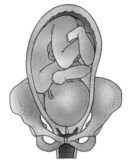

OCCIPUT POSTERIOR
Your baby's head is down with his or her back turned toward your spine.

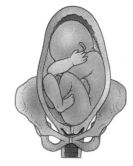

BREECH PRESENTATION
Your baby is presented bottom first, with his or her legs flexed at the knees and hips.

Q HOW WILL I FEEL DURING THE FIRST STAGE OF LABOR?

A You may feel a range of intense emotions. At one moment you may feel excited and joyful and the next you may feel despondent, afraid, and tired; or you may feel exhilarated throughout. You will probably be stretched to your physical limits, and at times feel that you cannot go on. Express your emotions and laugh or cry depending on how you feel; this can help you to relax, which can help the labor to progress. You may also be oblivious to your surroundings because your entire being is centered on pushing out and delivering your baby.

Q WILL I FEEL MUCH PAIN DURING THE FIRST STAGE?

A The degree of pain felt varies from woman to woman. The pain usually intensifies toward the end of the first stage of labor when your contractions are becoming stronger and your cervix is almost fully dilated.

Q WILL I NEED PAIN RELIEF IN THE FIRST STAGE?

A This will depend on the intensity of your contractions, also on how you, your midwife, or your doctor feel you are coping with the pain. If there is concern about your progress, they may ask if you want, or suggest that you try, some form of pain relief (see p. 154). If you do need relief, the first stage of labor is usually the best time for this.

Q DOES THE CERVIX START OPENING ONCE REGULAR CONTRACTIONS BEGIN?

A No, the cervix needs to soften before it can dilate. Labor doesn't always begin when your contractions start. You may have irregular, painful contractions for hours or even a day or two before your cervix dilates, especially if this is your first baby. So you may feel tired, nauseous, and be unable to eat properly while waiting for your cervix to dilate. This is called the "prolonged latent phase."

Q WHAT WILL HAPPEN IF MY CONTRACTIONS STOP DURING THE FIRST STAGE?

A Contractions can sometimes start regularly, but then die away halfway through your labor. If this happens and the progress of your labor halts for a few hours, your midwife or doctor may suggest breaking your water (if it has not already broken) or artificially stimulating your labor with oxytocin (see pp. 159 and 164).

HOW YOUR CERVIX OPENS

The first stage of labor begins with the onset of regular contractions. This causes the cervix to thin out, known as "effacement." Once the cervix has softened, the contractions cause the cervix to dilate (widen) progressively, so that your baby's head can pass through. Contractions draw the cervix up over the baby's head like a sleeve, toward the vaginal walls.

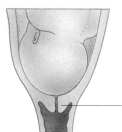

BEFORE LABOR
The cervix is thick and closed (known as "uneffaced") and your baby's head is engaged.

Cervix is closed

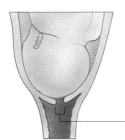

EARLY FIRST STAGE
The cervix thins and softens (effacement) before it can stretch and dilate.

The cervix starts to dilate

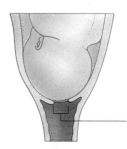

LATE FIRST STAGE
At about 5 cm, the cervix is said to be halfway to full dilatation.

Dilatation is proceeding

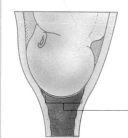

FULLY DILATED
The cervix is fully dilated when its opening measures about 10 cm in diameter.

The cervix is now fully opened

LABOR AND BIRTH

POSITIONS FOR THE FIRST STAGE

In the first stage of labor, when there is no urge to push yet, you are usually free to move around and find a comfortable position. Some women instinctively find a position that suits them and stay in this position for the entire first stage. Others prefer to walk around and keep upright as much as possible. Staying upright is beneficial because gravity helps your baby's weight to press down on your cervix, which, in turn, helps it to open. If you want to stay mobile, work out a small circuit in the delivery room and place chairs or cushions strategically so that you can stop and concentrate on breathing during a contraction. Try different positions until you find one that you prefer.

STANDING
Stand behind a chair, facing the back, and place your arms on the back for support. This can help you rest during a contraction if you are moving around during the first stage of labor.

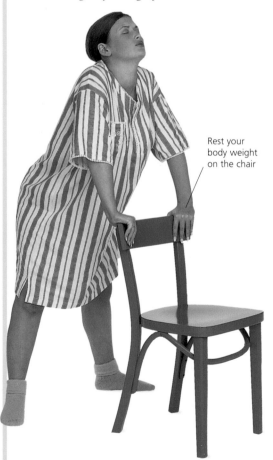

Rest your body weight on the chair

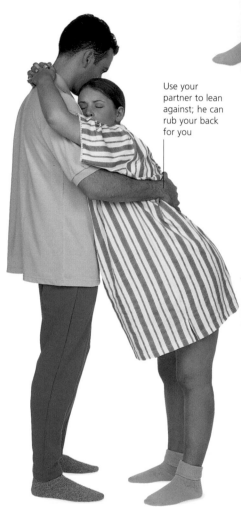

Use your partner to lean against; he can rub your back for you

LEANING
Stand facing your birth partner with your arms around him or her and lean forward so that your body weight is supported. Ask your birth partner for a lower back massage at the same time if this helps.

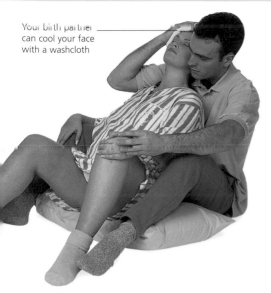

Your birth partner can cool your face with a washcloth

SUPPORTED SITTING
Get your partner to sit against a wall or sit on a bean bag or cushion. Sit in front of him or her, allowing your body weight to be supported. This position can also be used during the second stage.

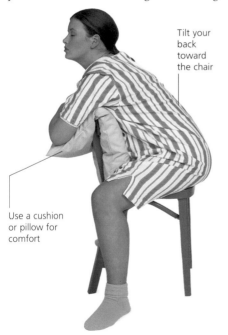

Tilt your back toward the chair

Use a cushion or pillow for comfort

SITTING
Sit on a chair, facing the chair back, and place your arms over it for support. Your birth partner can then stand in front of you and sponge your face, or stand behind you and massage your back and shoulders.

THE ROLE OF THE BIRTH PARTNER

Your role as a birth partner is to support your partner both emotionally and physically. Mop her brow or hold her during a contraction; you can also make helpful suggestions, and offer her encouragement and praise. Because she knows you best, the chances are good that she will take any anxieties or irritations out on you. Be prepared for this to happen, be understanding, and try not to take it personally! The following is a list of ideas that you could use to help your partner through labor:

■ Ask her what you can do to make her more comfortable. She may not know herself, so be ready to make suggestions. Don't get annoyed if she doesn't seem to want to take your advice.
■ Suggest a change of position if you can see that your partner is feeling tired or stressed.
■ Offer to massage her back, feet, or shoulders.
■ Talk her through the contractions and always try to praise her achievement.
■ Remind her how much closer she is than this time yesterday, or a few hours ago.
■ Encourage her to take little drinks every few hours.
■ Remind her to urinate every two hours or so.
■ For distraction, if she is agreeable, read to her, or play a game together.
■ If labor is very long and you are also feeling tired, have some refreshment so that you can recharge your batteries and be of maximum help to your partner.
■ Join your partner in breathing exercises.

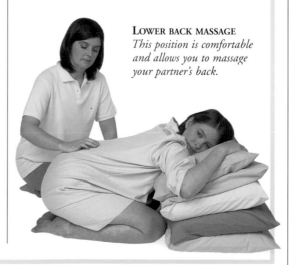

LOWER BACK MASSAGE
This position is comfortable and allows you to massage your partner's back.

As the First Stage Ends

Q WHAT HAPPENS BETWEEN THE FIRST AND SECOND STAGES?

A After the cervix has fully dilated there is often, but not always, a period before the second stage of labor – with its intense urge to push – arrives. You may find this interlude, called transition, one of the most difficult stages of labor.

Q WHY IS THIS A DIFFICULT TIME IN LABOR?

A Transition can last for a few minutes or for several hours, and can be confusing and hard to cope with for several reasons: your contractions may become more intense and frequent, which can make you nauseous or cause you to vomit; you may also feel shivery, or anxious and out of control. Transition usually occurs after you have already experienced several hours of strong contractions, when your strength is beginning to wane, and you feel tired and irritable, and think that you are getting nowhere. This low point can make some women wish they had never become pregnant in the first place!

Q HOW WILL I BE ABLE TO MAKE IT THROUGH TRANSITION?

A Despite being uncomfortable, the transition stage is a very positive sign that you are making progress – the time to push the baby out is about to begin. While you wait for the next stage to start, you could try: changing your position by sitting up if you have been lying down, or by standing up; walking around the room if you are able to; asking your partner to massage you gently, or sponge your face, or simply to ask you questions that require your concentration; changing partners for a while if you have more than one person with you; making eye contact with your partner.

Q WHAT HAPPENS IF I NEED TO PUSH AND MY CERVIX IS NOT DILATED ENOUGH?

A Your midwife will give you an internal examination to confirm that your cervix is fully dilated, so it will not be damaged. If you feel a strong urge to push but your cervix is not quite ready, your caregiver will ask you to slow things down by panting during contractions.

WHAT HAPPENS IF MY WATER DOESN'T BREAK NATURALLY?

Your water may break spontaneously at any time before labor (see p. 156); this can be a sign that labor may be about to begin. It can also happen as your baby's head descends into the birth canal during the first stage.

Does my water need to be broken?
Your water does not always need to be artificially broken unless there is a problem such as: a long labor not progressing satisfactorily – breaking your water could speed things up because your baby's head will then push on the cervix and help it to dilate; signs that your baby is distressed (see p. 176); the need to attach an internal monitor, called a fetal scalp electrode (FSE), to your baby's head.

How is my water broken artificially?
Your midwife or doctor will give you an internal examination, then use a long, thin, plastic hook to brush against the delicate membranes, which break, releasing the amniotic fluid.

Can I refuse to have my water broken?
Yes, but it is very unlikely that your midwife or doctor will suggest breaking your water unless they have a good reason to do so; if you are unsure about it, discuss it with them. No midwife or doctor should "routinely" break your water.

Are there reasons why my water should not be broken?
There are instances when breaking your water is not a good idea. One reason is if your baby's head is too high and is not yet engaged properly in your pelvis. In this situation, if your water is broken artificially, there is a risk of the umbilical cord coming down ahead of the baby (cord prolapse). Also, if your baby is very premature, it is better to deliver with the membranes intact, so that your baby has more protection during the birth. If you are carrying twins, your midwife or doctor may be reluctant to break your water artificially because doing this too early can complicate the delivery of the second twin.

THE SECOND STAGE OF LABOR

Q WHAT IS THE SECOND STAGE OF LABOR?

A The second stage begins when your cervix is fully dilated, and ends with the birth of your baby. This stage averages about one to two hours for a first baby. The second stage means that you can now bear down and push your baby out; this stage may start as soon as full dilatation is confirmed. If the head still has quite a way to come down through your pelvis, you may be discouraged from pushing immediately, so that you do not become exhausted. Therefore, the second stage is often divided into "passive" (you wait for the head to come down on its own) and "active" (you push with each contraction).

Q HOW DO I KNOW WHEN I'M IN THE SECOND STAGE?

A An internal examination will confirm full dilatation, but there are other signs that indicate the onset of the second stage, such as a strong urge to push, and involuntary grunting with contractions (you can get this urge before full dilatation). Your perineum may bulge because your baby's head is just behind it; you may feel a need to defecate and may do so. Don't be embarrassed; this is involuntary and your midwife or doctor will have seen it often. In fact, it shows that things are about to happen in earnest.

Q WHAT DETERMINES HOW LONG THE SECOND STAGE LASTS?

A Various factors can influence the length of the second stage: how strong your contractions are; the size and position of your baby's head; and the size of your pelvis. The second stage tends to be shorter with second and subsequent births.

Q ARE THE CONTRACTIONS THE SAME AS BEFORE?

A No, your contractions will change, often becoming less frequent and more intense. You may only have two every ten minutes but they will last longer and allow you more time to make the most of your pushing technique. Also, you will have a strong urge to push now. If your water has not yet broken, it probably will now, or it may be broken for you (see left).

Q AM I LIKELY TO BE TOO TIRED TO PUSH MY BABY OUT?

A If your labor has been long, and without adequate pain relief, you may be exhausted when the time comes to have your baby. However, careful, modern management of your labor should prevent this and you should have been able to rest, especially with good pain relief. This active second stage, when you push your baby out, can last up to two hours. If it lasts any longer, you may get tired, and your baby may become distressed.

Q HOW DO I PUSH?

A When you get the urge to push, take a deep breath at the start of the contraction, put your chin on your chest, and push down into your bottom for as long as you can. You can usually take several breaths with each contraction and, as you bear down, your baby will gradually move farther through your pelvis. Your partner's and caregiver's encouragement can help you to continue pushing for as long as possible with each contraction, even if it seems as if nothing is happening.

Q CAN I PUSH IF I HAVE HAD AN EPIDURAL?

A Just because you can't feel contractions doesn't mean you can't push! If your epidural is still working in the second stage, the midwife or doctor will put a hand on your abdomen, feel for contractions, and tell you when to push. Contractions can also be predicted from fetal monitor tracings. Alternatively, your epidural may be allowed to wear off partially, so that you can feel the contractions and start pushing.

Q WHO NEEDS TO BE THERE FOR THE BIRTH?

A If everything progresses normally, there can be just you, your partner, your caregiver, and possibly a nurse present. A specialist may be there if a problem is anticipated, and a pediatrician will be called if your amniotic fluid contains meconium, which can be an indication of fetal distress, and you are going to need an assisted birth.

LABOR AND BIRTH

POSITIONS FOR THE SECOND STAGE

The positions shown here are all suitable for the second stage of your labor. At this stage, when your contractions are lasting longer and you are likely to feel tired, you might be tempted to lie down – resist this, however, because lying flat is not a beneficial position and does not help gravity push your baby down the birth canal. The best position is one in which you are upright, so that gravity can assist the process; relaxed, with your pelvis as open as possible; and one in which your weight is supported. Some women stay in one position, others change position as and when they feel they need to.

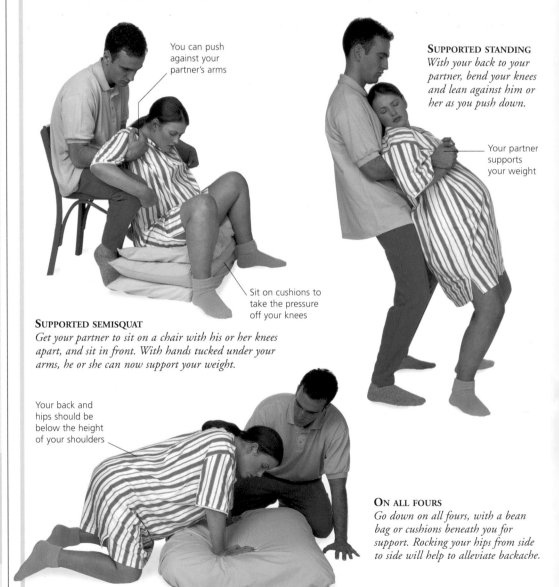

You can push against your partner's arms

Sit on cushions to take the pressure off your knees

SUPPORTED SEMISQUAT
Get your partner to sit on a chair with his or her knees apart, and sit in front. With hands tucked under your arms, he or she can now support your weight.

SUPPORTED STANDING
With your back to your partner, bend your knees and lean against him or her as you push down.

Your partner supports your weight

Your back and hips should be below the height of your shoulders

ON ALL FOURS
Go down on all fours, with a bean bag or cushions beneath you for support. Rocking your hips from side to side will help to alleviate backache.

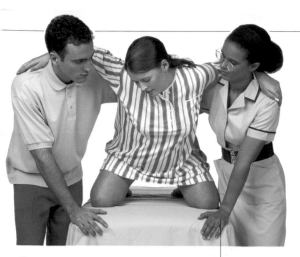

SUPPORTED KNEELING
Kneel on the bed between your birth partner and your caregiver. Place your arms around their shoulders for support, and concentrate on pushing down.

Your caregiver can help support you

THE ROLE OF THE BIRTH PARTNER

By the second stage your partner will probably be feeling very uncomfortable, very tired, and possibly overwhelmed as the baby begins the descent into the birth canal. As in the first stage, be quietly supportive and encouraging; remind her that she is nearly there, that the baby will be born very soon. You could also try the following:

- Help her to get into a position in which she is comfortable for the delivery.
- Talk her through her contractions and pushing; massage her back if required.
- Spray her face with water or apply cold washcloths if she wishes.
- As the baby is being born, communicate with your partner through touch, rather than trying to talk over the midwife's or nurse's instructions.
- Watch for the baby's head as it crowns (see p. 168). If you have brought a mirror, angle it so that she can also see the head.
- If you wish, you could cut the cord after delivery, and help lay the baby on your partner's abdomen.
- Take photographs! Celebrate life!

LYING WITH LEG SUPPORT
Place some cushions or a bean bag on the floor, lie on your side, and support your head on another pillow. Get your partner to lift your leg.

Your partner can support your upper leg

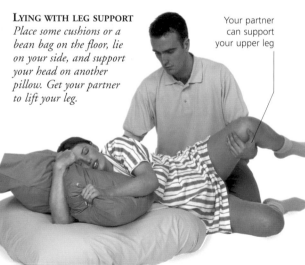

Keep as upright as possible

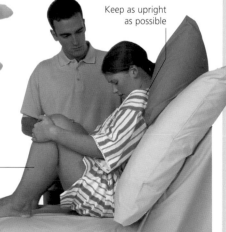

Legs wide apart

SITTING
Sit upright with pillows behind your back for support. Keep your legs apart and push down with contractions.

LABOR AND BIRTH

THE BIRTH OF YOUR BABY

The final countdown to the most exciting part of your delivery has begun: the actual birth of your baby. However exciting this is, though, you must now concentrate hard during contractions to push your baby out. Your caregiver will talk you through the next hour or so, while your partner provides support and comfort. Although you may have read or thought often about this moment, you may be unprepared for how you feel when you see your baby for the first time. Amazed by the completeness of this tiny human being, you will probably be engulfed in waves of emotion. For most, all the pain and effort will suddenly seem a small price to pay for such a miracle.

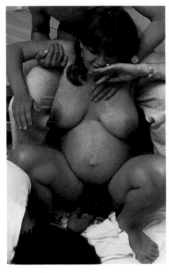

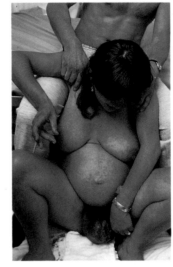

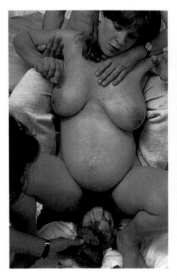

1 Now that the mother has begun to push with each contraction, the baby will move slowly through her pelvis until eventually the top of the baby's head will be visible at the entrance to the vagina. This process may take from a few minutes to two hours.

2 Initially, the baby's head slips back inside the vagina between contractions, but eventually it stays visible; this is called "crowning." The mother can put her hand down and feel the head or see it in a mirror. At this stage, as the tissues stretch, she may feel burning or stinging.

3 The caregiver may ask the mother to pant now to slow the head's delivery a little and to give the vaginal area time to stretch rather than tear. As the head appears, the mother may cry out involuntarily. The baby usually emerges face down but will turn to one side at once.

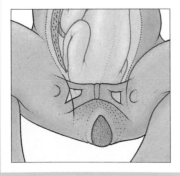

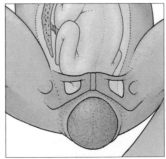

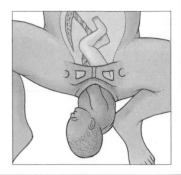

WHAT EFFECT DOES THE BIRTH HAVE ON MY BABY?

During the hardest part of labor your baby is squeezed and pushed down the narrow vaginal canal. This will cause your baby's heartbeat to slow intermittently, but this is not serious. When your baby arrives, it is a wonderful moment, but you may be concerned about the way he or she looks. Your baby will probably be covered in blood or the white greasy cream (vernix) that protected its skin while in the womb. Your baby's face may be bruised from the pressure of the delivery, and may appear blue or bright red from congestion caused during delivery. Although surprising, remember that these marks are only temporary and will soon disappear. Once you hold your newborn baby, all you will probably feel is an immense tenderness for him or her.

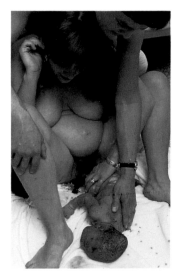

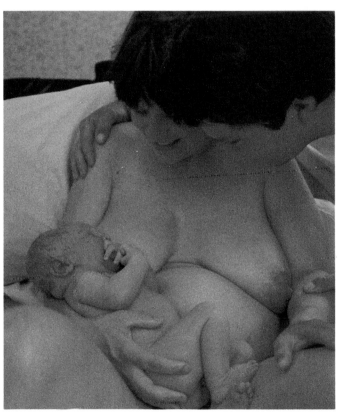

4 The midwife will wipe the baby's eyes, nose, and mouth clear of any mucus; if necessary, any fluid in the air passages will be sucked out through a tube. During the next one or two contractions the baby's shoulders, then body, will usually slide out quickly.

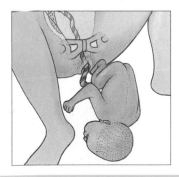

5 The baby may lie quietly or cry lustily right away. The baby's condition will be checked and, provided that all is well, he or she will be lifted onto your abdomen. The mother and her partner welcome and comfort the baby by stroking or touching, and the newborn may soon be put to the breast. At this stage, the cord will still be pulsating; it will now be clamped and cut, either by the caregiver or the mother's partner.

As Your Baby is Born

Q WILL I TEAR AS MY BABY'S HEAD COMES OUT?

A Not necessarily. In fact, this can be very difficult to predict, although tearing does tend to be more common with a first baby. If it seems likely that your baby's head cannot come out easily, or that you might tear badly, your caregiver will perform (with your permission) an "episiotomy," which is a small cut made with scissors at the entrance to your vagina (see below).

Q HOW COMMON IS IT TO NEED AN EPISIOTOMY?

A It is more common to need an episiotomy if you are having your first baby because the vaginal opening may not stretch on its own to accommodate the baby's head. With subsequent babies, the vaginal tissues are more likely to stretch sufficiently.

HOW IS AN EPISIOTOMY DONE?

When your baby's head appears, the midwife or doctor gets your permission to make a small cut at the entrance to your vagina, so that it will be easier for you to push your baby out without tearing. Your pelvic floor area will be numbed with an injection of local anesthetic, and the cut will be made from the bottom of the vagina, at the peak of a contraction. There are two types of episiotomy – midline and medio-lateral.

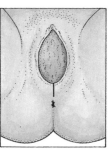

MIDLINE CUT
The cut extends directly backward from the vagina, stopping short of the anus.

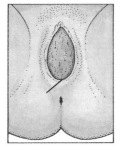

MEDIOLATERAL CUT
The cut starts off like the midline cut, but goes to one side to avoid the anus.

Q ARE THERE OTHER REASONS FOR HAVING AN EPISIOTOMY?

A There are other complications that may make it necessary to perform an episiotomy. You will need an episiotomy if:
■ There is a risk that you might tear badly and that this is likely to involve your anus.
■ It is anticipated that your baby is very large, and that there may be a problem delivering him or her.
■ Your baby is in the breech position.
■ You need to be delivered with the assistance of forceps or vacuum extraction.

Q IS THERE ANYTHING I CAN DO TO AVOID A TEAR OR AN EPISIOTOMY?

A Unfortunately, there is no certain way to avoid having either a tear or an episiotomy. As your baby's head stretches the outlet of the birth canal, the natural reaction is to tense the muscles of the pelvic floor, when what you really need to do is to relax them. The pelvic floor exercises suggested in Chapter 5 (see p. 107) help you to relax the muscles of the pelvic floor during labor. You may find that giving your body time to stretch can help: try to push down for as long as possible, so that the perineal area is encouraged to stretch. However, if you have an epidural, do not push down too hard as the baby's head is delivered. A warm washcloth placed on the perineal area between the vagina and the anus during labor can help this area to stretch more easily. Massaging the area during pregnancy with oils or creams (particularly vitamin E creams) may also help it to become more supple.

Q WHAT HAPPENS IF THERE IS A TEAR?

A There are different degrees of tearing during delivery; most, however, are not serious. It is more common to tear backward, toward your anus. Tearing toward the front is very painful, and is more likely to happen if you deliver in the all-fours position, because the pressure is more toward your labia or clitoris. If you have what is called a second-degree tear, this involves the skin as well as the muscles of the vagina, and those that lie beneath. Rarely, a tear may involve the muscles or lining of the anus, which is known as a third-degree tear. This will need to be repaired by a physician, sometimes under general anesthesia.

Q CAN MY PARTNER HELP TO DELIVER OUR BABY?

A This obviously depends on the circumstances of the birth, and whether or not the midwife or doctor supervising the delivery is happy with this. If the birth is progressing normally, with no complications, there is no reason why your partner cannot assist in lifting the baby out, as long as your midwife or doctor agrees.

Q AT WHAT STAGE IS THE CORD CUT?

A This depends on the methods of the doctor or midwife present, but the cord is usually clamped straight away. However, there is also a school of thought which holds that your baby can benefit from the blood and oxygen he or she receives from the placenta during the first ten minutes after the delivery, and that the cord should be left intact until it stops pulsating. The cord is then clamped and you or your partner can enjoy the ritual of cutting the cord if you want to. If you do not wish the cord to be cut immediately, be sure to state this in your birth plan (see p. 138) and discuss it with your midwife or doctor. Your baby's umbilical cord stump will drop off about ten days after the birth (see p. 196); the pediatrician will tell you what to do.

Q WHAT HAPPENS IF THE CORD IS WRAPPED AROUND MY BABY'S NECK?

A As soon as your baby's head is born, the midwife or doctor will check to see whether the cord is around the neck because this is quite common. If the cord has wound around just once, the midwife can slip it over your baby's head, which can sometimes cause a tiny bruise or a slightly bloodshot eye. If the cord is wound round more than once, or if it feels tight, the midwife will clamp and cut the cord immediately, to ensure that your baby is born without restriction, and to prevent the placenta from being pulled away from the wall of the womb.

Q WHAT IS THE SEQUENCE OF EVENTS AFTER THE CORD IS CUT?

A Immediately after your baby is born, the doctor or midwife will examine your baby and use the Apgar score (see p. 175) to assess his or her condition. If there are no problems and your baby is breathing properly, he or she will be handed to you at once. However, if your baby is not breathing satisfactorily, he or she will be treated immediately with the resuscitation equipment at hand. A pediatrician will be called to check your baby over, and you and your partner will be kept informed of your baby's condition.

IS IT BETTER TO TEAR NATURALLY OR TO BE CUT?

Tearing is a hazard of giving birth; most tears are minor and heal easily, but if your midwife thinks that tearing will be severe, she may feel that an episiotomy is necessary, and ask you for permission to perform one.

Cutting – cruel or kind?

The subject of episiotomy is still controversial. Many women fear that this procedure is still treated as a routine aid to getting the baby's head out, rather than as an emergency procedure when there are genuine complications. Clinicians in favor of episiotomy argue that it prevents the vaginal entrance from overstretching, and that it is much easier and neater to stitch a cut back together than an uneven tear. However, supporters of natural birth argue that if you are left to tear naturally – and only have a minor tear – then you may not need stitching at all, and that tears heal better and faster.

Can I refuse an episiotomy?

Unless there are complications in the labor (see below), you should be able to choose whether or not you are prepared to have an episiotomy. Careful clinicians will always try to avoid having to perform one unless it is absolutely necessary – although many first-time mothers will be encouraged to have one if the perineum is not stretching easily. If you are strongly opposed to an episiotomy, include your wishes in your birth plan (see p. 138), and tell your caregiver before or when you go into labor. If medical staff still insist that an episiotomy is necessary, there is obviously a good reason for one, and it is advisable to follow their advice.

Is an episiotomy ever essential?

Where the baby is in the breech position and where an assisted delivery is necessary, an episiotomy is essential, and will have to to be carried out.

THE THIRD STAGE OF LABOR

Q WHAT IS THE THIRD STAGE OF LABOR?

A This stage starts immediately after your baby's birth and concludes with the delivery of the placenta; it can take as little as 15 minutes or last an hour or more.

Q WHAT HAPPENS DURING THE THIRD STAGE?

A A few minutes after the birth of your baby you will begin to have mild contractions, which you may hardly notice. You will be asked to give a little push to deliver the placenta, and your caregiver may pull gently on the cord (see below).

Q IS IT NECESSARY TO ASSIST THE DELIVERY OF THE PLACENTA?

A In some births, a nurse or doctor will inject a drug into your thigh during a contraction immediately after birth to speed up the delivery of the placenta; this is known as an "active" third stage (see below). It also reduces the risk of postpartum hemorrhage (see p. 178).

Q IS THE INJECTION ALWAYS USED?

A In most cases, you will be allowed to wait for the natural delivery of the placenta. Some doctors prefer to use an injection of oxytocin, prostaglandin, or a similar drug, which causes the womb to contract rapidly and speeds up the delivery of the placenta. If, however, the placenta has not been expelled 30 minutes after the birth, your doctor or midwife may remove the placenta manually. You may wish to discuss management of the third stage of labor with your caregiver before labor begins.

Q CAN THE PLACENTA BE DELIVERED NATURALLY?

A If you do not want to be injected with drugs to assist the delivery of the placenta, you can tell the doctor that you would like to have a natural third stage. This does mean, however, that the delivery of the placenta can take considerably longer than with an active delivery – sometimes up to an hour or more.

HOW IS THE PLACENTA DELIVERED?

Usually, the midwife or doctor delivers the placenta (see right). This will not cause you any pain, because the placenta is soft and comes away easily with a contraction.

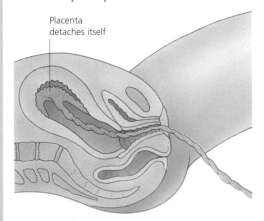

Placenta detaches itself

Speeding up the process
As soon as your baby is born, you may be given an injection of a synthetic hormone in your thigh, which encourages the womb to contract and the placenta to detach itself from the womb wall; this can also reduce the risk of a hemorrhage after the birth. When the womb has contracted to the size of a small melon and the placenta has peeled away, your caregiver will place one hand on your abdomen and gently pull on the cord to ease the placenta out; you may be asked to give a little push at the same time. Your abdomen will be checked to be sure that your womb has contracted tightly into a ball.

WHEN THE PLACENTA HAS SEPARATED
A small gush of blood, and a lengthening of the cord between your legs indicates to your midwife or doctor that the placenta has separated from your womb wall.

Q HOW DO I SPEED UP THE THIRD STAGE WITHOUT USING DRUGS?

A You can try to speed up the process by getting your baby to suckle at your breast. This sucking action stimulates the release of oxytocin, the hormone in your body that causes your womb to contract, thereby encouraging the placenta to shear away from the womb wall. If you prefer, or if your baby doesn't suckle immediately, you can roll your nipples between your thumb and forefinger, which should have the same effect.

Q WHAT ARE THE RISKS OF DELIVERING THE PLACENTA WITHOUT DRUGS?

A There is a greater risk of you having a hemorrhage during a natural third stage because part of the placenta may remain in the womb, or the placenta may not separate from the womb wall. In these situations you will probably be given a general, epidural, or spinal anesthetic and the placenta, or what remains of it, will be removed. Occasionally, this happens in an active third stage of labor.

Q CAN COMPLICATIONS ARISE DURING THE DELIVERY OF THE PLACENTA?

A There are certain factors that can make the delivery of the placenta difficult, for example, a full bladder. This is usually solved by passing a catheter into your bladder to drain the urine. A more serious, but rare, problem during the third stage of labor is the presence of large fibroids obstructing the placenta. In this situation, you would probably have the placenta surgically removed under general anesthesia.

Q WHAT HAPPENS TO MY PLACENTA?

A Once your placenta has been delivered, it is checked to make sure that it looks healthy, and that none of it is missing and has remained inside your womb. If there is no need to keep it for tests – and you do not wish to keep it for any reason – it will be disposed of by the hospital.

Q HOW MIGHT THE THIRD STAGE AFFECT ME?

A You will probably feel quite shaky after the birth of your baby and the delivery of the placenta. However, this is the point at which you can finally relax – you and your partner should be able to spend some quiet time together with the new addition to your family.

WHY MIGHT I NEED STITCHES?

Small tears, or cuts that only involve the skin of the vagina, will heal naturally and do not usually require stitches. However, larger tears, especially those affecting the muscles around the vagina, will be stitched to ensure that they heal properly, and to prevent hemorrhage.

When will I be stitched?
If you are bleeding, you will be stitched as soon as the placenta is delivered. Otherwise your doctor or midwife may leave you and your baby to rest first. Stitches are less painful if done straight after the placenta's delivery; the longer you wait, the more painful the procedure can be; also, pain relief used in labor will be wearing off.

What is the procedure for stitching?
The tear or cut is repaired in layers: first, the vaginal skin is stitched, then the underlying muscle, and finally the perineal (external) skin. You will be given a local anesthetic to numb the area; or your epidural will be topped off; you can also use gas and air. You will probably need to rest your legs in stirrups, however ungainly this may seem, because your legs will be very shaky after the delivery. It will take about half an hour to be stitched.

Will I need a catheter if I have stitches?
If the tear has affected your urethra, this can make it difficult to pass urine and you may therefore need a catheter. If you had an epidural, a catheter may be left in overnight or until feeling has returned to your bladder.

How long will the stitches take to heal?
Nowadays absorbable stitches that dissolve and fall out as you heal are used. The area around your vagina has an excellent blood supply; as long as no infections develop, the cut or tear should heal rapidly, leaving no scar.

How many stitches are normally used?
It is very difficult to be precise because the number of stitches depends on the length of the tear or cut. Technically, you will only have one stitch because they are made with one continuous length of material.

LABOR AND BIRTH

AFTER YOUR DELIVERY

Q HOW WILL THE BIRTH OF MY BABY AFFECT ME?

A At last, the moment has arrived when you can greet the little stranger that you've carried around inside you for the past nine months. You may feel a sense of instant recognition; when you look at your baby in those first euphoric seconds, you may find yourself saying, "Oh, there you are!" Not everyone feels an immediate bond, though; some women feel slightly surreal or detached at first, particularly after an exhausting, prolonged labor. This is also quite normal. You'll probably feel different after a meal, rest, or a good sleep.

Q WHAT HAPPENS IMMEDIATELY AFTER THE DELIVERY?

A You and your partner should be left alone for a little while so that you can enjoy some precious time holding and getting to know your baby before he or she is weighed and checked. This is an ideal time to begin the bonding process (see below).

Q HOW LONG WILL I HAVE TO STAY ON THE LABOR UNIT?

A You will probably remain on the labor unit a few hours after the birth. If you need to have stitches, these will be done and, if possible, you can have a bath; you will then be moved to a room. If you are only staying in the hospital for a few hours, the pediatrician will check your baby.

Q WHAT WILL MY BABY LOOK LIKE AFTER THE BIRTH?

A Most babies look quite normal, but don't be surprised if your baby looks blotchy and wrinkled. Some babies have bluish fingers and toes as a result of initial circulation changes, but this is not serious. If your baby's head took a while to come through, it may look pointed, and the face can look blue and engorged; if the delivery was assisted, there may be marks on the face and head. With a breech birth, the bottom may be swollen or bruised. These marks will lessen in a few days.

ENJOYING THOSE FIRST MOMENTS

As soon as your baby is born, you and your partner will probably want to spend some quiet, private time to greet and to bond with your new arrival because your baby is already alert and responsive to your voices, smell, and touch.

The origins of bonding

"Bonding" was a revolutionary idea in the 1970s; research discovered that the most sensitive period for establishing contact with your baby is during the first hour of life. But remember that bonding is not some magical process that guarantees a lifetime of closeness. Indeed, before the concept was codified, generations of parents formed perfectly loving relationships with their children.

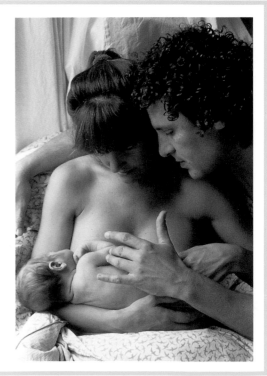

EVERYDAY CONTACT
As important as early bonding is the long-term daily contact of caring for, feeding, and loving your baby.

Q WHO CHECKS MY BABY AFTER HE OR SHE IS BORN?

A Your caregiver and possibly a pediatrician will check your baby after the birth. The check is usually swift but thorough and it is done to establish that your baby is normal, and to detect anything that is unusual or abnormal (see p. 190). Your baby will be weighed and measured. While doing this, the examiner will also observe your baby's color, breathing, heart rate, muscle tone, and any delivery marks.

Q WILL I NEED ANY CHECKS OR TREATMENT IMMEDIATELY AFTER BIRTH?

A Common problems in this early stage after giving birth include feeling dizzy, faint, and nauseous. Your blood pressure, temperature, and pulse rate will be recorded, and special attention will be paid to your bleeding, which will probably be very heavy. Your stomach will also be checked to confirm that your womb is contracting well because a relaxed womb can lead to postpartum hemorrhage (see p. 178). You will be encouraged to pass urine in the first few hours after the birth, because a full bladder can also prevent your womb from contracting fully.

Q CAN I PUT MY BABY TO THE BREAST RIGHT AWAY?

A Yes, you can. It may only be for a short while until you need to be stitched up but it is worth getting your baby to suckle as soon as possible; this helps you and your baby to bond, and also helps to stimulate the womb to contract and expel the placenta. Breastfeeding is not immediately possible if your baby needs to be given oxygen to help with breathing, or is taken to neonatal intensive care, or if you're still feeling sleepy after an anesthetic.

Q HOW LONG WILL MY PARTNER BE ALLOWED TO STAY WITH ME?

A Your partner can stay with you while you're in the labor unit; check with the hospital to see if partners are welcome overnight, too. You should, in any event, encourage your partner to go home and get some rest, as he'll probably be feeling emotionally drained; this will also give you a chance to get some rest. You should also remember when considering visits from friends and family that you will be very tired. Don't be afraid to limit visits to a brief period, or perhaps ask people to wait until you are at home before they come to see you and your baby.

WHAT DOES AN APGAR SCORE ASSESS?

Within one minute of birth, your baby's well-being is assessed by a simple test recorded by the doctor or midwife (see below). Called the Apgar score, this system evaluates a newborn's condition. Scores are given out of ten. An Apgar score of seven or over indicates a baby in good condition; a low score (between four and six) may mean that a baby needs help with breathing or resuscitation; under four means he or she could need lifesaving techniques. The Apgar is done again at five minutes, when a score of seven or more indicates a good outlook. If the score is low, the baby needs monitoring.

INSTANT APPRAISAL

The Apgar score was developed by an American doctor, Virginia Apgar, for short-term diagnosis of a baby's physical condition after the birth. It is of little significance in terms of assessing a baby's long-term development, so don't worry if your baby had low scores but recovered within the next few minutes; he or she will almost certainly turn out to be normal and healthy.

SIGN	0	1	2
Heart rate	Absent	Slow	More than 100/minute
Breathing	Absent	Slow	Good; crying
Muscle tone	Limp	Some tone	Active motion
Response to stimulus	None	Some response	Sneezes or coughs
Color of body	Pale/blue	Blue/pink	Pink all over

WHAT CAN GO WRONG?

Q WHAT PROBLEMS CAN OCCUR IN LABOR?

A Most labors are quite straightforward, but at any stage there may be complications – minor or major – that mean you or your baby require some form of medical help. Complications include a prolonged labor, unexpected bleeding during labor, premature labor, or fetal distress.

Q CAN LABOR TAKE TOO LONG?

A There are wide variations in the length of time labor takes. In fact, there is really no such thing as a "normal" length of time for labor. If it's your first labor it can last up to 20 hours, although this is unusual. If you are feeling particularly tired, the labor may be speeded up. There are also time limits for each stage to indicate when it seems necessary to lend a helping hand (see p. 160).

Q DOES LABOR TAKE LONGER IF IT IS MY FIRST BABY?

A Yes, first labors are usually slower than subsequent ones. After you have been through one labor your womb muscles tend to be more coordinated, and your cervix dilates more rapidly. There is no known scientific explanation for this.

Q WHY DO SOME LABORS TAKE LONGER THAN OTHERS?

A Labor can be slow for various reasons. The baby may be quite big, or his or her head may be in the wrong position (its back to your back, "OP" position, or sideways "OT" position, see p. 160). Your contractions may not be strong or coordinated enough to make labor progress efficiently, or it may be a combination of all these.

Q CAN ANYTHING BE DONE TO SPEED UP LABOR IF IT IS GOING TOO SLOWLY?

A If your contractions are not powerful or regular enough, your midwife or doctor may rupture the amniotic membranes (see p. 164) to speed up and increase the intensity of contractions. If this doesn't work, you may be given a drip containing oxytocin (see p. 159). The drip is regulated according to the rate of your contractions.

Q HOW EFFECTIVE IS OXYTOCIN?

A Oxytocin performs the same way as the endogenous hormone oxytocin, which regulates contractions. As long as it is given carefully, it is considered very effective and safe.

Q IS IT USUAL TO BLEED DURING LABOR?

A It is quite common to have a small amount of bleeding from your vagina during labor. As your cervix opens up (dilates), it bleeds slightly and as the membranes come away from the wall of your womb, this can also cause a small amount of bleeding. Too much bleeding during labor, however, may suggest that there is a problem and will always be taken seriously by your midwife and obstetrician (see below).

Q CAN BLEEDING IN LABOR BE SERIOUS?

A Severe bleeding during labor is called an antepartum hemorrhage and it may be coming from your placenta. If the placenta is "low" in your womb – near the cervix, known as placenta previa (see p. 128) – and you go into labor, it can cause heavy bleeding. (If it is so low that your baby can't pass it on the way down the birth canal, you may need a cesarean delivery. You will have been told that this is a possibility after an ultrasound.) Another cause of bleeding is when part of your placenta separates from the wall of your womb; this is known as placental abruption, and it produces pain and bright red bleeding (see p. 128). This is also potentially dangerous and may mean that your baby needs to be delivered imminently, or that you need an emergency cesarean. Whatever the cause, the bleeding is coming from you, not from your baby.

Q WHAT IS MEANT BY FETAL DISTRESS?

A Fetal distress usually occurs when the blood flow from the placenta to your baby is reduced so that your baby is not receiving enough oxygen. This may mean your baby will need to be delivered quickly. If it is severe, your obstetrician may decide to deliver your baby by cesarean.

Q HOW WILL THE DOCTORS KNOW THAT MY BABY IS IN DISTRESS?

A Your baby's heartbeat will be monitored regularly during labor via fetal monitoring (see p. 158), and any changes will be picked up. If there are irregularities, or your baby's heart beats persistently very quickly or very slowly, it can mean that your baby is short of oxygen. Another common sign of distress is if your baby passes dark green "meconium"; this drains out of your vagina in your amniotic fluid (see p. 62). Serious signs of distress indicate that your baby must be delivered quickly and treated if necessary.

Q WILL MY BABY BE AFFECTED IF HE OR SHE BECOMES DISTRESSED?

A Many babies show some signs of distress in labor because the baby's body endures high levels of stress and pressure, but usually the baby's heart rate returns to normal or you give birth before serious problems develop. Very rarely, a severe lack of oxygen to the baby can result in brain damage. In extreme situations, oxygen deprivation can be fatal. However, your midwife and doctor are trained to identify the signs of fetal distress and to minimize the risk of any complications developing.

WHAT HAPPENS IF I GO INTO PREMATURE LABOR?

In about five percent of pregnancies, labor starts before 37 weeks of pregnancy. If your baby is born between 34 and 37 weeks of pregnancy, he or she should be fine and will probably not need special care after the birth. However, if you go into labor before 30 weeks of pregnancy, your baby is likely to be very immature and will need to be cared for in a neonatal intensive care unit or special nursery (see p. 214).

Why might labor start early?

Premature labor is more likely to happen if you have had a premature baby before, if you have an infection that is giving you a high temperature, if you are having twins (or more), or if you are suffering from an infection in your womb.

Is the start of premature labor the same as normal labor?

Yes, the signs are often the same (see p. 156). However, if you are very early (24 to 28 weeks), it is possible that you will only feel low back pain and not experience strong contractions. If you think your labor is starting early, contact your midwife or doctor immediately.

What can be done to stop premature labor?

Nothing can actually stop your labor once it is underway, but your contractions can be temporarily slowed down with drugs. These are not very effective in the long term, and some have unpleasant side effects, so in general they are not given to you for longer than 48 hours.

What else can be done?

If there is any hint of an infection, doctors can give you antibiotics; if you are feeling very nervous, you may be given a mild dose of a pain reliever or an antianxiety drug. If you become dehydrated, you may also be put on an intravenous drip. Often these measures alone can calm your contractions down.

Will the hospital be able to cope if my baby is born prematurely?

If your hospital's intensive care unit is unable to cope, either because there is no more room or because it does not have the proper facilities to care for premature babies, you and your baby will be transferred to a nearby hospital that has the necessary resources.

Will my premature labor be any different from a normal full-term delivery?

Yes, in general, a premature labor is faster than a full-term labor, because the baby is smaller.

Is there anything that can help to prepare my baby for premature birth?

As immature lungs cause the most problems for premature babies, you will be given a course of steroids 24 to 48 hours before the delivery to improve your baby's chances. Steroids can be given to you via an injection or orally; the steroids cross the placenta to your baby and help your baby's lungs to develop more rapidly. If doctors know that you have a high risk of delivering early, you may be given steroids every couple of weeks or so during pregnancy; this is perfectly safe for you and your baby.

LABOR AND BIRTH

RARE COMPLICATIONS

Q WHAT CAUSES SEVERE BLEEDING AFTER DELIVERY?

A Severe vaginal bleeding after a delivery (called postpartum hemorrhage) occurs when your womb has not emptied completely and cannot contract tightly enough to stop the bleeding. Postpartum hemorrhage usually occurs because a small fragment of the placenta has been retained by the womb, or because the womb muscles are too tired to contract.

Q WHY IS POSTPARTUM HEMORRHAGE RARE?

A Postpartum hemorrhage is rare because your womb has a self-protecting device to stop it from bleeding. Once your baby has been born and the placenta has been expelled, your empty womb contracts down to the size of a grapefruit, quickly closing the uterine arteries so that they cannot bleed excessively.

Q WHAT CAN BE DONE IF I HAVE A HEMORRHAGE?

A You will be given an injection of a drug to help to expel the placenta and make your womb contract. If even after the injection the bleeding does not stop quickly enough, you may need another procedure to clear your womb under either a general or an epidural anesthetic. You may also need to be given a blood transfusion if the bleeding is serious.

Q HOW LIKELY IS IT THAT I WILL NEED A BLOOD TRANSFUSION?

A Your chances of needing a blood transfusion are very low, and an obstetrician will only suggest this if it is absolutely necessary. If you lose a lot of blood and your circulation is suffering, your blood pressure is dropping, and your pulse rate is increasing, a transfusion will be recommended. In certain situations, a transfusion of blood can save your life, so it is unwise to refuse one.

Q HOW CAN I BE SURE THAT I AM NOT RECEIVING CONTAMINATED BLOOD?

A Blood transfusion is a safe practice and carries virtually no risk of transmitting infections such as HIV or hepatitis. If you are advised to have one, it is because the doctor considers that the benefits will outweigh any slight risk of infection. To truly allay your concerns, your partner or a family member can donate blood for your labor and birth.

Q CAN I GIVE MY OWN BLOOD IN ADVANCE IN CASE I NEED SOME?

A This is both impractical and inadvisable. Although you might be able to donate up to one liter (two pints) of blood before you deliver your baby, if you do need a transfusion because of a postpartum hemorrhage (see above), you would need at least two liters (four pints) of blood. It is not possible to give this without compromising your pregnancy and making yourself seriously anemic.

CAN BEING HIV-POSITIVE AFFECT HOW MY BABY IS BORN?

Evidence suggests that your baby has less chance of catching HIV if delivered by a cesarean rather than vaginally because, as the baby makes its way down the birth canal, there is contact with your blood and fluids that may contain the virus. For this reason, the medical profession also believes that any procedures that can cause contamination, such as fetal blood sampling in labor, are best avoided. If the drug azidothymidine (AZT) is given before and during delivery, it may reduce the chances of passing on HIV.

Physical contact
While you can cuddle and kiss your baby as much as you wish, it is important not to allow any of your blood to come into contact with him or her. Unfortunately, because the HIV virus can also be transmitted by other body fluids, including breast milk, you should not breastfeed.

Confidentiality
If you request it, the fact that you're HIV-positive will not be written on your hospital notes and only those caregivers specifically looking after you need to know that you are HIV-positive.

WHAT IF MY BABY DIES?

When a baby you have carried for up to nine months and in whom you and your partner have invested countless hopes and dreams dies, the loss is immense and it will be hard to overcome the grief, anger, and depression that it causes. You will probably want to find out why and how this has happened, which is quite normal, yet you must also go on living and planning for the future.

How will I know if my baby has died?

When your baby dies in the womb after the twenty fourth week of pregnancy, this is called a stillbirth, and labor will usually start a few days thereafter. You may suspect that this has happened if your baby stops moving, or if you do not feel pregnant any more because any signs and sensations of pregnancy disappear as the pregnancy hormones diminish. You may also experience weight loss because the womb will shrink in size due to the re-absorption of the amniotic fluid.

What causes stillbirth?

It is not always possible to discover the cause. An autopsy may help to answer some questions but can be difficult for the parents. Common causes of death include severe fetal defects, or an unhealthy placenta that fails to nourish the baby, either because it hasn't developed properly, or because it is diseased. Less common causes include Rhesus incompatibility (see p. 129), diabetes, and autoimmune diseases.

How will I feel?

After the birth you will have all the physical effects of childbirth to recover from. Because of the sudden withdrawal of pregnancy hormones, which can cause a flood of emotional feelings, you may feel emotionally raw. While some women find this reassuring because it helps to remind them of their pregnancy, others find that it adds to their distress. Either reaction is possible.

Your recovery

It can take a long time to work through the grief of losing a baby. Life may seem very unreal for a while, and you and your partner will probably find yourselves asking, "Why us?" and "What did we do wrong?" You need to share your thoughts and feelings, but often your friends avoid the subject because they feel awkward reminding you of the loss or because they don't know if they will be able to cope with your grief. Perhaps the greatest support can only come from other people who have experienced such a loss. About six weeks after your baby's death, you and your partner should see your physician who will discuss any test results with you and try to answer your questions. Ask to be put in touch with a local support group (see p. 232). You will never completely get over your loss, but the intense pain and grief will ease in time.

Your partner's grief

Your partner may have trouble expressing his emotions unless you encourage him. He may even choose to hide his grief by throwing himself into his work or going out more with his friends, which can cause great tension in your relationship. However inappropriate his behavior may seem, try to recognize what is really going on. Your partner's pain is just as great as yours, and this is his way of trying to deal with it. Try to accept that there are stages to grief that you and your partner may experience in different ways and at different times, and allow yourself and your partner time to work through your grief.

Coming to terms with your loss

Certain rituals and procedures can help you to accept the loss of your baby more quickly and provide you with an occasion or memento by which you can remember your child. For example, you will be given the chance to hold your baby and take photographs, give him or her a name, and think about what kind of funeral you would like. One of the hardest things to come to terms with will be trying not to apportion blame and guilt, because often the reason remains unknown.

The legal position

If a baby is born after 24 weeks of pregnancy, a certificate is given by the hospital so that the baby's birth and death can be registered, and to allow you to make funeral or cremation arrangements. Before 24 weeks, most hospitals will have a patient advocate or chaplain who can help you to decide on funeral arrangements.

AN ASSISTED DELIVERY

Q WHAT IS AN ASSISTED DELIVERY AND WHY IS IT DONE?

A Instruments, such as forceps or a vacuum extraction cup (see below) may have to be used in the second stage if the cervix is fully dilated but your baby fails to make good progress down the birth canal. An assisted delivery may also be needed if your baby's head is facing the wrong way and is wedged in your pelvis, or if your baby is large, or is distressed and has to be delivered quickly.

Q WILL THE MIDWIFE OR AN OBSTETRICIAN ATTEND IF I HAVE AN ASSISTED DELIVERY?

A If forceps or a vacuum cup need to be used during your labor, an obstetrician will usually deliver your baby. Your midwife will remain with you and will also assist with the procedure. Your obstetrician's experience and personal preferences will probably dictate whether he or she completes the delivery by using forceps or a vacuum extraction cup.

WHAT DOES AN ASSISTED DELIVERY INVOLVE?

An assisted delivery is carried out if your labor is prolonged or if there is a delay in the second stage and you or your baby have become distressed. You may also need an assisted delivery if you have an epidural and cannot push properly or to deliver a breech baby. Occasionally, forceps are used to deliver a second twin. Forceps or vacuum extraction gently pull your baby out while you continue to push.

How are forceps used?

Forceps can only be used when the cervix is fully dilated and the baby's head is low in the pelvic outlet. There are various designs of forceps but all are based on the principle of two separate metal tongs that can be placed around the baby's head and linked together so that there is little pressure on the baby's head. A type of forceps called Kielland's forceps is used to turn the baby when the head is in the wrong position for delivery. Forceps called Neville Barnes' (or Wrigley's) are used when the baby is facing the right way and needs lifting out.

How does vacuum extraction work?

A vacuum cup can only be used when the cervix is fully dilated and the baby's head low in the pelvic outlet. The principle for the vacuum cup is very simple: a plastic or a metal cup is placed on the baby's head; a tube runs from the cup to a machine that uses either an electrical mechanism or a pump to build up suction in the cup. Once a good seal has been established on the baby's head, the obstetrician will gently pull on the cup while you continue to push, until the baby's head and body begin to emerge from the birth canal.

Delivery by forceps

Curved blunt sides, like salad tongs, cradle the baby's head

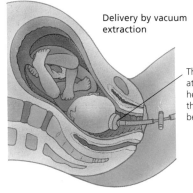

Delivery by vacuum extraction

The cup is attached to the head so that the baby can be pulled out

LABOR AND BIRTH

Q HOW LONG HAVE THESE METHODS BEEN USED FOR DELIVERING BABIES?

A Forceps were invented in the sixteenth century by a British surgeon, a member of the Chamberlain family, who kept the method a closely guarded secret for over a century. Vacuum extraction is a more recent invention that became popular in the 1950s and 1960s.

Q HOW LONG DOES AN ASSISTED DELIVERY TAKE?

A The delivery itself rarely takes longer than ten minutes but it can take about 45 minutes to get you ready for the procedure. You may need an epidural or spinal anesthetic, and you may be moved to a larger delivery room or operating theater if a cesarean delivery is necessary. You will also require a catheter in your bladder to drain away any urine beforehand.

Q I'VE HEARD SO MANY SAD STORIES ABOUT FORCEPS. ARE THEY TRUE?

A Such stories were associated with an early procedure called "high-forceps delivery," which involved reaching up into the maternal pelvis to extract the baby, causing much pain and internal bruising. This method is no longer used. Now, forceps deliveries are undertaken only when the baby's head has descended well into the pelvis or is in the pelvic outlet. If the baby's head is not well positioned, a cesarean delivery is indicated.

Q HOW MUCH PAIN WILL I FEEL WITH AN ASSISTED DELIVERY?

A You are usually given a spinal or epidural anesthetic so that you feel little of what is going on. If you already have an epidural anesthetic in position (see p. 152), it will be topped off, but if it is too late in labor for you to be given an epidural, a local anesthetic will be given to numb the perineum. Rarely, a general anesthetic is required.

Q WILL THE FORCEPS OR VACUUM CUP LEAVE ANY MARKS ON MY BABY'S HEAD?

A Forceps may leave two bruises or red marks on either side of your baby's head, and a cup commonly leaves a bump on top of the baby's head. The marks or bump should disappear within a few days, and the bruising within a week or so. Sometimes the swelling makes the head look elongated, but this isn't permanent.

Q WHAT IF MY BABY CAN'T BE DELIVERED BY FORCEPS OR VACUUM EXTRACTION?

A If there is any question about whether the baby can be delivered vaginally, you will be taken to the operating theater for a trial to see whether a vaginal delivery is possible. If it is not, because your baby is in the wrong position, or is too large, a cesarean will be necessary (see p. 182). If you are already in the operating room, this can take place quite speedily.

HOW SAFE ARE ASSISTED DELIVERIES?

The use of instruments to deliver babies has been common practice for centuries and has undoubtedly saved babies who would otherwise have died in the birth canal. It is a very safe method of delivery as long as it is undertaken by competent doctors with the facilities to perform a cesarean delivery, should the procedure fail.

Which method is safer for me?
Despite many clinical studies, noone is absolutely certain which is the safer method for the mother – forceps or vacuum extraction. The use of a vacuum cup can result in fewer tears and less need for an episiotomy than forceps, although it may be more traumatic for your baby than forceps.

Your baby and forceps
With the sides acting as a protective "cradle," forceps are a little gentler on the baby's head as it descends through the birth canal. But if a delivery is particularly difficult, the nerves to the baby's arms may be temporarily damaged. Permanent damage is very rare, however, and the majority of babies are absolutely fine after a forceps delivery.

Your baby and vacuum extraction
A vacuum extraction commonly leaves a swelling on the the top of the baby's head; this should, however, soon go down. A very large bump can sometimes turn into an extensive bruise and may even cause the baby to become jaundiced, but such complications are the exception rather than the rule.

A CESAREAN BIRTH

Q **WHAT IS A CESAREAN BIRTH AND WHEN MIGHT I NEED ONE?**

A A cesarean birth is the delivery of your baby by an operation on your abdomen. Instead of passing down your vagina, your baby is lifted out of your womb through your abdomen. You will have a cesarean if your doctors decide that a vaginal delivery could threaten the health of you or your baby, or that it is impossible to achieve.

Q **WHAT IS AN ELECTIVE CESAREAN?**

A An elective cesarean is a planned procedure decided upon before you go into labor. There are a number of reasons why your doctor may suggest before labor that you should have a cesarean, for example, if you have a medical condition, such as diabetes, or you are HIV-positive. There are other conditions that indicate that you will definitely need to have a cesarean; these include severe cephalopelvic disproportion (CPD), where your baby is very large and your pelvis very small, or when the placenta is completely covering the cervix, known as placenta previa (see p. 128).

Q **WHEN IS AN EMERGENCY CESAREAN NECESSARY?**

A An emergency cesarean takes place when a problem is discovered that threatens the life of the mother and/or her baby. This situation can arise before labor begins, for example, if you have an antepartum hemorrhage (see p. 176) or a cord prolapse. An emergency cesarean may also be decided upon during labor if the mother's blood pressure becomes dangerously high or if doctors see that the baby is showing signs of being in distress (see p. 176).

SOME COMMON WORRIES ABOUT CESAREAN DELIVERIES

Do my doctors want me to have a cesarean just because it's easier for them?
Obstetricians prefer vaginal deliveries. Although cesareans are safe, a vaginal birth is the safest, and you can recover more quickly. Cesareans are advised only if there is a valid medical reason.

If I have one cesarean, will I ever be able to have a vaginal birth?
About 75 percent of women who have had a cesarean can have a vaginal delivery with their next baby. Doctors used to worry that a cesarean scar could rupture in subsequent labors, but this risk is now known to be low. However, you may have a condition that makes a cesarean the safest way to have a baby, or have a very small pelvis that prevents a vaginal delivery.

My mother and sisters have had cesareans; will I need one, too?
This is not usually the case unless all of your family are small, with small pelvic bones. This is not common, and many women who look quite short and slim manage to have normal labors.

Will my baby have psychological problems if I cannot deliver him or her vaginally?
There is no evidence to suggest that this can affect your baby's psychological development. The best way for your baby to be born is the safest way, whether this is by a cesarean or by a vaginal delivery.

Will I be able to breastfeed?
Yes. In fact, breastfeeding is encouraged. However, if you have an elective cesarean (see above) and are not in labor, it can take a little more time for your breasts to produce milk. Also, if you have a general anesthetic, it will take a few hours for the drugs to wash out of your body, so it is better for you to wait a while before breastfeeding your baby.

Will I be able to see my baby immediately after the birth?
Unless your baby needs to be taken to a neonatal intensive care unit (see p. 214) or you had general anesthesia, you can hold your baby right away. The doctor or midwife will then check and weigh your baby before returning him or her to you.

Q WILL I HAVE TO HAVE A GENERAL ANESTHETIC IF I HAVE A CESAREAN?

A It used to be common to have a general anesthetic, but now you are likely to have epidural or spinal anesthesia (see p. 152). With an epidural, you are awake and can see and hold your baby when he or she is lifted out of your womb. You may feel sensations, but it is unusual to feel pain. With an emergency cesarean, you may be given a general anesthetic unless you had an epidural earlier.

Q HOW COMMON ARE CESAREAN DELIVERIES?

A Cesareans are far more common today than they were 50 years ago. This is because techniques for cesarean operations have greatly improved over the past few decades, and a cesarean is now considered an extremely safe way to have a baby. It is estimated that about 20 percent of babies are now delivered by cesarean section.

WHAT HAPPENS DURING A CESAREAN OPERATION?

You are prepared for a cesarean by being shaved below the pubic hairline and given anesthesia. An intravenous drip will provide you with fluids. Although this is a major abdominal operation, a cesarean is usually fairly quick, taking only about half an hour.

WHO CAN BE PRESENT

If you are awake, a screen will be set up so that you can't see the operation and, if your birth partner is squeamish, he or she can also sit behind the screen and remain with you without seeing the operation.

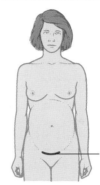

THE INCISION
A side-to-side cut is usually made below your shaved pubic hairline. This is better than a vertical incision from the navel downward because it heals more quickly.

Horizontal incision

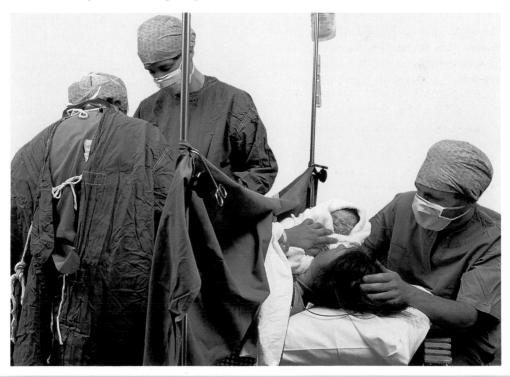

LABOR AND BIRTH

A BREECH BIRTH

Q WHAT IS A BREECH BABY?

A At around 32 to 34 weeks, most babies settle into position in the womb with their head down; this is called the cephalic position (see p. 63). If your baby is "breech," this means that your baby is bottom down inside your womb. If the baby stays in this position, this could cause complications during the birth, for example, if the baby's head becomes stuck during the second stage of labor (see box). You are therefore more likely to have a cesarean delivery. As the pregnancy progresses, most babies turn to the head-down position; at term, only about three percent of babies are still breech.

Q WILL I NEED AN EPIDURAL?

A It is not essential but, because you may need an assisted birth or a cesarean, your doctors may suggest an epidural so that you are already anesthetized for these procedures.

Q SHOULD I EXPECT A CESAREAN IF MY BABY IS BREECH?

A If it is your first baby, your doctor may suggest one. But if you start labor naturally, your baby is an average size, and there are no problems, you have a good chance of a vaginal breech delivery. If you want to try a vaginal birth, discuss the pros and cons with your obstetrician before labor.

HOW DOES A BREECH BIRTH DIFFER FROM A NORMAL ONE?

Breech deliveries are more complicated than cephalic ones, and therefore need experienced doctors and midwives. Recently, there has been a trend for breech babies to be delivered by a cesarean and, therefore, there are now fewer doctors who are sufficiently experienced to deal with a vaginal breech delivery.

What are the problems?
The main potential problem with a vaginal breech delivery is that your baby's head may become stuck in the pelvis in the second stage of labor, depriving your baby of oxygen, which increases the risk of fetal distress. Your labor may also be slower because your baby's head isn't pushing down on the cervix, and there is a higher risk of tears or bleeding.

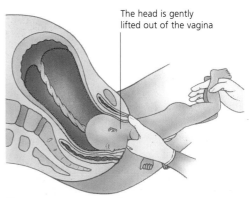

The baby's body is carefully supported

The head is gently lifted out of the vagina

DELIVERING YOUR BABY'S BODY
With a breech delivery, your baby's buttocks will be delivered first and then the legs will emerge. You may need an episiotomy before the head is delivered.

DELIVERING YOUR BABY'S HEAD
Once the rest of the body is delivered, the head will be drawn down the vagina. At this stage, forceps can be used to complete the delivery.

TWINS AND MULTIPLE BIRTHS

Q HOW DOES A TWIN DELIVERY DIFFER FROM THE DELIVERY OF ONE BABY?

A A twin delivery, like a twin pregnancy, is considered "high risk." Twin births nearly always take place in a hospital, and are done by one or more obstetrician, two pediatricians, and probably two nurses or midwives. Athough many twin deliveries do proceed without any complications, there is a higher chance that the birth will need assistance (see p. 180), or that you will need a cesarean delivery (see p. 182).

Q WHO WILL DELIVER MY BABIES?

A With a normal vaginal delivery, a midwife can deliver your babies with an obstetrician in attendance. If there are complications, the obstetrician will probably deliver your babies or carry out a cesarean section.

Q WILL I NEED TO HAVE AN EPIDURAL WITH TWINS OR TRIPLETS?

A This is not obligatory but sometimes it is advisable because, should you need help in the second stage of labor (such as forceps, vacuum extraction, or a cesarean), your pain relief will be in place and the delivery will not be further delayed.

Q ARE THERE LIKELY TO BE PROBLEMS WITH THE SECOND TWIN'S DELIVERY?

A After your first baby is born, your contractions may ebb away and there may be a pause before they pick up again, delaying the birth of your second baby. If this wait seems to be too long, you may be given oxytocin (see p. 159) to increase the regularity and strength of your contractions. Once this baby is coming down the birth canal, its waters are broken to speed up the delivery.

Q I'M EXPECTING TRIPLETS. WILL I NEED TO HAVE A CESAREAN?

A Yes. A cesarean is the least traumatic way for triplets to be delivered. This is because the babies may be in awkward positions, or are premature and very small, and therefore unable to cope with the extra strains involved in a vaginal birth. They may also need special neonatal care after the delivery.

PRESENTATION OF TWINS

The position of twins can influence the kind of delivery you have. If both are in the same position, the outcome is easier to predict. If in different positions, a different type of delivery may be needed for each twin; for example, your first twin may have a vaginal delivery, but a second, breech twin may get distressed and have to be delivered by cesarean section.

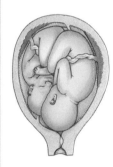

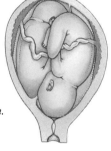

CEPHALIC TWINS (left)
With this presentation a vaginal delivery may be possible for both babies.

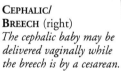

CEPHALIC/ BREECH (right)
The cephalic baby may be delivered vaginally while the breech is by a cesarean.

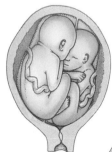

BREECH TWINS (left)
With both babies feet down, there is a strong chance of a cesarean.

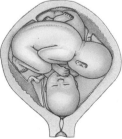

CEPHALIC/ TRANSVERSE (right)
The transverse baby may be delivered by a cesarean.

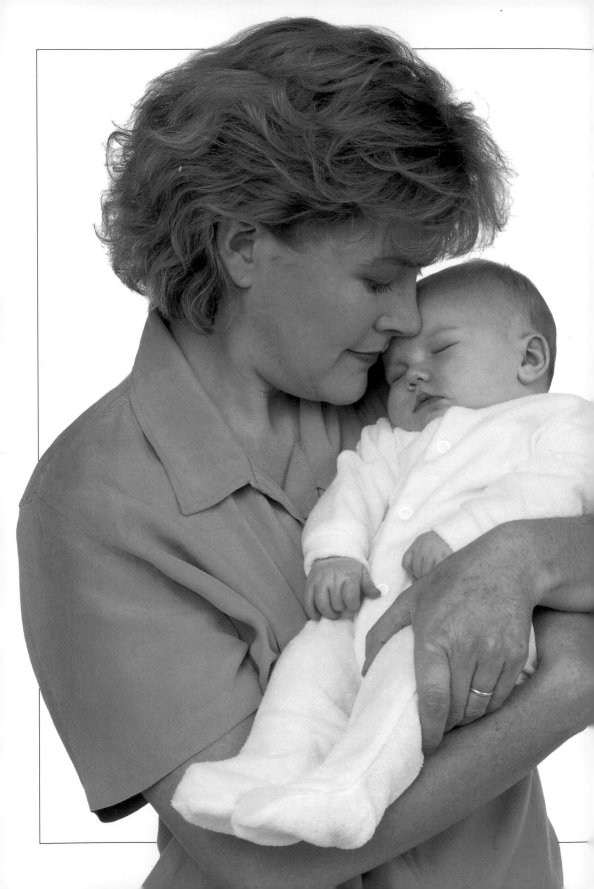

THE FIRST SIX WEEKS

A baby to hold, love, and care for is all a parent-to-be longs for. The arrival in your life of such a beautiful boy or girl is a wonderful thing – but you are now responsible for this tiny new life, and this can seem daunting at first. The baby's arrival will change your lives forever – but few would ever consider that the hard work, lack of sleep, and the ever-present demands of their baby were not worth it. In addition to answering your questions about your own recovery and the well-being of your newborn, this chapter offers practical advice and reassurance to help you and your partner find your way during the first few weeks following the birth.

YOUR FIRST 48 HOURS

Q WHAT CAN I EXPECT TO HAPPEN IN THE FIRST FEW DAYS?

A In the first 48 hours of your baby's life, your biggest concern will probably be your new baby! After that, you'll think about how tired and sore you feel. You may also feel relief and euphoria that it is all over (see below). Your baby will probably sleep a great deal at first, so make the most of this and catch up on your rest. If you had a home birth or go home within a few hours of a hospital birth, you will be able to relax in your own familiar surroundings.

Q CAN I DRESS MY BABY, AND WHAT KIND OF DIAPER SHOULD I USE?

A Hospitals expect you to bring clothes with you to take your baby home, but most often keep newborns in undershirts, diapers, tiny caps, and swaddling blankets while they're in the hospital. During these first few days after the birth most women opt for disposable diapers.

Q HOW OFTEN DOES MY BABY NEED TO BE FED?

A It is common for babies to feed little in the first 48 hours because they are quite sleepy; some forms of pain relief given to you before delivery can cross the placenta and make a baby even more sleepy. If your baby sleeps for much of the time, wake him or her up at least every four hours or so to feed, particularly first thing in the morning. Your baby may want to suckle frequently, probably more for comfort than from hunger. If you are bottle-feeding, feed about every three to four hours.

Q HOW MUCH WILL MY BABY TAKE IN AT EACH FEEDING?

A If you are breastfeeding, your baby will need relatively little of the colostrum that comes in the first two days, because it is so rich and high in protein. If bottle-fed, he or she will need more feedings as the food will be less rich.

HOW YOU FEEL EMOTIONALLY

Nothing quite prepares you and your partner for the mixed emotions and sudden mood swings that you will experience during the first few days after the birth of your child. One minute you feel on.top of the world, and the next exhausted and tearful. The arrival of a new baby creates conflicting feelings of joy, responsibility, and pride, possibly even fear. Or you may feel so overwhelmed by the whole event that you experience a sense of anticlimax. After a painful labor, you may feel resentful and detached – this, too, is quite common. Just remember that you have done an amazing thing – brought a new life into being.

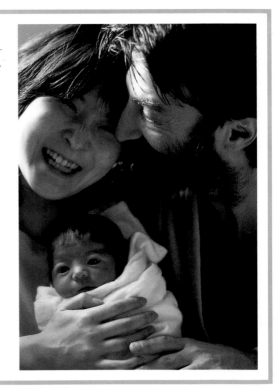

NOW COMES THE JOY
Who would have thought that such a small bundle could bring such joy and wonder.

What can I expect to happen in the hospital?

When you stay in the hospital after birth, you and your baby will be welcomed by the nursing staff and settled into bed. Some hospitals offer total or partial rooming-in, where the baby stays with you, and others require that newborns stay in the nursery. Check with your hospital prior to labor.

Can my partner come in to see me at any time?
Every hospital has its own visiting hours, but these do not usually restrict partners from visiting from morning until late at night. Some hospitals will not allow partners to stay overnight.

How is my baby identified?
Your baby will have a name band around each ankle. The details on the bands will include your name and other basic information, and the date and time of birth. When the time comes to remove the bands, keep one as a memento; when your baby has grown, you will be amazed to see just how tiny he or she once was.

Will I have to adapt to the hospital routine?
Most hospitals have a set routine that may not allow for as much rest as you would like, unless you have a private room. Your day can begin as early as 6:30 am, and each day might seem like an endless round of feeding, changing, checks, and visits from doctors and other staff, as well as from family and friends. Try not to let the first few days with your baby be marred by these irritations. Some hospital staff will try to be flexible if certain routines really don't suit you – ask.

I need a good night's sleep but can't stay asleep for long. Why?
Apart from a crying baby, there are several possible reasons for this: first, you may be on an adrenalin "high" from the delivery and need to calm down; you are finding that the hospital is too strange or noisy at night to allow unbroken sleep; or you may unconsciously fear sleeping too deeply in case your baby needs you. Talk to your midwife or doctor if you feel that this lack of sleep is a problem. You should also try to take naps in the daytime while your baby is asleep. Remember, once you're home, these long nights' sleeps may be a while in returning, as night feedings take precedence.

This is my first baby – where do I begin?
First, don't compare yourself with more experienced mothers, or feel inadequate when you see the confidence with which other women handle their babies. The nurses and midwives will help you feed, bathe, and change your baby, and you will be able to ask them questions; you should find them supportive rather than critical. There's much to be said for the companionship that exists between mothers; you can share your worries, experiences, and observations, as well as form lasting friendships.

How long do I have to stay in the hospital?
Doctors used to think that long stays were essential, but it is now recognized that a woman with an uncomplicated delivery does not need to stay in the hospital for long. Talk to your doctor or midwife about your options – which may well be determined in part by your insurance. Several states now require 48-hour insurance coverage to avoid the "drive-thru" deliveries that were becoming commonplace. If you're anxious to get home, and feel that you and your baby are well, you may wish to go home earlier. If not, you should be able to stay for at least 48 hours after the birth. When it is agreed that you can go, your baby will be examined again (your baby should have been examined shortly after birth by your pediatrician). This is a routine part of the discharge procedure and does not mean that anything is wrong. Ask the pediatrician when you should bring the baby in for a first office visit; the doctor may want to check your baby fairly soon after discharge for signs of jaundice.

Why am I so anxious about going home with my new baby?
Taking a newborn baby home for the first time can be a stressful experience. Before leaving the hospital, make sure that you are comfortable about dealing with basic baby care; if there's anything you're not sure about, ask a nurse or your midwife. You'll need suitable outdoor clothing for you and your baby to travel home in, as well as a car seat if you are going home by car. At home, there should be a supply of diapers and other basic items (see p. 196). It is a good idea to have someone – either your partner, your mother, an aunt, or a friend – available to help you for at least the first few days.

THE FIRST SIX WEEKS

YOUR NEWBORN BABY

The labor is over and you are holding the baby you have dreamed about for so long. But your baby's appearance may be a shock. Instead of the beautiful baby you imagined, your baby emerges with visible signs of the birth, from bloody hair and minor bruising to blotchy, wrinkled skin; it takes a little time for your baby to "smooth out" and become a perfect baby. Your baby will be checked for any problems (see opposite).

WHAT MIGHT MY BABY LOOK LIKE?

Besides being covered with blood and vernix, your baby may be bruised and marked from the birth, especially if a fetal scalp monitor was attached or forceps were used. The skin can be an alarming, dull bluish gray in the first minutes after the birth, but soon becomes pinker. Add to this a red, wrinkled face and a strangely shaped head from the pressure of birth, and you have a realistic picture of a newborn. The body's systems are not effective yet, so you will notice blotches, and color changes that may worry you, but are perfectly normal. Most blemishes will disappear by the time your baby is two weeks old.

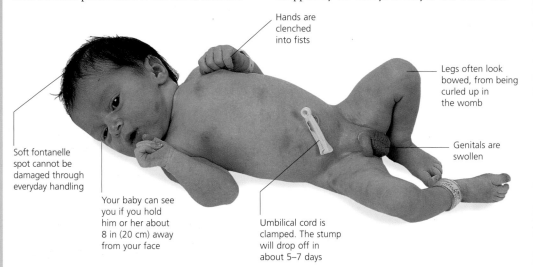

Hands are clenched into fists

Legs often look bowed, from being curled up in the womb

Genitals are swollen

Soft fontanelle spot cannot be damaged through everyday handling

Your baby can see you if you hold him or her about 8 in (20 cm) away from your face

Umbilical cord is clamped. The stump will drop off in about 5–7 days

The head
Pressure exerted during the birth can distort the shape of the head for the first two weeks. The bones of the soft spot (fontanelle) on the top of the head have not yet knitted together; this will not happen until about 18 months.

The hands and feet
If your baby's circulation is slow to start, the hands and feet may appear bluish, but should turn pink if you move your baby into another position. Fingernails can be long at birth.

The eyes
Often blue at birth; true eye color may not develop until your baby is six months old. Puffy eyelids are caused by the pressure of birth, and squinting is common. Your baby may even look cross-eyed at times in the first months.

The skin
The thick white grease (vernix) that protected the skin in the womb is absorbed or rubbed off. Pimples, rashes, and dry skin should clear naturally. Body hair (lanugo) rubs off in two weeks.

The breasts
Your baby boy or girl may have swollen breasts and even leak a little milk. This is normal in both sexes. The swelling should go down within two days. Do not try to squeeze the milk out.

The genitals
Swollen genitals are common in both sexes. A baby girl may have a clear or pinkish vaginal discharge but this should soon disappear. The testicles of a baby boy are often pulled up into his groin and will descend later.

What is the doctor looking for?

A pediatrician will examine your baby from head to toe at least once after birth. Besides checking for any physical abnormalities, the doctor looks for signs of infection or other problems.

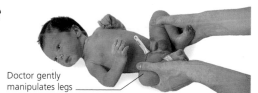

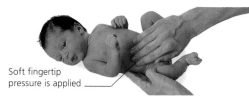

Doctor gently manipulates legs _____

Hips
The hips are checked for signs of dislocation by bending the legs up and gently swiveling them.

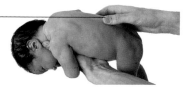

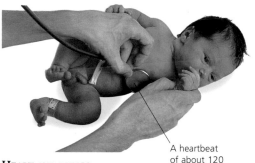

A heartbeat of about 120 beats a minute is normal

Heart and lungs
A stethoscope is used to listen to the heart and lungs.

Soft fingertip pressure is applied _____

Abdominal organs
The abdomen will be gently palpated so that the size of the abdominal organs can be checked.

Blood test
A few days after the birth, a blood sample is taken by pricking your baby's heel. The sample is tested for phenylketonuria (PKU, a rare cause of mental handicap) and for thyroid deficiency.

Any spinal problems can be detected at this stage _____

Spine
The doctor runs his or her thumb along the length of the back to check that the vertebrae are in the correct place.

What can my baby do?

Although newborn babies are entirely dependent on an adult for food and warmth, they are not completely helpless: they can breathe for themselves, cry to get your attention, grasp with their fingers and toes, see your face at close range, and hear and possibly distinguish your and your partner's voice from other voices. They can also eat reflexively and startle in response to stimuli.

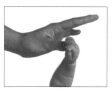

Grasp reflex
A newborn's grasp can be tight enough to support his or her whole weight – although you should never try this.

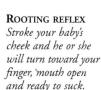

Rooting reflex
Stroke your baby's cheek and he or she will turn toward your finger, mouth open and ready to suck.

Hands reach out as if to hold something _____

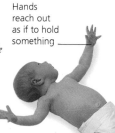

Startle reflex
If you let your baby's head flop back, the baby will think he's falling and stretch out his arms and legs.

Stepping reflex
Your baby will perform a walking action when supported under the shoulders in an upright position, feet touching a firm surface.

Reflex stepping movements

THE FIRST SIX WEEKS

YOUR RECOVERY

Q WHY DOES BREASTFEEDING GIVE ME STOMACH PAINS?

A You are probably experiencing afterpains, firm contractions of your womb that feel like menstrual cramps. Afterpains are more pronounced during breastfeeding because nipple stimulation provokes the release of oxytocin, the hormone that causes contractions. These contractions mean that your womb is shrinking and returning to its normal position in your pelvis. For severe spasmodic cramps, you may need to take pain relievers before starting to breastfeed.

Q I HAVEN'T HAD A BOWEL MOVEMENT SINCE THE BIRTH. IS THIS A PROBLEM?

A Many women find that they cannot move their bowels for three to four days after delivery. This is normal: you probably passed some feces while in labor, and haven't had much to eat since the birth. If you're concerned about being constipated, increase the fiber content in your diet.

Q WILL A BOWEL MOVEMENT TEAR MY STITCHES?

A If you are scared to use the toilet because you're worried about tearing your stitches, try to relax – your stitches are tough enough to cope with this. Ask your doctor or midwife to prescribe a soothing cream or some pain relievers to help with any discomfort. You could also try making a pad of toilet tissue and supporting your vaginal area with this during your bowel movement – it will give you reassurance that your stitches are not about to burst.

Q I'M PASSING A LOT OF BLOOD SINCE THE BIRTH. IS THIS NORMAL?

A The bleeding that you see after the delivery is lochia that is discharged via your vagina as your womb contracts. For the first few days or weeks, the lochia is heavily bloodstained, and thereafter, over the following few weeks, it becomes pinkish and finally colorless. Occasionally, you may pass blood clots in the first day or so; bring this to the attention of your midwife as it sometimes means that a small piece of placenta or membrane is left behind in your womb. Usually, however, the bleeding clears up on its own.

POSTPARTUM CHECKS

Shortly after the baby is born, you will have a postpartum checkup. Your doctor or midwife will ask you questions and examine you to confirm that you are recovering from the birth, that you show no signs of infection (for example, in your womb or breasts), and that you are well emotionally. Such checks will be daily while you're in the hospital, and your progress recorded. If you had an assisted delivery, or a cesarean delivery, or a medical problem, such as high blood pressure, a physician will check your recovery during routine rounds.

What do the checks entail?
■ You will be asked questions about your breasts, your bleeding (lochia, see below, left), how you feel, if you are urinating and defecating easily, how your stitches feel, your contraceptive plans, and any concerns you have.
■ Your breasts, nipples, and womb will be examined, any stitches looked at, your legs checked for swelling, and your temperature, pulse, and blood pressure taken.
■ Your hemoglobin level and, if necessary, your immunity to rubella will be checked.

Problems to watch out for
■ You have a temperature soon after delivery.
■ You experience pain on urination, or if your bleeding smells odd.
■ You have a persistent gush of heavy bleeding.
■ You feel faint and fall, or lose consciousness for a few seconds.
■ You can't pass urine despite feeling really uncomfortable, as if your bladder is too full.
■ You feel breathless or develop chest pain.
■ Your calf or leg becomes tender and swollen.
■ You are concerned about your baby.
■ Your breasts are particularly painful, warm to the touch, and engorged (possible mastitis).

WHY IS MY ABDOMEN STILL LARGE AND MY HANDS AND FEET STILL SWOLLEN?

Your baby was only part of your overall weight gain in pregnancy; you also gained extra fat and probably have significant fluid retention – which is why your fingers, toes, and possibly legs are still swollen. This swelling (called "edema") can last for several days, but it will go down gradually as you pass more urine. To speed up this process, try to rest with your feet up whenever possible, and avoid standing for long periods.

IS IT NORMAL TO HAVE A HEADACHE AFTER AN EPIDURAL?

You may get a mild headache after you've had your baby, but there is no concrete evidence as to whether this is due to the epidural or the delivery itself. Very rarely (this occurs in less than one percent of epidurals), you may get a severe headache because the epidural needle has made a hole in the thin membrane of the spinal cord and caused a leakage of cerebrospinal fluid (CSF). This is not dangerous, but it is uncomfortable.

WILL I NEED TREATMENT FOR A SEVERE EPIDURAL HEADACHE?

You will be advised to lie flat, drink fluids, and take a recommended dose of pain relievers, such as acetaminophen, for at least two days, while the puncture heals itself. If the symptoms are severe, an anesthesiologist may perform a simple procedure called a "blood patch." Using a needle, he or she will squirt a few drops of your blood into your spine where the hole is; this forms a clot and plugs the hole. Recovery is normally rapid after this.

DOES THE CATHETER REMAIN IN AFTER AN EPIDURAL?

If you have had a catheter inserted into your bladder during the epidural (see p. 152), it may stay in for a few hours after the epidural is removed. This allows time for the nerve supply to your bladder to return to full working order; while these nerves are still numb, you can't tell whether or not your bladder is full, so the bladder may get distended and damaged. Once the epidural wears off, you should urinate within a few hours.

AFTER A CESAREAN BIRTH

When can I go home after a cesarean?
The normal length of stay in hospital after a cesarean is five to seven days, but you may be able to go home earlier. Ask your midwife or doctor about this. After six to seven days, your stitches will be removed by your doctor or midwife. While the removal of stitches is not painful, it may be uncomfortable.

What kind of discomfort might I experience?
Your first few attempts at getting out of bed and walking will be painful, and you may feel dizzy, but don't give up – the more you try, the sooner you will be able to move around without any assistance. Although you will not be able to lift your baby right away, you can cuddle and breastfeed by placing a pillow on your lap to support your baby (see p. 202). It may take a few days before you have a bowel movement, and you may suffer with trapped gas, which can cause considerable discomfort as it presses against your incision. The best solution is to let out as much gas as possible to reduce this discomfort. Coughing can also hurt quite a bit.

Why are there lumps on my scar?
The skin around your incision can feel lumpy for days, or maybe even weeks, after a cesarean operation. These lumps will eventually become bruises and the skin will return to normal. The lumps are caused by slight bleeding under the skin after the operation.

Why is the skin around my wound numb?
Small nerves just beneath your skin were cut during the operation, and this causes numbness just around the scar. These nerves will grow back over the next couple of months, and normal sensation will return.

How can I look after my incision at home?
Just keep it dry and ventilated; it may leak a little in the first few days, but this is nothing to be concerned about. You can bathe once the dressing has been removed by your doctor, but dry the incision with a separate clean towel. If the scar becomes tender or red, show it to your midwife or doctor; you may have developed a mild infection that needs antibiotics.

AT HOME WITH YOUR BABY

Q HOW AM I GOING TO COPE WITH MY FIRST FEW DAYS AT HOME?

A It's only natural to feel anxious about your new responsibilities when you arrive home with your new baby. You're obviously not going to be able to run the home quite the way you've been accustomed for a few weeks or months – your main priority is to look after yourself and your baby. Don't struggle with the day-to-day domestic chores at the expense of your own well-being. Get help. If your partner is entitled to some paternity leave he may be able to help you for a week or two, or perhaps your mother or a friend can stay for a while. If a generous friend asks what you need, be honest and ask for help!

Q MY BABY WAS WEIGHED TODAY AND HAS LOST WEIGHT – IS THIS NORMAL?

A This is entirely normal. If you think of the tiny amounts your baby has eaten, and of the contents of all those diapers, it is not surprising that your baby has lost weight. Newborn babies are expected to lose up to ten percent of their birth weight in the first few days after delivery. Your baby should regain this lost weight and will probably be back to birth weight by about ten days after the birth.

Q MY BABY VOMITED BITS OF DRIED BLOOD AFTER FEEDING – IS THIS SERIOUS?

A What you are seeing is mucus mixed with blood from the delivery which your baby has swallowed and cannot digest. The best thing for your baby to do is to bring it up. Try to feed your baby again and tell your midwife or doctor about the incident. Sometimes a "stomach washout," which involves her running warmed sterile water through a tube into the baby's stomach to bring out any residue of mucus or blood that may be lying there is recommended.

Q WHEN I CHANGED MY BABY'S DIAPER, IT WAS STAINED PINK – IS THIS BLOOD?

A Pink stains are simply urates (acids in the urine), which a newborn baby passes at first and this is quite normal. However, blood in the urine is very uncommon and should always be reported to your doctor.

POSTPARTUM VISITS AND CHECKS

What the midwife or doctor does
The midwife's role after the birth is to establish that you are recovering physically and emotionally from the birth and that your baby is thriving. An obstetrician will mainly be concerned with your health, a pediatrician with the health of your baby. For breastfeeding questions, you may wish to seek help from a lactation consultant.

Your baby's health checks
The postpartum checks establish that your baby is well or pick up any problems. The pediatrician asks about your baby's feeding, sleeping, and toilet habits and will weigh your baby at regular intervals (see below); the umbilical cord will be checked, and any delivery marks.

Looking after your baby
Ask the midwife or doctor questions about your baby, or about any aspects of baby care, from sterilizing your feeding equipment to what type of diapers to use and how often to feed your baby.

How often should my baby be weighed?
This can vary, but the usual practice is for your baby to be weighed about twice a month for the first few weeks of his or her life. Because babies lose and regain ten percent of their birth weight during the first ten days of life, your caregiver may not be concerned with the baby's weight gain as long as he or she is feeding well, until after ten days.

Why was my baby given vitamin K?
This is because newborn babies are low in vitamin K and this helps blood clot and protects against hemorrhage (especially into the brain). Vitamin K can be given by mouth or injection but if you had a forceps, vacuum extraction, or cesarean delivery, or gave birth prematurely, your baby should be given the injection.

Q MY BABY'S BOWEL MOVEMENTS ARE GREENISH BLACK. IS ANYTHING WRONG?

A Your baby is completely normal! The first few bowel movements are made of meconium, the sticky, dark substance that lined your baby's bowel during the pregnancy and is now being excreted. This may take up to 48 hours to pass through, after which your baby's stool will be more solid, and yellow in color, especially if you are breastfeeding.

Q HOW OFTEN SHOULD MY BABY PASS URINE AND EMPTY HIS OR HER BOWELS?

A How much a newborn baby urinates varies, but as long as there are six wet diapers every 24 hours, all is well. Usually, however, because their bladders are so tiny, newborns urinate every hour. Bowel movements also vary greatly but again should occur at least once a day. It may be that your baby had a big bowel movement just before,

during, or after birth and so may not need to have another bowel movement for some time. The first bowel movement is significant because it confirms that the anus is open. The same goes for urinating: it shows that the baby's kidneys, bladder, and all the other plumbing is working properly.

Q WHEN WILL MY BABY SETTLE INTO A ROUTINE?

A You will end up feeling very frustrated if you try to make your baby conform to a set pattern at this stage. Just go with the flow in these early weeks, taking each very different day as it comes. Old-fashioned ideas of imposing discipline and a routine on very young babies serve no real purpose and usually fail. Babies have different sleep patterns (see p. 200); some sleep for long periods of time, others sleep fitfully, but after a few weeks or months a sleeping and waking pattern will gradually emerge.

HANDLING YOUR NEWBORN

You may be afraid to handle your newborn baby at first because he or she seems so small. The important thing is to support the baby's head, because the neck muscles are still quite weak. Because it is reassuring and helps you to develop a relationship with your baby, talk to your baby when changing a diaper or giving a bath. You will soon gain enough confidence to relax and enjoy handling your baby.

PICKING UP YOUR BABY

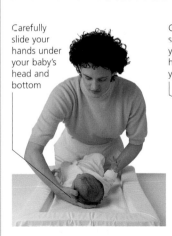

Carefully slide your hands under your baby's head and bottom

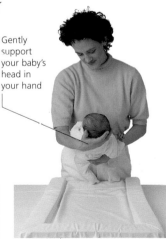

Gently support your baby's head in your hand

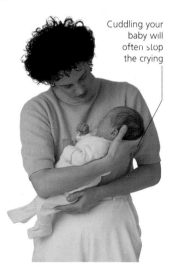

Cuddling your baby will often stop the crying

1 Lift your baby by placing one hand under the head and one under the bottom.

2 Lift slowly and gently while supporting your baby's body and head with each hand.

3 Turn your baby so that the head and the back are cradled by your arms.

BABY CARE

Q HOW CAN I MAKE SURE THAT MY BABY IS COMFORTABLE AND CONTENT?

A Your baby has simple but time-consuming needs during the first few weeks of life. Making sure that your baby is warm, comfortable, and satisfied will keep him or her content. You'll be feeding and holding your baby constantly, and spending a lot of time changing diapers after feedings, when your baby wakes, and before your baby sleeps. These basic tasks can be enjoyable for both of you if you play games, talk to, and cuddle your baby as you do them.

Q I DON'T LIKE TOUCHING MY BABY'S CORD. DO I HAVE TO CLEAN IT?

A Your baby's cord will dry up, wither, and drop off naturally about five to seven days after the birth. However, keep the cord as dry as possible, even if you do not actively clean it: make sure that the diaper isn't covering the cord and dry the cord thoroughly after bathing your baby. Some pediatricians recommend applying alcohol or antiseptic powder, or will give you sterile swabs to clean the stump. If the cord or navel area gets swollen, red, smelly, or weepy, tell your pediatrician.

ESSENTIALS FOR YOUR NEWBORN BABY

Preparing for the arrival of your baby can be one of the most enjoyable parts of your pregnancy, as you shop for clothes and equipment. Remember, when buying baby clothes, that your baby will grow quickly, so buy only a few of the smaller sized items to begin with. Below are some suggestions for the basic items you will need.

PRACTICAL ITEMS

- Several packs of disposable diapers (or 2 dozen cloth diapers with plastic pants and liners, diaper pail, and some safety pins)
- Baby wipes
- Barrier cream (e.g., vitamins A & D cream or petroleum jelly)
- Plastic changing pad
- Cotton balls
- Baby soap/shampoo/liquid soap/baby lotion/oil (for dry skin)
- Waterproof apron
- Baby tub
- Sponge/washcloth
- Large, soft towel
- Baby brush

Shaped fabric diaper

Cotton balls

Cream

Disposable diaper

SLEEPING

- Crib, cradle, or bassinet
- Crib and mattress (when your baby is older)
- 4 cotton sheets
- 2 soft, lightweight blankets
- Baby monitor (optional)

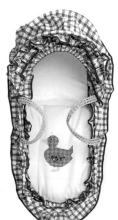
Bassinet

CLOTHES

Choose machine-washable clothes in natural fabrics
- 4 sleepers/rompers
- 3 undershirts/bodysuits
- Light cotton nighties (if too hot to sleep in bodysuit; makes it easier to change diapers)
- 4 pairs of socks and booties
- Shawl (optional)
- Scratch mittens, bibs
- In winter: cardigan, warm hat
In summer: light summer hat

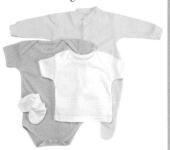
Sleepers, shirts, and mittens

Q WHAT TYPES OF DIAPERS ARE AVAILABLE AND WHICH SHOULD I CHOOSE?

A There are two types of diaper: cloth, which you can wash and is reusable; or disposable. Disposable diapers are more costly over a period of time, but are also more convenient to use. There is a wide range of disposable diapers available for boys or girls and from newborn to toddler sizes. Occasionally, babies are sensitive to disposables and develop a mild rash, so you may need to change your brand. Although cloth diapers involve more work, they do work out less expensive in the long run. And you can choose between using a diaper service or washing the diapers yourself. If you wash them, you will need to buy two dozen diapers and a diaper pail for soaking cloth diapers until laundry day.

Q DO I NEED TO USE DIAPER CREAM EACH TIME I CHANGE THE BABY?

A After the birth, using a gentle cream, like petroleum jelly, can make it easier to clean off meconium (see p. 62) from your baby's bottom. After a few days you may need to use a small amount of cream if your baby develops a rash or soreness. Avoid zinc oxide cream unless your baby has a rash.

Q SHOULD I HAVE MY BABY BOY CIRCUMCISED?

A This is an emotional issue. Circumcising boys is done primarily for religious and cultural reasons. Circumcision is also done to reduce the risk of infection. However, it has also been suggested that, during the early years, the foreskin can protect the tip of the penis.

CHANGING YOUR BABY'S DIAPER

Keeping everything you need in one place will make the task much easier. When putting on a fresh disposable diaper, avoid touching the front of the diaper if you have cream or oil on your fingers; the ointment can keep the tapes from sticking.

Cleaning a boy
Wipe gently; don't drag on the skin of the penis or pull the foreskin back.

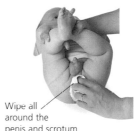

Wipe all around the penis and scrotum

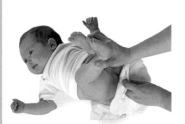

1 Open the soiled diaper and remove feces with a cotton ball or baby wipe, then discard.

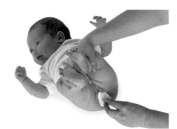

2 Clean the bottom: wipe in the skin creases using a wipe or wet cotton balls. Dry carefully.

Cleaning a girl
To prevent the spread of bacteria from the anus to the vagina, always wipe from the front to the back.

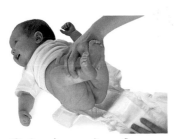

3 Lay the new diaper flat under your baby, and line the top up with your baby's waist.

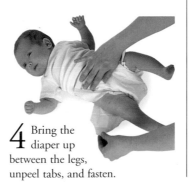

4 Bring the diaper up between the legs, unpeel tabs, and fasten.

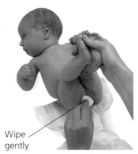

Wipe gently

BATHING AND DRESSING YOUR BABY

With a little care and planning, washing your baby can be a playful experience, and dressing your baby in snug-fitting clothes can be a simple procedure. Gather everything you need before you start because you should never leave your baby unattended (see p. 196). If you have to move away to retrieve something you forgot or to answer the telephone, take the baby with you. As you clean and change your baby, always remember to keep talking to and cuddling him or her.

GIVING YOUR BABY A SPONGE BATH

Your baby's face, hands, and bottom are prone to irritation from sweat, urine, and feces, and must be cleaned daily. A sponge bath allows you to clean these areas without giving your baby a full bath. To reduce the risk of infection, start with the face and work your way down.

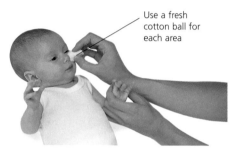

Use a fresh cotton ball for each area

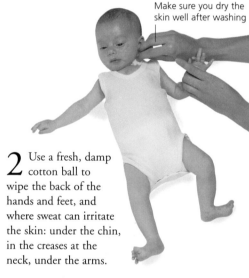

Make sure you dry the skin well after washing

1 Set out a bowl of warm water. Wipe each eye from the corner out, using a new cotton ball for each. Wipe over and behind, but not inside, the ears, and then clean the face and around the nose.

2 Use a fresh, damp cotton ball to wipe the back of the hands and feet, and where sweat can irritate the skin: under the chin, in the creases at the neck, under the arms.

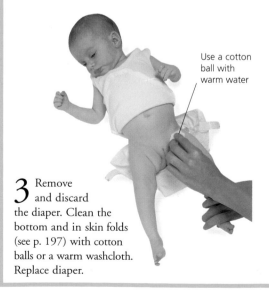

Use a cotton ball with warm water

3 Remove and discard the diaper. Clean the bottom and in skin folds (see p. 197) with cotton balls or a warm washcloth. Replace diaper.

Cleaning the cord
Using a cotton ball, clean in the creases around the stump. Dry with a fresh, dry cotton ball.

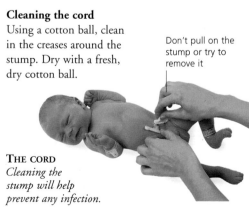

Don't pull on the stump or try to remove it

THE CORD
Cleaning the stump will help prevent any infection.

BATHING YOUR BABY

Put cold water in the tub, then hot. Test the temperature with an elbow: it should be warm, not hot. Keeping the undershirt on, clean the face and neck. Remove the undershirt to wash the hair, then remove the diaper and bathe your baby.

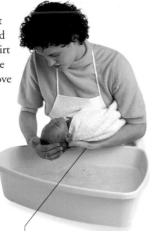

1 With your baby wrapped in a towel, lower the head over the tub and gently pour water over your baby's hair. Gently rub shampoo into the hair and rinse away with water, avoiding the face.

Support your baby's body with your arm, and the head and neck with your hand

2 A baby can lose a lot of heat through his or her head, so dry your baby's head immediately by gently patting it with a towel.

Comfort your baby by talking or singing to him or her

3 Remove the towel and the diaper, and gently lower your baby into the bath. Support the head above the water with one hand and splash water over your baby. Softly soap the body (or use liquid bath soap) and then rinse away.

Keep the head above the water

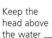

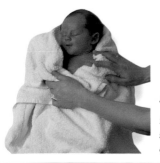

4 Wrap your baby in a soft, dry towel. Pat your baby dry, making sure there is no water in the skin creases. If you wish, apply cream or baby cornstarch, and dress.

DRESSING YOUR BABY

You can ease your baby gently into close-fitting clothes, such as undershirts and bodysuits, by stretching and rolling the neck and arm openings. Babies often cry while being dressed, but this is usually because they don't like to feel air on their skin. Never lay your baby on the edge of a surface because he or she could roll off.

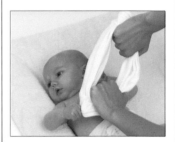

1 Roll the undershirt up and pull the neck wide so that it can slip over your baby's head.

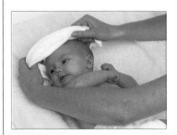

2 Bring it over the baby's head, making sure that it doesn't drag over your baby's face.

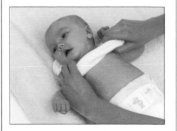

3 Stretch the armholes and guide the arms through; roll the shirt down over the body.

SOOTHING YOUR BABY

Q **HOW CAN I HELP MY BABY ESTABLISH A ROUTINE?**

A As your confidence in your ability to take care of your new baby grows, the way you approach some tasks can help your baby recognize a pattern. For example, if your baby needs feeding in the night, try to do it swiftly, and don't "play" with your baby. He or she will then begin to associate play and stimulation only with the day and will sleep more easily if he or she does not expect this kind of attention at night.

Q **SHOULD I ATTEND TO MY BABY EVERY TIME HE OR SHE CRIES?**

A Yes, you should always attend to your crying baby. At this very early stage your baby will cry for specific reasons; crying is your baby's only means of communicating his or her discomfort or distress to you. Your baby has not yet learned that by crying he or she can always get your attention.

Q **WHAT IS THE MOST LIKELY REASON FOR MY BABY'S CRYING?**

A Apart from hunger or a diaper change, your baby may be uncomfortable because he or she is suffering from colic (see p. 213). Once older, your baby may cry for less concrete reasons, like to win your attention or get a quick cuddle.

Q **MY BABY ISN'T HUNGRY OR WET, SO WHY IS HE OR SHE STILL CRYING?**

A Your baby could be too hot or too cold. Feel the chest or the base of the neck; if the skin feels either flushed and hot, or chilled, add or remove layers of clothing as needed. If your baby has been fed recently, he or she may have gas; place your baby against your shoulder and gently pat on the back (see p. 208). If none of these measures help, try rocking with or singing to your baby to offer comfort. If nothing seems to work, your baby may be unwell; contact your pediatrician.

HELPING BABY SLEEP SAFE AND WELL

When you put your baby to bed, you obviously want him or her to be safe and comfortable. To allay your own fears, there are some general precautions that you can take to help your baby to sleep safe and well. These precautions are also recommended in order to reduce the possibility of crib death.

- Put your baby on his or her back or side to sleep, not on the front. When your baby is big enough to be in a crib (around three months), make sure you lay him or her in it correctly (see below).
- Make sure your baby's room is warm, ideally about 70°F (20°C), and well ventilated.
- Be sure that your baby does not overheat, keep the bedclothes light, and remove layers as needed.
- Never allow anyone to smoke near your baby.
- If you feel happier, let your baby sleep in your room for the first six months.
- Make sure that your baby's mattress is firm and also that it is clean and well aired, so that your baby is not breathing dust.
- Breastfeed if you can; it has been suggested that this reduces the risk of crib death.

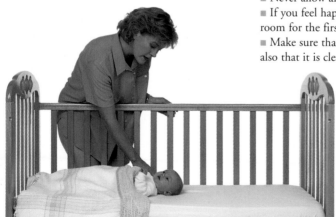

LAYING YOUR BABY DOWN
Be sure that your baby's feet touch the end of the crib so that he or she can't wriggle under the covers. Use light blankets and sheets so that you can add or remove layers.

PUTTING YOUR BABY TO SLEEP

Your new baby is unlikely to get into a sleep routine right away, but instead will sleep whenever he or she feels the need to, especially after a satisfying feeding. Most young babies tend to sleep for three or four hours, then wake for a change or a feeding. Try to establish a bedtime routine early on, so that your baby associates certain events with the day's end.

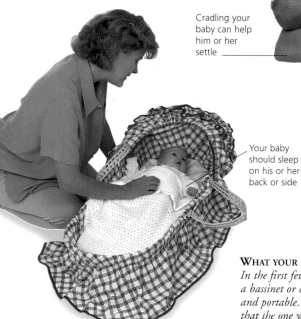

Cradling your baby can help him or her settle

Your baby should sleep on his or her back or side

RELAXING YOUR BABY
To help your baby fall asleep, try gently rocking in your arms, which will have a soothing effect. You can also try singing or gently rubbing your baby's back.

WHAT YOUR BABY SLEEPS IN
In the first few weeks of life, your baby is so small that a bassinet or cradle is perfectly adequate; it is also cozy and portable. Later on you will need a crib; make sure that the one you buy conforms to current safety standards.

YOUR BABY'S SLEEP PATTERN

The chart below shows how, in the first weeks, your baby's sleep pattern may be erratic. Babies sleep an average of 18 hours out of 24 – and not necessarily at night. In the next few months, your baby should establish a more regular sleep pattern, sleeping more at night and less during the day.

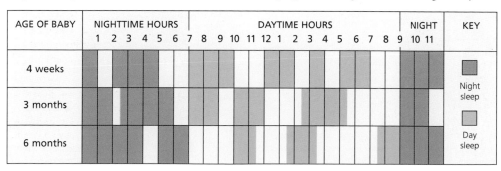

AGE OF BABY	NIGHTTIME HOURS 1 2 3 4 5 6	DAYTIME HOURS 7 8 9 10 11 12 1 2 3 4 5 6 7 8 9	NIGHT 10 11	KEY
4 weeks				Night sleep
3 months				
6 months				Day sleep

BREASTFEEDING YOUR BABY

Q I DON'T KNOW IF I CAN DO IT – HOW WILL I LEARN HOW TO BREASTFEED?

A As the subject is usually covered in prenatal classes, you'll have some idea of what to expect, and the midwives or nurses in the hospital will show you what to do. For many mothers, breastfeeding is uncomplicated, but for others it can prove difficult. It can take several weeks before you feel confident with the process but once you do, it should become second nature. There are support groups with lactation consultants to help mothers who are finding it hard to breastfeed (see p. 232).

Q CAN I NURSE MY BABY RIGHT AFTER GIVING BIRTH?

A As long as your baby is able to suck, yes, you can and should breastfeed immediately after delivery to trigger milk production. The sucking action on your nipple stimulates the hormone oxytocin, which causes the muscle fibers in the milk glands to contract, squeezing milk into the ducts. This is known as the "let-down reflex." Most babies do not need to feed much in the first 48 hours because the first milk, colostrum (see opposite), is very rich.

GETTING STARTED

When you start to feed your baby, make sure you are comfortable and can sit without having to get up for at least 30–45 minutes. Your baby will feed best when cradled in your arms, his or her body held close to yours; the head should be level with your nipple. Brush your nipple along your baby's lips to trigger the "rooting reflex," which makes your baby open his or her mouth wide to accept your nipple.

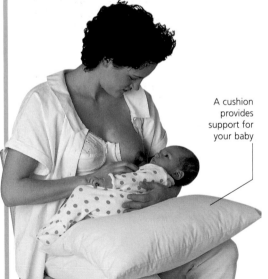

A cushion provides support for your baby

SIT COMFORTABLY
Get into the habit of settling yourself comfortably before a feeding, perhaps with a drink by your side; try not to hunch over your baby.

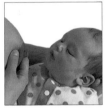

OFFERING YOUR NIPPLE
Cup your breast and offer – rather than push – your nipple to the side of your baby's mouth or brush it across his or her lips. Your baby should open his or her mouth wide to take it.

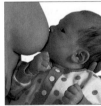

LATCHING ON
To prevent your baby from chewing on the sensitive tip of the nipple, encourage him or her to take the whole nipple and areola into the mouth. Your baby should suck hard and rhythmically.

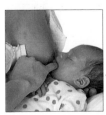

REMOVING YOUR NIPPLE
When finished with one breast, place your little finger in your baby's mouth and push gently down on the lower jaw. This will break the suction and avoid painful pulling on your nipple.

Q WHAT IS COLOSTRUM AND WHY IS IT SO IMPORTANT?

A Colostrum is the thick yellow "premilk" that your breasts produce for the first few days after delivery. This premilk contains water, protein, and minerals in the correct proportion to take care of a newborn's nutritional needs at this early stage. It is also high in antibodies and rich in lactoferrin, a substance that is, in effect, a natural antibiotic.

Q WHEN WILL I START PRODUCING REAL BREAST MILK?

A By the third day after delivery, your breasts will produce real white breast milk, high in protein, fat, and carbohydrate, all vital for your baby's growth, as well as maternal antibodies that protect against disease and infection. When the milk first comes in, your breasts may expand, which causes discomfort. This is normal, and usually only lasts for 24 hours. Your body then adapts to your baby's needs, producing just enough milk for your baby.

Q SHOULD I GIVE MY BABY BOTH BREASTS AT EVERY FEEDING?

A Breast milk is different at the beginning and end of feeds; the watery "foremilk" is thirst-quenching and the "hindmilk" has far more fat and is nourishing. So, when you alternate, make sure that your baby gets both kinds of milk from one breast rather than just the foremilk from both; emptying a breast usually takes five to ten minutes.

Q FOR HOW LONG AND HOW OFTEN SHOULD MY BABY FEED?

A There's no official time limit; it can be as little as five minutes or as much as 15–20 minutes. It depends how hard your baby sucks and how quickly he or she swallows the milk, which depends on how alert your baby is (which varies at different times of the day), and how comfortable. Time is not a good yardstick. You will learn to tell when your baby is content because the sucking will dwindle or the baby may release the nipple. Also, your breasts will feel less full. How often you feed your baby depends on your milk and your baby's appetite.

Q WHY IS IT IMPORTANT TO BE COMFORTABLE AND RELAXED?

A Feeling tense can stop the let-down reflex. You are also likely to be in one position for a while, so find a comfortable one: lie on your side facing your baby; sit up with your baby resting in the crook of your arm; or rest back on cushions.

CAN I BREASTFEED AFTER HAVING A CESAREAN?

Yes, you can breastfeed your newborn baby after having a cesarean delivery. Indeed, if you are both fine, you will be encouraged to breastfeed as soon as you can. But you will have to wait for a while if you are feeling groggy after a general anesthetic, or if your baby needs special care.

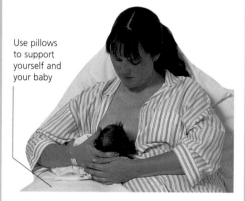

Use pillows to support yourself and your baby

FEEDING WITHOUT PAIN
It is often uncomfortable to breastfeed after a cesarean delivery, because of the pressure on the incision, and sore stomach muscles. To alleviate this, place a pillow on your lap under your baby for support.

Q DO I HAVE TO EAT AND DRINK MORE THAN USUAL IF I'M BREASTFEEDING?

A Yes, you do. The quality of your breast milk depends on your diet; you will also probably be feeling thirstier and hungrier. Make sure that there are enough nutrients both for making milk and for your own needs. Eat a varied and well-balanced diet of about 2,500 calories a day and make sure that you include plenty of fluids and protein (see p. 100).

Q WILL BREASTFEEDING CAUSE MY BREASTS TO SAG AND WILL IT RUIN MY FIGURE?

A If you always wear a good support bra while pregnant and breastfeeding, your breasts should return to their normal shape when you stop breastfeeding. Your figure will return to its prepregnant size quicker if you breastfeed because it uses your body's fat stores laid down in pregnancy.

THE FIRST SIX WEEKS

BREASTFEEDING AND YOU

Q CAN I MAKE BREASTFEEDING EASIER OR LESS DEMANDING?

A Breastfeeding can present physical and practical problems. Expressing your milk and knowing how to deal with sore breasts can help.

Q WHY MIGHT I WANT TO EXPRESS MY MILK?

A Expressing breast milk into a bottle gives you flexibility, allowing you to store your milk and enabling your partner or other carer to help with feeds. For a baby in intensive care, expressed milk ensures that the mother's natural immunity is passed on via her breast milk. Expressed milk is useful when you and your baby cannot be together: if you go out for an evening, or later, if you return to work.

Q WHEN IS THE BEST TIME TO EXPRESS – BEFORE OR AFTER FEEDING MY BABY?

A It is best to express milk between feedings. If you express before feeding, there may not be enough to satisfy your baby, and if you express afterward there may not be much milk left. Or you could feed with one breast entirely and express the milk from the other one.

Q HOW DO I STORE EXPRESSED MILK?

A The safest storage is in the freezer, where frozen milk will keep for up to three months. Refrigerated, breast milk must be used within 24 hours or discarded. Try storing frozen milk in the sterilized plastic bags used with baby bottles.

HOW TO EXPRESS YOUR MILK

There are two ways to express your breast milk: either with your hands or by using a pump (see below). Expressing by hand is fairly easy and painless but very slow, whereas a pump is often quicker and less tiring. Hand expressing may help to relieve sore, engorged breasts, and may be less painful than expressing by pump.

By hand
Wash your hands, have a sterile bowl ready, support your breast in one hand and massage around the entire breast, including the underside, at least ten times. Stroking and gentle pressure toward the areola squeezes the milk out through the nipple.

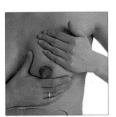

MASSAGE FIRST
In order to encourage the flow of milk though the milk ducts, massage around the entire breast at least ten times.

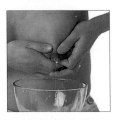

SQUEEZE LAST
Squeeze areola with the thumbs and forefingers together, while pressing back; the milk should begin to spurt out. Continue this action for several minutes.

By pump
Pumps are manual, battery operated, or electric. All pumps vary slightly but work on the same principle: a funnel forms a seal over your nipple, then you pump the milk out by suction. The milk collects in the bottle attached to the pump.

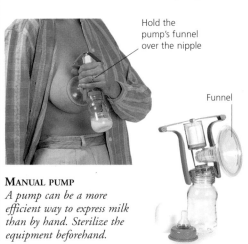

Hold the pump's funnel over the nipple

Funnel

MANUAL PUMP
A pump can be a more efficient way to express milk than by hand. Sterilize the equipment beforehand.

IF YOU HAVE PROBLEMS

If you have any difficulties with your breasts or breastfeeding, you should seek professional help as soon as possible. Never struggle on alone or give up – persevere, because it will be worth it. Ask your midwife or doctor for advice or talk to a support group (see p. 232).

CARING FOR YOUR BREASTS

Let the air get to your nipples often, and wash your breasts every day – but don't use soap, which can be drying. Gently pat yourself dry. Support your breasts with a good nursing bra, and wear it day and night in the early weeks. If milk leaks between feedings (this is common), buy some breast pads and wear them inside your bra for protection. Change the pads frequently.

LEAKING BREASTS
A disposable breast pad will absorb any drips and small leaks.

Front-opening
maternity bra

Engorgement
The production of milk is a finely tuned "supply and demand" process, but when your milk first comes in, it takes a while to achieve a balance. Your breasts may become hard, swollen, warm, and sore (known as engorgement) because they are producing too much milk; this can raise your temperature and make you feel feverish and weepy.

Can expressing milk relieve engorgement?
If your breasts are engorged, nursing is difficult for your baby and painful for you. Expressing large amounts of milk is not the answer because your body will keep producing milk to this capacity. However, expressing a small amount of milk can bring relief. You could also try applying alternate warm and cold compresses, or use the shower to play warm and then cold water on your breasts. A pain reliever such as acetaminophen may help.

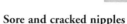

NIPPLE CREAM
A calendula-based cream may help to relieve the soreness.

Sore and cracked nipples
Tender nipples are normal for the first few days; it takes time to get used to the baby's strong sucking. If your baby isn't latching on properly (see p. 202), he or she may be chewing your nipples and damaging soft tissue, even making them bleed. If you are not in too much pain, it is safe to continue feeding. Your milk contains natural antiseptics, so after every feeding, rub some of your milk around the nipple and allow it to dry naturally. You may need to use a special nipple cream, such as a calendula cream; consult your midwife or doctor.

Breast inflammation
If one or both breasts become red, patchy, and very sore, you may have a condition called mastitis, when a milk duct is blocked, causing stagnation. The milk and surrounding tissue may become infected by bacteria that have entered the milk ducts through your nipple.

Can breast inflammation be relieved?
In its early stages, this condition may respond to antibiotics and pain-relieving drugs. It is important to continue breastfeeding in order to empty the breasts and relieve pressure. If you have a high temperature and feel nauseous and dizzy, and have a hot, firm lump in your breast, this is an abscess; you need to call your midwife or doctor immediately.

Pain-relieving drugs and breastfeeding
It is safe to take most drugs that are based on acetaminophen, because only a very small amount passes into the milk and reaches the baby. However, aspirin is best avoided because it has been linked to a rare condition (Reye's syndrome) that can affect babies.

THE FIRST SIX WEEKS

BEGINNING BOTTLE-FEEDING

Q I HAVE DECIDED NOT TO BREASTFEED. DO I NEED TO TELL MY CAREGIVER?

A If you are having a hospital birth, tell your caregiver, who will advise hospital staff. They will provide bottle-feeding equipment and formula and show you how to use it. Many hospitals send new parents home with a few days' supply of formula, but you should stock up on your own, especially if you give birth at home.

Q WHICH FORMULA SHOULD I BUY?

A Most of the wide variety of baby formulas now available are based on cows' milk and contain vitamins and minerals. If you don't want your baby to have animal products or your baby develops an allergy to cows' milk, there are soy milk formulas. Dry powder formulas are cheaper, but liquid formulas are more convenient.

Q IS IT SO IMPORTANT TO KEEP ALL THE EQUIPMENT CLEAN?

A Clean equipment is crucial because formula is an ideal breeding ground for the bacteria that cause gastroenteritis, a disease that can be life-threatening in a young baby. Keep everything that comes into contact with the formula clean.

Q HOW DO I MAKE SURE THAT THE EQUIPMENT IS STERILE?

A If your pediatrician advises you to sterilize the equipment, wash everything in warm, soapy water. Scrub bottle rims, clean to the bottom of the bottles, and turn the nipples inside out to wash them. If milk collects in the nipples, rub it away with salt, and rinse well. Sterilize the equipment either by placing it in a steamer, boiling it, immersing it in sterilizing fluid, or microwaving it. Keep equipment below water level, and remove air bubbles.

WHAT EQUIPMENT DO I NEED?

Essential equipment for bottle-feeding includes four to six bottles and nipples. You also need a measuring cup, a funnel, a plastic spoon, and a plastic knife for leveling off the formula. To sterilize equipment you need a bottle brush, salt, and/or a steam sterilizer.

Other equipment

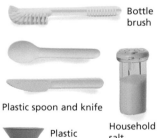

Bottle brush

Plastic spoon and knife

Household salt

Plastic funnel

Measuring cup

Feeding equipment

Cap

Ring top

Nipple

8 oz (250 ml) bottle

TYPES OF BOTTLE AND NIPPLES
Bottles are usually made of plastic. One system consists of disposable bags that fit inside a plastic tube. Nipples can be made of latex or silicone and come in several shapes: experiment to find the one that suits your baby best.

Wide-necked bottle with silicone nipple

4 oz (125 ml) bottle

With this system, only the nipple needs to be sterilized

Disposable plastic bottle liner

CARING FOR THE EQUIPMENT
Keep all equipment scrupulously clean. Rub the inside of nipples with salt, clean bottles with a bottle brush. Sterilize all equipment if your pediatrician advises.

HOW DO I MAKE UP A FEEDING?

When making up your baby's feeding, it is important to follow the directions on the can (or package) exactly. Don't add extra scoops, or dilute the formula further, or add cereals to your baby's bottle. To do so changes the specific concentration and could lead to obesity or even serious illness in your baby. Always use boiled, cooled tap water.

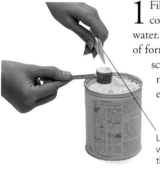

1 Fill a cup with the correct amount of water. Open the can of formula and use the scoop provided to measure out the exact amount.

Level each scoop with the back of the knife

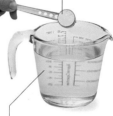

Level scoop

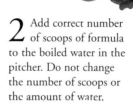

2 Add correct number of scoops of formula to the boiled water in the pitcher. Do not change the number of scoops or the amount of water.

Boiled tap (not mineral) water

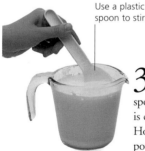

Use a plastic spoon to stir

3 Stir the formula well with a plastic spoon until the powder is completely dissolved. Hot water will help the powder dissolve faster.

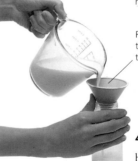

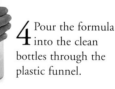

Pour the formula through a funnel to avoid spillage

4 Pour the formula into the clean bottles through the plastic funnel.

STORING BOTTLES

You can make up a batch of bottles that can be stored for 24 hours; this is particularly useful for night feedings. Make up several bottles of formula and pour into bottles. Put the nipples on upside down, but don't let them dip into the milk. If they do touch the milk, put the nipples the right way up. Cover with the tops to keep the bottles clean. Cool the bottles and refrigerate them immediately (but not in the door). Breast milk expressed into bottles can also be stored in this way.

Do not let the nipple touch the milk

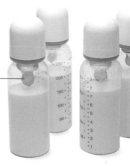

TIME LIMIT
Store formula in the refrigerator for no longer than 24 hours.

THE FIRST SIX WEEKS

BOTTLE-FEEDING YOUR BABY

Q HOW OFTEN SHOULD I FEED MY BABY?

A Bottle-fed babies should be fed, like breastfed babies, on demand, not at set times; this can vary from day to day, depending on how big your baby is, and how hungry. You will not spoil your baby by answering his or her hunger cries. A baby's feeding clock works on a 24-hour basis; most have an average of six to ten feedings during that time. Since your baby will expect to be fed as often during the night as during the day, you will probably get no more than two to three hours of sleep at a stretch.

Q HOW LONG SHOULD A FEEDING TAKE?

A Just as there are no set times for feeding your baby, there is no set time for how long a feeding should take. Always let your baby set the pace. Sometimes he or she will be feeling playful and will want to pause to look around or touch the bottle; when this happens, a feeding can take up to half an hour. When your baby lets go of the nipple, or finishes all the milk, take the bottle away. If he or she still wants to suck, offer your clean little finger.

GIVING YOUR BABY A BOTTLE

Before you feed your baby, check that the milk is at the correct temperature by shaking a little onto your wrist; it should feel just warm.

FEEDING YOUR BABY

It is always best to feed your baby while cradling him or her in your arms, with the head tilted slightly back. Make sure the nipple is always full of milk and that there are no air pockets. To give your baby the comforting feeling of skin-to-skin closeness, you could remove your blouse during the feeding.

HOLDING THE BOTTLE
Hold the feeding bottle firmly so that your baby can pull against it slightly to get a good sucking action.

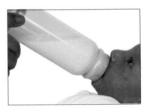

AVOIDING GAS
To stop your baby sucking in air, keep the milk level up.

BURPING

Bottle-fed babies need burping more often than breastfed babies because there is a tendency to gulp down air or milk if the rate of flow is not quite right.

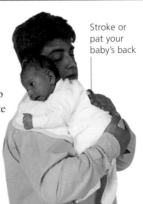

Stroke or pat your baby's back

OVER THE SHOULDER
Burp your baby over your shoulder. Some milk may come up ("cheesing"), so protect your clothes.

SITTING UP
Sit your baby upright and support the head under the chin, gently rubbing or patting on the back. If a burp does not come up after a minute, then give up. It is not necessary to burp after every feeding.

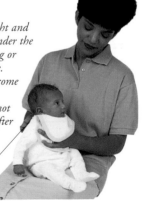

Always be gentle, or the entire feed can come back up

Q CAN MY BABY AND I STILL ENJOY A SENSE OF CLOSENESS IF I BOTTLE-FEED?

A Yes, you can enjoy the same intimacy as a breastfeeding mother enjoys with her baby. Hold your baby close (if you like, against your bare skin) and smile and talk to your baby. Never leave your baby to drink from a bottle propped up in the crib or stroller; this can cause choking.

Q WHAT IF MY BABY FALLS ASLEEP WHILE BOTTLE-FEEDING?

A If your baby dozes off, it may be because he or she has had enough milk, or gas has made your baby feel full. Take the bottle away, burp your baby (see opposite), then start to feed again. Burping is not always needed; your baby will usually seem uncomfortable when he or she needs to burp.

Q MY BABY RARELY FINISHES THE BOTTLE, IS HE OR SHE GETTING ENOUGH MILK?

A This may be the result of making too much milk per feeding. Ask your midwife or pediatrician how much milk your baby should have according to his or her weight, and have your baby weighed. It is possible to overfeed a bottle-fed baby but not a breastfed one because the strength of breast milk varies and it is thirst-quenching. If you bottle-feed, give your baby cooled, boiled water between feedings if he or she seems thirsty. Poor feeding may signal an illness that needs attention. If your baby gains weight, he or she is probably feeding well.

Q HOW DO I CHANGE FROM BREAST-TO BOTTLE-FEEDING?

A Make a gradual transition by replacing one breastfeeding every third day; replace a lunchtime breastfeeding with a bottle. If your baby won't take the bottle, try again at the same feed the next day. You may need to try different types of nipple, or moisten the bottle nipple with breast milk to encourage your baby. After three days with a bottle-feeding each day, replace a second daytime feeding with a bottle; do this for another three days before tackling a third feeding, until eventually your baby is being bottle-fed. If your baby persists in not taking the bottle, get someone else to give the bottle so that your baby can't smell you, or your milk.

Q HOW LONG WILL MY MILK TAKE TO DRY UP ONCE I STOP BREASTFEEDING?

A You may be uncomfortable for a few days while the milk dries up. Take acetaminophen if your breasts are full and sore, but they should return to normal after about five to ten days.

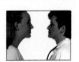

DISCUSSION POINT

IS BREAST OR BOTTLE BEST?

Protecting your baby from illness
An important argument in favor of breastfeeding is that the thick yellow "premilk" (colostrum) produced immediately after delivery, and breast milk itself, contain antibodies to protect your baby against certain types of illness (especially stomach, respiratory, and viral infections), and may protect against allergies such as asthma. Today's baby formulas are unable to reproduce these antibodies.

Preparing for a feeding
Breast milk is convenient because it's always available, already sterile, and is the correct temperature and strength for your baby, whereas if you bottle feed, you need to spend time ensuring that the equipment is scrupulously clean so that your baby is not exposed to gastrointestinal infections.

Bonding with your baby
Breastfeeding with regular skin-to-skin contact allows you to share a special closeness with your baby. If your partner feels excluded from this process, expressing your milk into a bottle will allow him to help with feedings.

Making a choice
Breastmilk is preferable because it contains all the nourishment your baby needs. It has also been suggested that breastfeeding may reduce the risk of crib death. However, you may have reasons why you do not wish to breastfeed; for example, breastfeeding may simply not be comfortable, or bottle-feeding may be more convenient for you if you are planning to return to work. If you are HIV-positive, it is best not to breastfeed because of the increased risk of passing the infection to your baby (see p. 124).

FAMILY CONCERNS

Q HOW DO WE KNOW IF WE WILL MAKE GOOD PARENTS?

A How can any of us know whether we will make good parents? This is something you have to learn "on the job," so all you can do is take each day at a time until your confidence grows through experience. Your insecurity may have something to do with the fact that you feel isolated at the moment. Once you have the opportunity to get out more, join a local mothers' group so that you can share your experiences with others.

Q HOW DO WE COPE WITH EVERYONE GIVING US ADVICE?

A Friends and relatives who have already survived the trials of parenthood naturally assume that you will benefit from their experience. This advice is well-intentioned and often useful but may also be old-fashioned or conflict with your own ideas of parenthood. It is hard to tell those who mean well that you want to do things your own way, but you must make yourself clear from the outset.

ADJUSTING TO FATHERHOOD

The enormous responsibility of fatherhood, and the fears this evokes, can prevent you from getting the most out of family life initially, but if you learn to play an active role, helping with diapering, bathtime, or bedtime, you will soon feel relaxed and confident with your baby.

Feeling neglected
It's a simple fact that newborn babies can take up every second of a mother's time in the early weeks, and that fathers can feel neglected or even jealous of the baby. This is only natural because your partner now has a new focus to her life, and it is not you. Tell your partner how you feel before this builds up into resentment and causes harm to your relationship. You could also take a more active role in caring for your baby.

Feeling left out
Many new fathers wrongly assume that their partner is coping perfectly well without any help from them, but you may be surprised to learn just how much she needs you. Just knowing that you are there helps your partner. If you feel excluded because you cannot share in breastfeeding, perhaps your partner could express some milk into a bottle so that you can help with the feeding, too, including in the middle of the night.

Being scared of your baby
Babies seem to be fragile little creatures, and many men are scared to do anything other than hold them unless they have had younger brothers and sisters. Babies are quite resilient to inept handling, as long as you don't drop them on their heads! Try to overcome your fears by watching your partner and then offer to help bathe and change your baby to give your partner a rest.

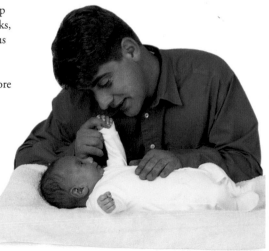

GETTING TO KNOW YOUR BABY
You will come to feel close to your baby through the daily loving contact and care: by changing diapers, giving baths, cuddling, stroking, and talking.

Q HOW WILL OUR OTHER CHILD/ CHILDREN REACT TO THE NEW BABY?

A Other children often see a new arrival as an exciting event. Alternatively, the new arrival may inspire feelings of jealousy in your other offspring; these jealous feelings may not be evident, as you may have expected, right after the birth, so be prepared to deal with them if they emerge later. There should not be too many problems as long as your children still get their share of attention and do not feel excluded (see below).

Q HOW CAN WE BE SURE THAT OUR OTHER CHILDREN DO NOT FEEL LEFT OUT?

A As soon as you bring your baby home, try to include your other child or children in everything that's going on by explaining what you are doing, and why, and getting their help with simple chores. However demanding your new baby is, you should try to make some special time for your other offspring – without the baby – and to honor some of their established routines. For example, if you always read bedtime stories, you or your partner should continue to do so.

Q I FEEL MOODY AND LOW. IS THIS NORMAL?

A In the first few days after the birth you may not feel like your usual self; your partner may also be worried that you seem depressed. However, this is quite normal and is probably just a case of the "baby blues" (see p. 218). Physically, you may be tired and sore, and you may be mentally overwhelmed by your new responsibility. Your body has undergone an hormonal upheaval, and you may also be anxious about your ability to care for your new baby. Talk to your partner about your feelings, so that he understands how you feel. He too, may be feeling a little exhausted or low as he adjusts to the ups and downs of a newborn baby in his life.

Q I'VE BEEN FEELING DEPRESSED FOR WEEKS. IS THIS NORMAL?

A Although mixed feelings are the norm soon after giving birth, if these feelings persist beyond the first week, you may be suffering from postpartum depression (see p. 218), which can be serious. You and your partner should talk to your caregiver or a therapist about your symptoms, so that you can both understand what you are going through and discuss ways in which you can work together to overcome the depression.

Q HOW CAN MY PARTNER AND I REKINDLE OUR ROMANCE?

A In all the excitement and stress caused by the arrival of your baby, it is easy to neglect each other's needs. It can be difficult to feel romantic in the hectic early round of feeding, diapers, and interrupted sleep, but once you have established a routine of caring for your baby, you can begin to think of simple ways to recapture the closeness you and your partner enjoyed before the birth. Ask someone you trust to babysit occasionally so that you and your partner can go out for a walk or a meal. Set aside time to express all the feelings you've both had since the arrival of your baby; just cuddle if you are too tired to make love; have a nap or a bath together at the end of the working day; try to make time to give each other a relaxing massage. Be prepared, though, for interruptions!

Q HOW WILL OUR NEW BABY AFFECT OUR SOCIAL LIFE?

A Your baby's demands will naturally take precedence over your social life in these early weeks, although you will probably find that you have plenty of visitors, and that it is also relatively easy to see friends with your new baby. You may also find that you make new friends through your baby as you meet other parents with young children. Most mothers, however, do not have the energy for late nights at this early stage. Rest assured, your social life will eventually return to a semblance of normality once you all settle into a routine together.

Q WILL WE EVER SETTLE DOWN AGAIN?

A The first six weeks after the birth are a continual round of bathing, changing, and feeding, and you will constantly feel tired. This is the downside of having a newborn baby, but you'll soon begin to experience the joys of parenthood as new patterns become established, your confidence in handling your baby increases, and your body begins to recover from the rigors of pregnancy, labor, and birth. You'll also find that your baby will start to distinguish between night (time to sleep) and day (time to wake up and be sociable), which gives you more time for rest. As your energy returns, your family life will begin to live up to your expectations, and you and your partner will be able to focus on all the positive aspects of parenthood.

CONCERNS ABOUT YOUNG BABIES

Q MY BABY'S FACE IS VERY PIMPLY. IS THIS NORMAL?

A Babies often have pimples, but they are rarely serious. Your baby's face may also have small, white spots (milia) caused by hormonal changes. These do not need treatment, and should disappear within a few days or weeks. If they get infected and red, leave them alone unless they burst; if this happens, gently clean them with cool, boiled water and apply antiseptic cream. If the infection persists or spreads, consult your pediatrician.

Q MY BABY'S BOTTOM LOOKS RED AND SORE. WHAT SHOULD I DO?

A Diaper rash is usually caused by the ammonia in urine irritating the skin, so change your baby's diaper often. A young baby's skin is very sensitive, especially to perfumed, chemical products; if a rash (not caused by wet diapers) develops, it may be due to the overuse of, or your baby's sensitivity to products such as baby cream or wipes (especially if they are not hypoallergenic), and you may have to change or stop using the product. Wash your baby's bottom gently with unscented baby soap and water and pat it dry. A barrier cream can ease soreness and protect against further irritation.

Q MY BABY OFTEN BRINGS UP SOME MILK AFTER A BOTTLE. AM I OVERFEEDING?

A Young babies don't realize when they have had enough milk and often just keep on feeding until they are too full, and then bring up some of their milk. It is also common for babies to vomit when they are trying to burp.

Q MY BABY VOMITED WITH GREAT FORCE. IS THIS NORMAL?

A This may be "projectile vomiting." If it happens only once or within 72 hours of the birth, when your baby may have mucus in his or her stomach, then it is probably not serious; feed and burp your baby well (see p. 208). If it happens after every feeding, consult your pediatrician. Your baby may have a blockage in the stomach's outlet, known as pyloric stenosis, which needs medical attention. However, this is a very rare condition.

Q WHY IS THERE A BLISTER ON MY BABY'S UPPER LIP?

A This is probably a "sucking" blister, caused when the lips tighten around the nipple. The blister is not serious and needs no treatment; just leave it alone and it should disappear.

HOW DO I KEEP MY BABY'S FACE FROM GETTING SCRATCHED?

Since babies tend to wave their fists and touch their faces a lot, they can scratch themselves with the sharp edges of their nails. These scratches are very superficial, and unlikely to cause your baby any lasting harm; they probably cause you more concern because they look sore. To stop this from happening, you can buy "scratch" mittens; some sleepers have sleeves that cover your baby's hands.

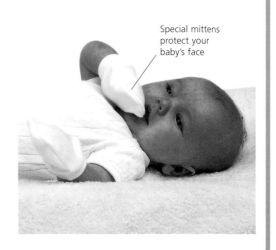

Special mittens protect your baby's face

CUTTING YOUR BABY'S NAILS
Your baby's fingernails are not yet growing beyond the fingertips, so are not ready to be cut.

Q MY BABY CRIES A LOT AND SEEMS VERY UNCOMFORTABLE. WHAT'S WRONG?

A This may be a condition called colic. Colic makes babies cry hard, pull their knees up to their abdomen, and also makes them reluctant to feed or to settle. You can help relieve the pain by massaging the abdomen, or putting your baby against your shoulder and rubbing the back. Ask your pediatrician for advice, and take comfort in the fact that colic is a symptom of early infancy – this, too, shall pass.

Q MY BABY'S STOOLS ARE VERY LOOSE, IS THIS NORMAL?

A Loose stools are quite common, although babies who are breastfed are much more likely to have loose stools than those who are bottle-fed. However, if your baby's stools are green as well as watery, your baby may have diarrhea. This could be serious because it means that your baby is losing fluids, which can lead to dehydration, and this may need medical attention. If your baby has severe diarrhea, a dry mouth, is lethargic, refuses to feed, and the fontanelle is sunken, contact your doctor at once or go to an emergency room.

Q WHAT CAN I DO IF MY BABY'S SCALP IS DRY AND SCALY?

A This is a condition called cradle cap, which often occurs in young babies. It looks unpleasant but is not at all serious and shouldn't cause your baby much discomfort. Cradle cap can spread to other parts of your baby's body, but usually clears up within a few days. You can treat it by gently rubbing baby oil onto the scalp; leave the oil on for up to 24 hours before using a baby comb to comb the hair and loosen the scales. If, after washing your baby's hair, the scaliness persists, consult your doctor.

Q WHY ARE MY BABY'S EYES STICKY AND "GLUED UP"?

A It is possible that your baby has conjunctivitis, which is a mild eye infection. This can occur in newborn babies if fluid or blood gets into the eye during the delivery. Gently wipe your baby's eyes with cotton balls soaked in cool, boiled water; make sure that you use a different cotton ball for each eye. If the condition persists, your doctor can prescribe an antibiotic cream. Some young infants may not yet have mature tear ducts, which can lead to sticky eyes. Ask your pediatrician to check on this.

Q IS OUR SMOKING HARMFUL TO MY YOUNG BABY?

A Yes, a baby's lungs and nose are very sensitive to irritants. Smoke is an irritant, and although your lungs may be used to nicotine, carbon monoxide, and other noxious fumes, your baby's are not. The fumes from cigarettes paralyze the lining of fine hairs in the nose, throat, and lungs that constantly sweep foreign particles out of the chest and help keep the lungs clear. There may be a link between a very smoky environment and crib death, but smoking around your baby will certainly increase his or her chances of developing respiratory problems such as asthma, chronic cough, and chest infections later on in childhood.

WHEN TO CONSULT A DOCTOR

On occasions your baby is likely to give you cause for concern, but you will soon learn to deal with most situations. However, in any of the situations listed below, your baby will need treatment, and should be taken to a doctor.

Contact your doctor if your baby:
- Is passing green, watery stools.
- Wheezes and has a dry, rasping cough.
- Has an unusually low temperature.
- Has a skin rash.
- You suspect an infection is present.
- Has been vomiting more than usual.
- Is very lethargic.
- Is generally irritable and is not feeding well.

Contact your doctor, EMS, or go to the emergency room immediately if your baby:
- Is breathing either very quickly, with a noisy grunting sound, or very slowly and irregularly.
- Seems to be having a seizure: his or her back is arched and/or the limbs are moving jerkily.
- Has turned blue.
- Is acting strangely and doesn't recognize you, or becomes unrousable or extremely sleepy.
- Has a sunken fontanelle.
- Develops a high temperature, especially in conjunction with any of the above.

If you can't contact your doctor, go straight to your local hospital's emergency room or, if you have no transportation, call for an ambulance.

213

THE INTENSIVE-CARE BABY

Q MY BABY HAS TO GO INTO INTENSIVE CARE – WHAT DOES THIS MEAN?

A It may be a confusing and frightening moment for you if your baby goes into intensive care immediately after the birth, but there are many reasons why this care may be needed, and it does not necessarily mean that the problem with your baby is serious. Intensive care can range from the observation of a minor problem such as breathing difficulties, to (very rarely) intensive life support. The time a baby needs to spend in intensive care varies from a few hours to a few weeks, depending on the seriousness of the condition, and the age and weight of your baby.

Q WHY MIGHT MY BABY NEED INTENSIVE CARE?

A Intensive care is needed if your baby is born with any problem that requires immediate observation or treatment. Most premature babies (babies born under 37 weeks of pregnancy) are placed in intensive care. If your baby has a problem related to the delivery itself, or arising after the birth (for example, jaundice) or if your baby has inhaled meconium, intensive care will also be needed.

Q WHERE DOES MY BABY GO FOR INTENSIVE CARE?

A Your baby may need to spend some time in neonatal intensive-care, which is a separate unit staffed by specialist nurses and pediatricians. In this unit there are more nurses available to attend to and observe babies than there are in a conventional nursery, so if your baby requires treatment or tests, this unit is the best place to be. Your baby may be placed in a regular crib or in an incubator.

Q WHO DECIDES WHETHER MY BABY NEEDS INTENSIVE CARE?

A If the doctors caring for your baby believe that intensive care is needed, they will suggest this, although the ultimate decision rests with you. It may be hard to separate from your baby at this point, but the important consideration is to do what is best for your baby.

Q WHY DOES MY BABY HAVE TO BE IN AN INCUBATOR?

A Incubators may look very frightening, but they are really just beds with lids that provide controlled conditions (see right). A small baby (particularly if premature) loses heat quickly and is vulnerable to bacteria; an incubator shields the baby from these and provides an environment in which a baby can develop and get stronger.

Q WHAT IS A VENTILATOR, AND WHY DOES MY BABY NEED IT?

A A ventilator (or respirator) is a machine that helps your baby breathe. Your baby may need this help if he or she is born with respiratory problems due to underdeveloped lungs (premature babies), or suffers from a diaphragmatic hernia, where the intestines put pressure on the lungs. Other breathing difficulties can occur during, or after the birth, such as a chest infection, or if there are drugs still in your baby's system from the delivery. Depending on the seriousness of the condition, the type of ventilator required can range from an enclosed oxygenated incubator to full artificial mechanical ventilation.

Q WHY DOES A PREMATURE BABY NEED TO GO INTO INTENSIVE CARE?

A A premature baby is usually placed in intensive care because the internal organs and lungs are not sufficiently developed to function independently; he or she may also have difficulty in maintaining body temperature. A baby's immature lungs may need help from a ventilator (see above) and the baby must be kept warm in an incubator (see opposite). Another problem is that milk or other fluids cannot be taken by mouth, so he or she may need to be fed via a drip or through a nasogastric tube.

Q HOW LONG WILL A PREMATURE BABY BE IN INTENSIVE CARE?

A This depends on how developed your baby was at birth, and if there are other complications. Premature babies may remain in intensive care until their original due date. A rule of thumb is: if your baby is born at 28 weeks, he or she may spend up to 12 weeks (three months) in intensive care, until he or she is stronger and more mature.

Q WHO CAN WE DISCUSS OUR CONCERNS AND WORRIES WITH?

A The pediatricians and neonatologists taking care of your baby will be able to answer all your questions concerning the medical condition and the outlook for your baby. They may not always be available, but you can always voice your concerns to nurses and other members of the staff. Do not be afraid to ask questions. No one expects you to be able to cope all the time: counselors and social workers attached to the unit are available to listen and to help you through this difficult and distressing period.

Q CAN WE HELP CARE FOR OUR BABY IN INTENSIVE CARE?

A Except in rare situations when your baby may be too ill or fragile to be touched, and there is a danger of infection, you and your partner will be encouraged to play a very important part in the well-being of your baby. Touching, cuddling, and talking to your baby can comfort and reassure him or her (see right). It may even be possible to help feed, clean, and change your baby.

Q CAN I BREASTFEED MY BABY WHILE HE OR SHE IS IN INTENSIVE CARE?

A You can usually still breastfeed your baby. However, if your baby cannot suck properly because he or she is too small, a tube will be passed into your baby's stomach and your breast milk fed through this tube. To feed your baby this way, you will have to express your milk first, either manually or with a pump (see p. 204).

Q CAN I STAY IN THE HOSPITAL WHILE MY BABY IS IN INTENSIVE CARE?

A You can spend as much time as you want with your baby, although you will usually sleep in a regular hospital room where you can receive postpartum care. If your baby has to be in intensive care for some time, especially if born prematurely, you will be discharged, but you can still visit your baby daily.

Q MY BABY HAS BEEN IN AN INCUBATOR FOR WEEKS. WILL THIS CAUSE PROBLEMS?

A Parents are often worried that their baby will be unable to bond with them once he or she is released from the incubator. However, there is no evidence to suggest that he or she cannot bond perfectly well with you and your partner once you are all at home.

Q HOW FAR WOULD DOCTORS GO TO SAVE MY BABY?

A Where there is any hope at all, doctors will try to help your baby. Advances in fetal and neonatal medicine have been spectacular in the past ten years, and those caring for your baby will use every available option to help him or her survive. In some circumstances, this may mean transferring you and your baby to another neonatal unit with more expertise and facilities.

CAN I TOUCH MY BABY?

Your baby may be put in an incubator to help maintain his or her body temperature and to monitor breathing. Some babies also need to be fed through a nasogastric tube.

Physical contact
Although you may not be able to hold your baby, most incubators have special portholes in the side through which you can put your hands to touch or stroke your baby so that he or she knows you are near. Tiny babies (especially premature ones) are much less able to cope with bacteria and viruses than adults and children. Because there is a risk of infection, you will have to clean your hands with special soap, and possibly wear a gown and gloves.

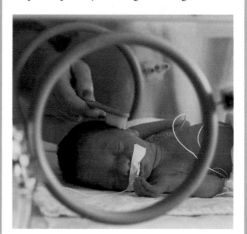

CARING FOR YOUR BABY
You can help care for your baby while he or she is in intensive care. Touching, stroking, and talking to your baby will help him or her during this time.

IF YOUR BABY HAS A CONDITION AT BIRTH

Q WHAT IF MY BABY IS BORN WITH A MEDICAL CONDITION?

A There are medical conditions that result in a baby needing special attention and medical care after birth. A minor problem, such as jaundice, may only need short-term intensive care, or your baby may have a serious condition that requires surgery, such as a hole in the heart, or a long-term disablility, such as cerebral palsy or Down syndrome (see opposite).

Q WHAT IS JAUNDICE?

A Jaundice is a blood condition that commonly affects newborn babies. It occurs for many reasons: usually, when red blood cells are broken down, the yellow pigment, bilirubin, is produced and is rapidly cleared by the kidneys and liver. If the bilirubin builds up, the body is unable to expel it and instead deposits it in the skin, causing the skin to develop a yellowish hue. Jaundice is more common in premature babies because their livers are not fully developed. It can also occur if your baby's head was bruised during a forceps or vacuum extraction delivery. A mild form of jaundice is linked to breastfeeding.

Q IS JAUNDICE SERIOUS?

A Not usually. Mild jaundice, known as physiological jaundice, typically occurs about four days after birth, and commonly disappears without any treatment within ten days. More rarely, however, jaundice may be a sign of a more serious underlying condition such as a blood disorder, for example, anemia, or an infection, or a thyroid or liver problem. This type of jaundice is known as pathological jaundice.

Q WILL MY BABY NEED TREATMENT FOR JAUNDICE?

A This depends on how severe it is. Severe physiological jaundice is treated by photo-therapy: your baby is exposed to ultraviolet light for a few hours every day to break down the bilirubin beneath the baby's skin. Pathological jaundice requires further investigation (especially if anemia is present) and your baby may need a blood transfusion. In certain situations drugs are given to stimulate the liver to get rid of excess bilirubin.

Q MY BABY HAD A SEIZURE AFTER BIRTH, IS THIS SERIOUS?

A There are many causes of seizures, most of which are not serious. These include low blood sugar levels in a baby if the mother is diabetic (see opposite); a temporary shortage of oxygen; a traumatic delivery; an infection; or a high temperature. Very rarely, a seizure happens because bleeding has occurred in the baby's brain, and this can cause lasting damage. Behavior such as a reluctance to feed, lethargy, or extreme agitation may alert doctors to this possibility, and an ultrasound scan of the baby's brain will be taken a few days after the birth.

Q MY BABY NEEDS SURGERY. WHEN WILL IT TAKE PLACE?

A In many situations, surgery is most successful and least dangerous when the baby has matured a little and put on some weight, so surgery will only be carried out immediately if the situation is extremely serious or life-threatening. Minor abnormalities, such as club foot and extra fingers or toes, are not life-threatening and will normally be repaired within a few weeks or months of the birth. A severe cleft palate may be dealt with sooner because it can cause feeding and, more rarely, breathing problems. A life-saving operation may be needed within a few days of birth if your baby has a hernia, either internal (affecting the lung) or external (around the umbilicus); hydrocephalus (water on the brain); heart problems; or, more rarely, problems of the bowel or windpipe.

Q DO I HAVE THE RIGHT TO SAY NO TO AN OPERATION ON MY BABY?

A Yes, it is your right to say no to any operation on your baby. If your baby has a very severe problem that is life-threatening, and an operation may well not be successful, you will have to make a decision (with the advice and guidance of the pediatric staff and the surgeon) whether or not to go ahead with the operation. In some situations, it may be more humane to hold off surgery and save your baby from further unnecessary pain. Unfortunately, many procedures are considered experimental by insurance companies, so be sure you understand the potential economic burden, as well as the medical and emotional issues.

Q I'M DIABETIC. WILL MY BABY HAVE DIABETES?

A No, but your diabetes can cause extra blood sugar to cross the placenta while in your womb. In response to this, your baby's pancreas will have produced high levels of insulin to keep his or her own blood sugar levels under control in the womb. This supply of sugar stops at birth, but your baby's pancreas takes hours, or days, to adjust to the new, lower sugar levels. During this time, he or she will need to be closely monitored.

Q MY BABY WAS BORN WITH A HEART MURMUR. WILL THIS NEED TREATMENT?

A Most heart murmurs occur because of changes in the baby's circulation at or just after the birth. Usually, with this type of benign murmur, a baby is a healthy pink color, feeds well, and the murmur disappears within a few days or weeks. Rarely, a murmur is present because of a structural problem in the heart, which causes a baby to turn blue and become ill. In this case, a cardiac scan is arranged, and your baby may need surgery.

WHAT DOES HAVING A DISABILITY MEAN FOR MY BABY?

Disability is a term that covers everything from minor learning disorders to severe cerebral palsy. Your baby's disability may be mild, such as a degree of deafness or, more rarely, your baby's condition may be severe and include paralysis or mental disability. An increasing number of problems are detected before birth and successfully treated.

When will we know how severely our baby is affected?

Many disabilities can be detected at birth, but it is often some time later before the extent of your baby's problem can be calculated. Once a problem is suspected, degrees of deafness or blindness can be picked up with tests and, if possible, treated immediately, whereas speech and learning difficulties naturally take time to surface. If your baby is suffering from a condition such as cerebral palsy or Down syndrome, he or she will have a more serious form of mental or physical disability and may need extensive help through childhood and in later life.

What is cerebral palsy?

Cerebral palsy is a rare disability that affects the baby's movements. It is caused by damage to the baby's brain late in pregnancy, or during or after the birth, due to lack of oxygen or flow of blood to the brain. It usually affects the baby's muscle control, often causing a degree of paralysis of the limbs.

What is Down syndrome?

A Down syndrome baby suffers from an inherited chromosome defect causing some mental disability and various physical abnormalities (see p. 132).

Will my baby get better?

With the recent advances in treatment, particularly in sight and hearing defects, a baby with an illness or a disability now has a better prospect of leading a more normal life. If your baby has a relatively minor problem, there is a good chance that he or she can be successfully treated. However, where the brain has been irreversibly damaged, the condition is essentially incurable, although much can be done to alleviate suffering and enhance quality of life. Surgery and physical therapy can help physical problems, while sympathetic teaching and support can help those with disabilities.

How will we cope with a disabled baby?

Due to the extra needs involved, a disabled baby can be very hard and stressful work. He or she may take longer to feed, cry a lot, and show little or no response to you or his or her surroundings. You will need to look into what professional care is available to help you and your baby, and plan ahead for any special educational needs. Try not to blame yourself for your baby's condition: it is extremely unlikely that anything you did while pregnant could have affected your baby.

Where can we seek advice and support?

Talking to someone about how you feel can be a great comfort, and will help you and your partner to come to terms with what has happened. Friends and relatives may be your first thought, but it can also be helpful to talk to a pediatrician or pediatric nurse, who can offer practical advice. There are also a number of groups where you can meet other parents of disabled children and receive advice and support (see p. 232).

LIFE AFTER BIRTH

Q HOW CAN I EXPECT TO FEEL IN THE FIRST FEW WEEKS AFTER THE BIRTH?

A In short, shell-shocked! Nothing can prepare you for the reality of having a baby, and the first few weeks will subject you to a barrage of new experiences and sensations. Powerful emotions will be evoked as you realize just how helpless and vulnerable your newborn is. The arrival of a new baby turns your whole world upside down, especially in the first few weeks, as you adjust to the demands of parenthood. Your baby will take up all your time and attention – for 24 hours a day – and you will feel tired and possibly tied down. Housework might pile up, social life and relationships could suffer, and your partner may feel neglected by your preoccupation with your baby.

Q MY BABY TAKES UP ALL MY TIME AND ENERGY. WILL IT ALWAYS BE LIKE THIS?

A Bringing up a new baby is hard work, especially in the early weeks. All the attention that was focused on you while you were pregnant is now being lavished on the baby – at a time when you could really use some of it yourself. It is important to talk about your needs with your partner primarily, and also with your caregiver, family, and friends. This early phase of adjustment and chaos will not last too long. You will soon master the new skills of motherhood and, more importantly, how to balance your needs, those of your partner, and your baby all at the same time. In turn, you will gain in confidence and find the way to enjoy family life.

WHY AM I DEPRESSED?

Most women expect to feel euphoric once their baby is here, but many feel low for several days after giving birth; this is known as "baby blues." Doctors are not entirely clear why this happens, but it is probably due to the adjustments that your body undergoes after the birth, and the sudden change in hormone levels, which can deeply affect your emotions. You may be more likely to get the blues if you experience premenstrual depression, if you were depressed during the pregnancy, and/or if this is your first baby.

How will the blues affect me?
You may feel miserable and tearful, and you may even feel strangely distant from your baby. This can happen when your milk first comes in, or because your sleeping and eating routines are disturbed. At times your spirits will lift – only to plummet again. These emotional highs and lows usually last for a day or two. You will be more able to cope if you understand what is causing this. You will need lots of support from your partner and family. Your doctor or midwife can also be a source of advice.

What is postpartum depression?
About one in ten women experience a prolonged bout of serious sadness that usually starts a week or two after the baby is born. Often you are home and the new-baby euphoria has faded. You may feel weepy, irritable, confused, have difficulty concentrating, and be tired, and even doubt your ability to look after your baby.

Why does it happen?
However much you longed for the event, the reality of having a baby can take some getting used to. Depression can result from the difficulty of adjusting to motherhood, or be the expression of a grieving process for the loss of your previous lifestyle. In your new, changed life you still need to feel that you are a person in your own right, and not merely an appendage of your baby.

How long does postpartum depression last?
The symptoms of postpartum depression usually diminish within a few weeks, but if they persist you may be suffering from severe depression and should see your doctor. You may benefit from seeing a therapist or, in extreme situations, from antidepressant drugs. Joining a mothers' group or support group may also be helpful.

Q HOW CAN I MAKE SOME TIME FOR MYSELF?

A Try not to make the mistake of neglecting yourself at this time, or you'll soon feel as if you have reached the end of your rope. You need to be fit and rested to cope with a newborn baby, especially if you are breastfeeding, so make an effort to schedule some time for your own needs, perhaps by asking your partner to help out with some of the baby care chores. Your baby will probably sleep for an average of 18 hours a day. Try to rest when he or she is asleep; do not be tempted to use this time to catch up on housework or any other tasks that you feel you may have neglected. If you learned any relaxation techniques in your prenatal classes, practice them now to help you relax and to reduce stress. It is essential to have some time to yourself. As your baby gets older, perhaps you can set up a reciprocal arrangement with a friend to look after each other's baby for a few hours each week.

Q I HAVE HAD TWINS – WILL I BE ABLE TO MANAGE ON MY OWN?

A Inevitably, looking after two babies is going to be hard work and is often more work than one pair of hands and one person's stamina can reasonably cope with. But don't panic. It is possible that you will stay in the hospital for longer than usual, until you are certain that you can manage your babies' feeding, bathing, changing, and sleeping routines. Having someone to help you on a daily basis in the early days will make a big difference once you are back at home, so try to arrange this if you can. You should, as parents, plan ahead by making lists and writing things down. And learn to delegate – do not be afraid to ask friends and relatives to help with shopping and cleaning. If you have other children, ask someone to entertain them occasionally, to allow you to rest and recuperate. You and your partner will soon develop the routines that will allow you to cope sucessfully.

RESUMING SEX

Relationships change in many ways when you have a baby. Your partner is no longer just your lover – he is also your companion in parenthood. Sex can become a problem in the first few months after the birth, and this can make you both feel depressed.

When to begin?

The best time to start making love again is when you both feel ready. It's quite normal to experience a temporary lack of interest, or to feel too sore and tender to resume sex before your postpartum checkup. If you had an episiotomy, your partner should not attempt intercourse until you are comfortable with this. Foreplay will be important because the glands that lubricate the vaginal area may not function well for a short time after delivery and you may need a lubricating cream or jelly.

Feeling unattractive

Many women feel unattractive after giving birth. Your body is probably still bloated or overweight, and it is difficult to feel sexually attractive if you are breastfeeding, and have sore nipples and leaking breasts. Starting postpartum exercises (see p. 220) to get back into shape will improve your self-esteem.

Partner's loss of interest

It is not uncommon for new fathers to lose their sex drive for several months after childbirth, especially if the baby is sleeping in the parents' bedroom, a seemingly constant distraction. Your partner may also feel neglected because the baby takes up most of your time and energy. Both of you must be prepared for these distressing reactions, and try not to take them personally. Being open and talking about any problems is often the best solution but if, after several months, one of you is still feeling reluctant to resume your sexual relationship, seek professional advice. You'll be surprised how easy it is to talk about your problems with a third party. Ask your doctor for a referral to a therapist.

What about contraception?

Even if you are breastfeeding or your periods have not begun again, you can get pregnant during this period. You and your partner will therefore need to use some form of contraception. Some contraceptive methods are recommended over others at this particular time, and your midwife or doctor will discuss these with you after the birth, and again at your six-week checkup (see p. 224).

GETTING BACK INTO SHAPE

Q WHAT CAN I DO TO GET BACK INTO SHAPE?

A It is probably the last thing on your mind in the first few days after the birth, yet beginning gentle exercises for your pelvic floor and abdomen is important if you want to get back into shape as soon as possible. For a few weeks, while you are getting used to your new life, you will certainly feel and look very tired, but if you make time for a regular exercise routine (see p. 222), you will find that it is doing far more for you than just reducing your waistline and rebuilding your muscle tone – it also increases your energy levels and enhances your emotional well-being.

Q HOW LONG WILL IT TAKE ME TO GET MY FIGURE BACK?

A Getting back into shape after having a baby doesn't happen overnight – you will have to work at it steadily and regularly. With daily exercise, your figure can return to normal in as little as three months after the birth, so begin exercising as soon as your caregiver approves.

Q WHY ARE PELVIC FLOOR EXERCISES SO IMPORTANT AFTER BIRTH?

A As described in Chapter 5, the pelvic floor is the hammock of muscles that supports your bowels, bladder, and womb. These muscles, which you tighten to help control your bladder and bowels when they are full, have been stretched and weakened by pregnancy and labor, so you may find that you leak urine involuntarily when you cough, sneeze, or laugh. You may also experience decreased satisfaction during intercourse. Both these problems can be improved by toning your pelvic floor muscles with special exercises (see p. 107).

Q HOW LONG WILL IT TAKE TO STRENGTHEN MY PELVIC FLOOR?

A With regular exercise, the pelvic floor muscles should have regained their strength after a month or two. You can test this by jumping up and down with a fairly full bladder, and coughing. If you don't leak any urine while doing this, then your pelvic muscles are in good shape. Another good test is to grip your partner's penis with your vaginal muscles when you make love, and ask him if he can feel this.

Q I USED TO GO TO EXERCISE CLASSES. WHEN CAN I START AGAIN?

A Wait until you have stopped bleeding, your pelvic floor muscles have strengthened, and you have had your postpartum checkup at six weeks. Don't expect to be as energetic as you used to be at first. You'll have to start slowly again, perhaps in a beginners' class, to build up your fitness level.

Q HOW SOON CAN I EXERCISE AFTER A CESAREAN?

A You can begin pelvic floor exercises immediately but should attempt nothing more until your postpartum checkup has given you the all-clear and your wound has fully healed. You should avoid any exercises that involve your abdominal muscles, such as sit-ups; also avoid any competitive sports for at least three months. Do not lift heavy weights, including groceries or even a toddler, for at least six weeks. When recovering from a cesarean, listen to your body. Stop if an exercise causes discomfort or you feel exhausted. Never exercise if you feel unwell.

Q CAN I START TO LOSE WEIGHT BY WATCHING MY CALORIE INTAKE?

A Much of the weight you gained during your pregnancy is nature's way of providing fat stores for you to draw on while breastfeeding, so it is not advisable to go on a diet until after you have stopped breastfeeding and even then you may not need to. Breastfeeding certainly helps you lose weight in the long run, but you will also find that you need to eat and drink more (about 2,500 calories a day) to maintain your energy level, as well as provide a good flow of milk.

Q IS MY DIET IMPORTANT EVEN IF I'M NOT BREASTFEEDING?

A Even if you are not breastfeeding it is essential that your diet be nutritious. You are recovering from the birth and now have a demanding baby to cope with. Try to start your day with a good breakfast; carbohydrates provide a good, steady supply of energy, and protein gives you a solid base (see p. 100), so choose whole wheat cereals, yogurt, or eggs, fruit, and whole grain breads or muffins. Later in the day, healthy sandwiches or snacks can keep you going; simple pasta or rice dishes are quick and easy to prepare in the evening.

Is there a special diet for breastfeeding?

Most women find that they have a larger appetite when breastfeeding. In order to provide milk without taking from your own energy requirements you will need about an extra 500 calories per day. Eat nutritious foods rather than sugary or salty snacks.

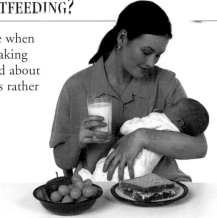

Eat more often
However tired or busy you are, it's important that you do not skimp on your meals. It may suit you to eat several lighter meals or snacks during the day, rather than one larger main meal that is harder to digest. Keep a stock of ingredients to make yourself quick, nutritious snacks.

Eat well
You need to eat plenty of protein and calcium, which are provided by eggs, dairy products, meat, or fish. (If you're a strict vegetarian, you will get your protein from whole grains and legumes.) Be sure to include fresh fruit and vegetables to avoid constipation, carbohydrates such as rice, pasta, or potatoes for energy, and iron-rich foods such as red meat, sardines, green leafy vegetables, or dried fruit.

Take extra fluids
Always drink plenty of fluids when breastfeeding, preferably water, milk, fruit juices (except citrus), or herbal teas instead of caffeinated drinks (see below).

FAST BUT NUTRITIOUS FOOD
You will need snacks and meals that require a minimum of preparation, for example, whole grain bread sandwiches, fresh fruit, and a glass of milk.

Quick healthy snacks

- Baked potatoes with toppings such as cheese.
- Whole grain sandwiches with healthy fillings.
- Cheese and pita or crackers.
- Pasta with melted butter or grated cheese.
- Milkshakes made with whole milk.
- Granola with yogurt and fresh fruit.
- Soups and wholegrain bread.

What should I avoid?

Although you should avoid consuming any nonessential drugs, including alcohol while breastfeeding, many other ideas about what you can or can't eat are myths.

Drugs and alcohol
Drugs and alcohol enter the bloodstream and can be passed on to your baby through your milk, so it's vital that you tell your pharmacist or doctor that you are breastfeeding when prescribed any drugs. Avoid alcohol, as your baby's system is unable to cope with it in the way that yours can.

Spicy foods, garlic, and caffeine
It is often said that certain foods, such as citrus fruits, chocolate, onions, garlic, and spicy foods such as curries, should be avoided because they can cause a baby to have loose stools or gas. This will not necessarily happen because the food you eat does not pass directly into the milk, but is first broken down by your digestive system. However, certain foods may change the acidity or taste of your milk. If you notice that a specific food upsets your baby, do not eat it. Try to avoid strong caffeinated drinks because caffeine could well affect your baby.

Empty calories
Even though you are short of time, try not to substitute fatty or sugary snacks – such as potato chips, candy, cookies, and cakes – for real meals. These snacks are usually high in calories but devoid of nutrients, and they can only give you a short burst of energy.

GETTING BACK YOUR FIGURE

With gentle daily exercise, your figure could return to normal within three to six months. Begin to strengthen the abdominal and pelvic floor muscles soon after the birth, unless you had a cesarean, in which case just practice the pelvic floor exercise until your doctor or midwife says you can be more active.

PELVIC FLOOR EXERCISE

Imagine that you are trying to stop yourself from passing gas, and at the same time trying to stop your flow of urine midstream. Squeeze and lift to close and draw up the perineal area, hold for as long as you can, then rest for about four seconds. Don't tighten your stomach or buttocks, or hold your breath. Try to do about ten every hour.

PELVIC TILT

Lie on the floor with your knees bent, feet flat on the floor, head and shoulders supported on a pillow. This is a good exercise for the first week after birth.

BEFORE YOU EXERCISE

■ While you can begin these gentle exercises immediately, do not attempt any vigorous exercise until your bleeding has ceased and your pelvic floor has strengthened (see p. 107).
■ If you have had a cesarean, wait until you have had your six-week postpartum checkup before starting any active exercise.
■ Never exercise if you feel exhausted or unwell.
■ If you have had back problems, consult your doctor about the suitability of these exercises.
■ Exercise little and often. Start with just one or two repetitions and build up to ten or more.
■ Do not attempt sit-ups or double-leg raises with your legs straight.
■ Remember to "exhale on the effort": breathe out when you tighten your stomach muscles.
■ Stop if an exercise hurts.

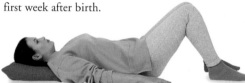

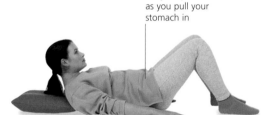

Tilt your pelvis as you pull your stomach in

1 Pull in your stomach, pressing the small of your back into the floor. Hold for four seconds, but don't hold your breath; then gently let go.

2 As you get stronger, you can work your stomach muscles harder by holding the flattened position while you curl forward and lift your head.

CURL-UPS

In the second or third week, you can try this more advanced position. Lie on the floor with your head on a pillow, knees bent, and feet slightly apart.

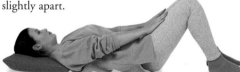

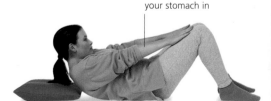

Always exhale when you pull your stomach in

1 Breathe in, and begin the exercise by stretching out your arms and trying to reach your knees with your hands.

2 As you breathe out, pull in your stomach muscles and lift your head. Try to hold for a few seconds, and then rest.

DIAGONAL REACHES

Tighten your stomach muscles before you reach over, and relax them between reaches.

Tighten your stomach muscles

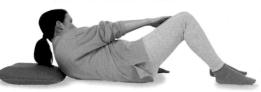

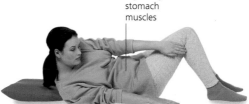

1 Lifting your head and right shoulder, reach the right arm across the body toward the left ankle.

2 Lie back and rest for a moment, then repeat the exercise on the other side.

LEG LIFTS

This exercise tones the hips and thighs. Use your hands and abdominal muscles for support and balance. Keep the leg straight but the knee soft.

1 Lie on your side, both legs directly in line with your hip and shoulder.

Foot faces forward

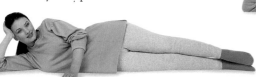

2 Keep the knees facing front, raise the upper leg more or less to shoulder height, and then lower the leg.

CAT STRETCHES

This is an excellent exercise for your back. Simply arch your spine toward the ceiling, like a cat having a good stretch.

Keep your back straight

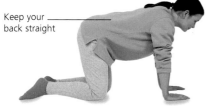

1 Get into position on all fours; make sure you start off with your back straight.

Arch your back like a cat

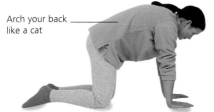

2 Slowly arch your back upward without making yourself uncomfortable.

SIDE BENDS

Stand with your feet apart. Slowly and smoothly, bend sideways, keeping your hips steady and facing front, with your feet flat on the floor. Exhale as you bend.

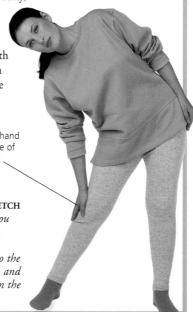

Rest your hand on the side of your knee

BEND AND STRETCH
Move as far as you comfortably can. Hold for a few seconds, return to the upright position, and inhale. Repeat on the other side.

THE FIRST SIX WEEKS

YOUR POSTPARTUM CHECKUP

Q WHY DO I NEED A CHECKUP AFTER SIX WEEKS?

A Your recovery from pregnancy and labor should be almost complete six weeks after the birth, and your midwife or doctor will want to check that everything is returning to normal. By now, your stitches should have healed, your bleeding stopped, and your breasts adapted to feeding, or returned to normal if you are bottle-feeding. If you feel that anything is not quite right, this is an opportunity to get it checked by your caregiver.

Q WHEN ARE MY PERIODS LIKELY TO START AGAIN?

A This date varies depending on individual circumstances. Your periods may begin before the postpartum checkup; if you are bottle-feeding (or you breastfeed only for a short time), your periods should return between two and four months after the birth. If you breastfeed for longer, your periods may not return until your baby starts to take solid food, or possibly even later.

Q WHEN DO I NEED TO START THINKING ABOUT CONTRACEPTION?

A Immediately. Even if your periods haven't started yet, it is important to realize that it is possible to become pregnant again within a month or two of giving birth. Ovulation can occur *before* your first period. Although breastfeeding reduces the likelihood of this, it cannot be regarded as a reliable form of contraception.

Q WHAT METHODS OF CONTRACEPTION CAN I USE?

A Condoms, diaphragms, and all barrier methods of contraception are safe to use at any time. You can take oral contraceptives if you are bottle-feeding, but not if you have chosen to breastfeed; estrogen can inhibit milk production. The "minipill" (containing only progesterone) is compatible with breastfeeding, but must be taken at the same time every day to be effective. There is also an electronic monitor available; this tests your urine for hormones, and shows the days when you are ovulating and those when you are not. However, this system should not be used if you are breastfeeding.

WHAT HAPPENS AT THE POSTPARTUM CHECKUP?

Besides a physical examination to check that you are fully recovered, the postpartum checkup is an ideal time to discuss any problems or incidents that occurred during your pregnancy or labor and why these occurred, and to express any other concerns you may have (see opposite). The postpartum checkup is normally carried out in the doctor's or the midwife's office. Your midwife or doctor will also discuss your choice of birth control method with you, and fit you for a new diaphragm or cervical cap, if needed.

Checks and advice
Any or all of the following checks will be carried out and appropriate advice given:
■ Your urine is tested for protein, to check your kidney function and for urinary tract infection.
■ Your weight is recorded.
■ Your blood pressure is noted.
■ Your breasts and nipples are checked, especially if you are breastfeeding.
■ Your abdomen is examined to check that your womb has shrunk back to its normal size.
■ Any wounds (cesarean or episiotomy) are examined.
■ Your vagina and perineum are examined.
■ You may be offered a Pap smear if you have not had one recently, or if the last one had an abnormal result.
■ If there is any suspicion that you are anemic, blood will be taken to test hemoglobin levels.
■ If you are not immune to rubella (German measles), you will be offered a vaccination.
■ You will be given advice about contraception: depending on your preference, you can have a new IUD inserted or a new diaphragm or cervical cap fitted; you can go on the "minipill" (see left) or be given condoms.

I'M WORRIED ABOUT...

This is an excellent time to discuss any health issues that you are concerned about with your caregivers, or any embarrassing problems that you are experiencing – from soreness to your sex life. It will also put your mind at ease to discover that your fears and problems are very common and also easily remedied.

I am still sore in the perineal area

If you had an episiotomy or tear in the perineal area during the birth, the stitches should have dissolved and the wound should have healed by now. If the area is still red or feels sore, there may be an infection present, and this will be examined; you may need to take an antibiotic to help clear up the infection. Sometimes, if the stitches haven't dissolved properly, they have to be removed.

My vagina feels different

It is common to feel that your vaginal area is "different" after having a baby. To some extent, this is true: your pelvic floor muscles have been stretched and need to be exercised to regain their original elasticity (see p. 222). Some women fear that they have not been "stitched back together" properly. Although this is most unlikely, in extremely rare cases where the stitches have healed badly, the result can interfere with the ability to urinate and defecate, and may even mar your sex life. In this case it may be necessary for you to have an operation, called a "restructuring of the perineum," to return things to normal.

I am leaking urine

Many women experience urine leakage (stress incontinence) after childbirth; don't be embarrassed to talk about it. Most commonly it stops within a few weeks. The sooner you bring it to your doctor's attention the sooner you will be referred to a specialist if necessary. Usually it is the result of damaged or weak pelvic floor muscles. Sometimes exercises can help, or a simple treatment is all that is required. Infection can also make you leak, so a urine specimen is often requested, or a course of antibiotics prescribed.

I feel weak after my cesarean

If you had a cesarean delivery, your stomach muscles can take some time to knit back together again and you will not have much strength in your abdominal area. You should avoid any lifting or driving for the first six weeks to give the wound time to heal properly. It will be at least three months before you can lift heavy objects, run, or take up sports again. Apart from the pelvic floor exercise and pelvic tilt (see p. 222), avoid any exercise until after six weeks.

I feel so tired

Many women feel exhausted in the weeks following the birth. If your fatigue is accompanied by breathlessness and pallor, you may be anemic. This can be caused by a lack of iron, or a loss of blood during labor. Normal blood loss does not cause a problem because your body is able to make it up rapidly. If you had a cesarean, however, you may have lost twice as much blood as in a vaginal delivery, so you will need to take iron supplements to replenish your body's stores.

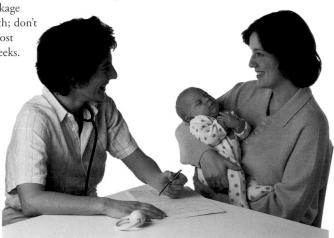

A SYMPATHETIC EAR
Your doctor will be ready to discuss any problems you are experiencing during your recovery.

YOUR BABY'S SIX-WEEK CHECKUP

Q HOW HAS MY BABY DEVELOPED OVER THE FIRST SIX WEEKS?

A You will find that your baby has become a more responsive individual, and less of a noisy, demanding bundle. You may also find that he or she does not cry as much as before, and that there is a longer wakeful period during the day. Control over the limbs has increased and the fists have unclenched, enabling objects to be grasped more easily. You will notice how your baby enjoys kicking his or her legs in the air. When lying face down, your baby may be able to lift his or her head momentarily, but will remain unable to do this when sitting.

WHICH IMMUNIZATIONS AND CHECKS WILL MY BABY NEED?

The six-week checkup is the first part of your baby's medical history and is followed by checkups and vaccinations up to four years old. Some vaccines are long-lasting, others need to be boosted at regular intervals. Call your local department of health for a schedule.

Immunizations

AGE	IMMUNIZATION
2, 4, 6, 15–18 months	DTP – Diphtheria, tetanus, whooping cough
12 months	MMR – Measles, mumps, rubella
2, 4, 18 months	Polio, hepatitis b, hemophilus influenzae b (Hib)

Checkup highlights
■ At eight months, your baby's hearing, growth, and development are tested.
■ At two years, your baby's walking, talking, comprehension, and coordination (fine motor skills) are assessed.
■ At three-and-a-half years, physical development, speech, and hearing are checked.

Q DOES MY BABY RECOGNIZE ME OR MY PARTNER YET?

A Yes, one of the biggest thrills for you and your partner is that your baby now has a range of facial expressions and can respond to you both. Your baby's head turns upon hearing your voice, and he or she will stare at your face when you are talking, meeting your eyes and smiling at you.

Q IS IT NORMAL FOR A PREMATURE BABY TO BE REALLY DIFFICULT AT FIRST?

A Premature babies can be especially difficult during the first six weeks, crying incessantly and refusing to be comforted, no matter how hard you try, or be very sleepy and reluctant to feed. He or she needs extra care, more frequent feeding, and lots of warmth – but because there is less response, you may feel discouraged. As your baby matures, you will see a reaction to your care. The checkup is a good time to ask about any issues or concerns that are causing you anxiety.

Q CAN IMMUNIZATIONS REALLY CAUSE BRAIN DAMAGE?

A There have been alarming stories about the side effects of vaccinations, but these cases are rare. There is no firm evidence that immunizations cause brain inflammation (encephalitis) and brain damage. Some babies and children develop seizures and subsequent brain damage shortly after being immunized, but since these problems afflict some babies anyway – even if they are not immunized – it is uncertain whether the immunizations received only a few days earlier are culpable.

QUESTIONS TO ASK

Is my baby developing normally?

Can my baby see and hear properly?

How do I get information about immunization?

Can I delay the start of the immunization program?

Do I have to remember checkup dates or will I be reminded?

WHAT IS THE DOCTOR LOOKING FOR?

The six-week checkup is the first of the major developmental assessments for a new baby. Your pediatrician will carry out the checkup in relaxed surroundings. This is a good time to raise any questions you may have about the daily care of your baby.

ROUTINE CHECKS

Your baby is undressed so that the doctor can observe how he or she moves her limbs. Your baby will be examined in detail from head to foot to be sure that physical progress is normal. You will be asked questions about your baby's feeding and toilet habits, as well as general well-being.

General assessment

The head circumference is measured to check for normal growth, and the fontanelles (soft parts of your baby's head at the front and back where the skull bones meet) are checked for abnormalities. The baby's eyes, ears, and mouth are examined; the chest and breathing are checked, and the genitals inspected. The doctor will also feel your baby's abdomen to check that the liver, stomach, and spleen are all developing normally; by manipulating your baby's legs, the hips are checked for possible dislocation.

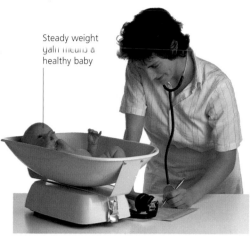

Steady weight gain means a healthy baby

WEIGHING
Your baby will be weighed regularly and the weight gain compared with the birth weight. Normal weight gain usually means a healthy baby; the weight chart will be an important record for months to come.

TONE AND GRASP
The doctor will observe your baby's muscle tone and how the limbs are working. She will also check the "grasp reflex," which demonstrates that your baby can now grasp a finger and hold on.

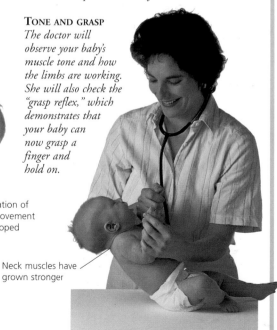

Neck muscles have grown stronger

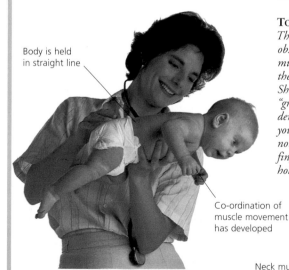

Body is held in straight line

Co-ordination of muscle movement has developed

HEAD CONTROL
Now that your baby has some control over the neck muscles, the doctor will see if he or she holds the head in line with the body while being held in the air, and even when moved into a sitting position.

THE FIRST SIX WEEKS

Enjoying Life With Your Baby

Q I'M FINDING IT HARD TO ESTABLISH A ROUTINE. WHEN WILL THIS GET EASIER?

A The first weeks following the birth of your baby will have been a period of great upheaval as you juggle the needs of the new baby and those of daily life. So much has had to be learned in a short time, and all your time and energy have been focused on the new arrival. Rest assured, whatever your experience or lack of it, you will eventually establish a way of life that suits your family and gives you more breathing space. Nights of broken sleep will become easier to cope with or become less frequent. Your baby will soon begin to know the difference between night and day, and become more responsive to you and your partner, making baby care easier and more fun.

Q AM I RIGHT TO WANT TO SPEND ALL MY TIME WITH MY BABY?

A You may feel that the helpless little bundle that you have brought into the world demands all of your time – time you will naturally want to give. What you should do, however, is to try to give your own well-being a high priority; being fit and rested is particularly important if you are breastfeeding. Remember to keep things in perspective. Spend as much time as you want with your baby, but don't forget about yourself and your partner. When you feel ready, ask a family member, friend, or neighbor to stay with your baby for an hour or so, so that you can spend time on your own or with your partner.

Q HOW CAN I KEEP IN CONTACT WITH FRIENDS AND FAMILY?

A Once your baby has arrived, it is important to keep in touch with your friends and family for adult conversation, support, and advice. The constant care of a baby can be quite a burden to shoulder without company, especially if your partner has returned to work. There are usually local "mother and baby groups," which you may already know about through your prenatal classes. If not, your pediatrician or hospital should be able to give you information and addresses. If your prenatal group has a reunion, it can be a good time to find out how everyone else is coping with parenthood.

Q WHEN CAN WE HAVE A NIGHT OUT AND LEAVE THE BABY WITH SOMEBODY ELSE?

A It depends on your confidence. It may be a few weeks or months before you feel relaxed enough to allow others to look after your baby. An evening out with your partner is a major step, but the break from the constant caring for your baby and the return to normality will probably be greatly appreciated by you both. If you are breastfeeding, expressing your milk allows you to leave your baby for a few hours knowing that he or she can be fed.

Q WHAT DO I NEED TO THINK ABOUT BEFORE GOING OUT WITH MY BABY?

A If you use public transportation, you will need something lightweight, portable, and easy to assemble and collapse; a stroller that adapts into a fully reclined position can be ideal (see opposite). An old-fashioned "pram" is sturdy and excellent for walks, but it is difficult to manage on steps, buses, or trains. If you use a car, be sure that whatever you use fits into the trunk. Also consider whether you and your partner are very different heights; if so, an adjustable stroller is probably more practical. If you have twins, you can choose either a side-by-side or back-and-front stroller. A side-by-side is wider and therefore more difficult to maneuver; both have advantages and disadvantages.

Q WHAT CAN I LOOK FORWARD TO IN THE COMING MONTHS?

A Babies are hard work, but they are also great fun. Watching your baby grow, develop, and discover the world around him or her makes parenthood a journey of learning that is probably one of the most satisfying experiences that life can offer you and your partner. Your baby will also be learning from you and can detect your mood. The more confident and relaxed you become, the happier he or she will be. As a parent you will have a major influence on the life and personality of your child. The year ahead will be one of unequaled development for your baby and, looking back at the end of the year, it will be difficult to imagine that the laughing, boisterous one-year-old was ever a helpless little infant.

GETTING OUT

There is no need to feel marooned at home with your young infant – a wide range of strollers, carriages, and car seats are available. Before buying any equipment, check that it is safe and comfortable for your baby, as well as easy to use and store.

CONVERTIBLE STROLLER

This is ideal for a newborn because your baby can lie flat. The bed can be removed from the chassis and used for sleeping. At six months, a seat fits on instead.

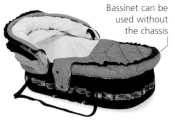

Bassinet can be used without the chassis

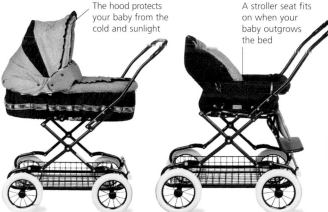

The hood protects your baby from the cold and sunlight

A stroller seat fits on when your baby outgrows the bed

CARRYING YOUR BABY

Instead of a stroller or carriage, you could use a front-carrying sling or a car seat to carry your baby, giving yourself more freedom of movement.

Head support for newborn

FRONT-CARRYING SLING
This convenient sling leaves your hands free.

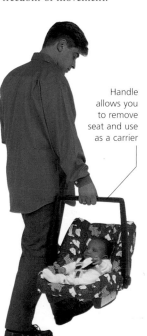

Handle allows you to remove seat and use as a carrier

Always strap your baby in

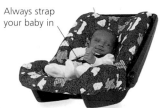

REMOVABLE CAR SEAT
Most car seats can be used as a carrier or baby seat. Check that it's the right size for your baby's weight.

THE DIAPER BAG

This is invaluable when you are out and about because it contains everything you need to change and, if necessary, feed your baby.

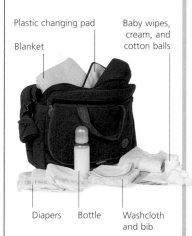

Plastic changing pad

Baby wipes, cream, and cotton balls

Blanket

Diapers   Bottle   Washcloth and bib

WHAT TO PACK
You need the essentials for feeding and changing your baby's diapers (see p. 197), a blanket, a change of clothes for your baby, and later, a favorite toy.

YOUR RIGHTS AND BENEFITS

MATERNAL AND PARENTAL LEAVE

Ideally, every pregnant woman should be able to take time off from the pressures of outside work both before and after the baby arrives. The reality, however, is that few working women have such a luxury of time and financial resources. Nevertheless, in Canada, permanently employed women are legally entitled to both paid and unpaid maternity leave, and parental leave for biological and adoptive parents is also provided within the law. While these rights are available, it is important to do your research before approaching your employer to discuss your leave of absence. It pays to know your entitlements.

PAID LEAVE

Federally, the new Employment Insurance Act, implemented in 1997, provides for paid maternity and parental leave based on a percentage of your current salary. A maximum of 15 weeks maternity benefits are available to biological mothers in a period surrounding the birth of the child; a maximum of 10 weeks parental benefits are available to natural and adoptive parents.

It is important to arrange your leave with your employer well in advance of the anticipated birth. The law states that on your return to work you must be reinstated in the same position that you left, or be promoted, at the same or higher salary.

UNPAID LEAVE

The Employment Standards branch of your provincial ministry of labour will provide you with information regarding your rights to unpaid pregnancy and parental leave. Not only are there provisions for unpaid leave for adoptive and natural parents, but there are also provisions for such leave if you suffer a miscarriage or stillbirth.

GOVERNMENT ASSISTANCE AND SOCIAL SERVICES

Your health card ensures that you are covered for all basic medical needs when you are pregnant. It is important to remember, however, that you must apply for a health card for your baby once he is born. Hospital staff or your midwife will provide you with the forms; consult your provincial health ministry for more details. A health card number will be assigned immediately for your new baby; a card will be mailed to you separately.

The government of Canada also provides what is known as the National Child Benefit, a program specifically designed to assist low-income families, linked to the Canada Child Tax Benefit, which is a universal program. Forms to apply for one or both of these benefits are available through your hospital or midwife.

At the community level, there are many publicly funded agencies providing assistance over and above the generally available government programs. Education, milk, food and housing for single mothers, for instance, are staples in communities across Canada. Look in the telephone book "blue pages" for government-funded programs. There are also programs funded by charitable organizations and private assistance that can be of use to pregnant women in need. Hospitals, medical clinics and midwives can provide the necessary information.

DAY CARE

Subsidized day care is an area in which Canadian municipalities are attempting to become better equipped to serve public requirements. For details on availability, contact your local day care services department under Community Services in the blue pages of the telephone book. It is generally recommended that, if you qualify for subsidized day care, you apply for a space well in advance, since waiting lists can be very long.

REGISTERING YOUR BABY'S BIRTH

You must register your baby's birth with the municipality, county or district in which she was born. This is done by giving the Office of the Registrar General of your province a Statement of Live Birth – papers that will be provided by the hospital or your midwife. Once this form is fully completed, you can proceed to obtain a birth certificate for your child. Get one or two copies of the certificate; you will need them periodically, most notably for school registration.

RIGHTS AND BENEFITS SUMMARY

WHEN	WHAT TO DO	WHY
Before you are pregnant	■ Check with your local government offices and your employer to determine maternity leave benefits and policies	■ To maximize your employee benefits
After 12 weeks or after the amniocentesis results are back	■ If you are working, inform your employer	■ As a consideration, to give your employer time to prepare
About 12 weeks before your due date	■ Discuss your maternity-leave plans with your employer	■ To negotiate the best possible maternity-leave package
About 10 weeks before your due date	■ Give your employer a letter summarizing your maternity-leave plans and what you have agreed upon	■ To clarify your and your employer's expectations, giving both of you time to fine-tune plans ■ To avoid misunderstandings
At least 30 days before going on maternity leave	■ Inform your employer in writing	■ To protect your rights under the Employment Insurance Act and your provincial employment standards provisions
1–2 days after birth	■ Submit information for birth certificate ■ Apply for Canada Child Tax Benefit ■ Apply for National Child Benefit, if you qualify ■ Apply for baby's provincial health card	■ More straightforward than waiting until later
6–8 weeks after birth	■ Purchase a copy or copies of baby's birth certificate and put in safekeeping ■ Receive baby's health card	■ For easy recordkeeping ■ For all medical needs

USEFUL ADDRESSES

MIDWIVES

To date, only British Columbia and Ontario have recognised midwifery and integrated it into their health care systems. In these provinces, a midwife must pass certain tests, continually upgrade her skills, and attend a minimum number of births per year. In provinces where midwifery is not recognised, there are no regulations governing the profession, though there may be self-regulating or voluntary associations of midwives.

Association of Ontario Midwives

102–562 Eglinton Avenue E,
Toronto, ON M4P 1P1
Tel (416) 481-2811
Fax (416) 481-7547
email: midwives@interlog.com
Information; assistance in locating a midwife in Ontario

Canadian Confederation of Midwives

Tel (403) 432-7645/email:
sgjames@gpu.srv.ualberta.ca
Information on midwifery in Canada; assistance in locating a midwife in your community

Midwife Association of British Columbia

219–1675 W 8th Avenue
Vancouver, BC V6J 1N2
Tel (604) 736-5976
Fax (604) 736-2152
email: mabc@bc.sympatico.ca
Information; assistance in locating a midwife in British Columbia

ADOPTION

Adoption Council of Canada

Box 8442, Station T
Ottawa, ON K1G 3H8
Tel (613) 235-1566
Referrals, counseling, information for adoptive and biological parents

BEREAVEMENT

Bereaved Families of Ontario

562 Eglinton Avenue E,
Suite 401
Toronto, ON M4P 1P1
Tel (416) 440-0290
Toll-Free 1-800-236-6364
Fax (416) 440-0304
email: bfo@inforamp.net
http://www.inforamp.net/~bfo/
Support after loss of a child, including pregnancy and/or infant loss; support for children who have lost a parent or sibling

The Canadian Foundation for the Study of Infant Deaths

586 Eglinton Avenue E,
Suite 401
Toronto, ON M4P 1P2
Tel (416) 488-3260
Toll-Free 1-800-END-SIDS
Fax (416) 488-3864
http://www.sidscanada.org/sids.html
email: sidscanada@inforamp.net
Research, education and support

BREASTFEEDING

La Leche League of Canada

18C Industrial Drive,
PO Box 29
Chesterville, ON K0C 1H0
Tel (613) 448-1842
Fax (613) 448-1845
Breastfeeding referral line
1-800-665-4324
email:laleche@igs.net
http://www.lalecheleague.org
Breastfeeding information, mother-to-mother support, publications on breastfeeding and child care

DAY CARE SERVICES

Check Community Services or Community and Social Services in the phone book "blue pages".

The Canadian Daycare Registry

http://www.canadian
daycare.com
Provides free (unscreened) listings of daycare providers in Canada

DISABILITES

The National Information Center for Children and Youth with Disabilities

PO Box 1492
Washington, DC 20013
Tel (202) 416-0300
Toll-Free 1-800-695-0285
email: nichcy@aed.org
http://www.nichcy.org
Information on disabilites and disability-related issues, focuses on children and youth, birth to 22

Easter Seal Society

1185 Eglinton Avenue E,
Suite 706
North York, ON M3C 3C6
Tel (416) 421-8377
email: info@easterseals.org
http://www.easterseals.org
Practical assistance, information and research on child disabilities

March of Dimes Birth Defects Foundation

1275 Mamaroneek Avenue
White Plains, NY 10605
Tel (914) 428-7100
http://www.modimes.org
Nonprofit organization fighting birth defects

FAMILY PLANNING

Infertility Network

160 Pickering Street
Toronto, ON M4E 3J7
Tel (416) 691-3611/email:
102137.3465@compuserve.com
Education, seminars, audiotapes, pamphlets, support groups

HEALTHCARE

AIDS and Sexual Health Infoline

Toll-Free 1-800-668-2437
Information, counseling, referrals

Canadian AIDS Society

130 Albert Street, Suite 900
Ottawa, ON K1P 5G4
Tel (613) 230-4998
Fax (613) 563-4998
email: CASinfo@cdnaids.ca
http://www.cdnaids.ca
Advocacy, programs, services, resources and information

Canadian Diabetes Association

15 Toronto Street, Suite 800
Toronto, ON M5C 2E3
Tel (416) 363-3373
Toll-Free 1-800-226-8464
Fax (416) 363-3393
email: infor@cda-nat.org
http://www.diabetes.ca
Information, support and advice on living with diabetes

Depression After Delivery

PO Box 278
Belle Mead, NJ 08502
Tel 1-800-944-4773
email: dt@infotrail.com/ http:
//infotrail.com/dad/dad.html
Information, support on postpartum depression

Epilepsy Canada

1470 Peel Street, Suite 745
Montreal, PQ H3A 1T1
Tel (514) 845-7855
Toll-Free 1-800-860-5499
Fax (514) 845-7866
http://www.epilepsy.ca
Information on epilepsy and associated risks in pregnancy

Infant and Toddler Safety Association

Tel (519) 570-0181
Information on product safety, regulations, recalls, child safety and childproofing homes.

Motherisk™ Program

Hospital for Sick Children
555 University Avenue
Toronto, ON M5G 1X8
Tel (416) 813-6780
http://www.motherisk.org
Information on prescription and over-the-counter medications, chemicals, etc., and their effects on pregnancy and breastfeeding.

Public Health Unit

Check telephone book government lists.
Resource for new mothers; counseling before and after birth

Safe@Home

email: safety@safebaby.net
http://www.safebaby.net
Supervised by: Childproofers Inc. Barbara Skala, R.N.
Extensive information on childproofing your home, child safety, child development, safety regulations, products and car seat safety

Society of Obstetricians and Gynecologists of Canada

774 Echo Drive
Ottawa, ON K1S 5N8
Tel (613) 730-4192
Toll-Free 1-800-561-2416
Assistance locating an obstetrician in your community

The Toronto Cord Blood Programme

The Toronto Hospital
General Division
200 Elizabeth Street
Toronto, ON M5G 2C4
Tel (416) 340-3323
Information on packages and counseling for parents interested in banking their unborn child's stem cells against future illness

LABOUR AND BIRTH

Cascade Birthing Catalogue

141 Commercial Street NE
Salem, OR 97301
Tel (503) 877-8266
Toll-Free 1-800-443-9942
Birthing supplies; baby products

Informed Homebirth and Parenting

3555 Pratt, PO Box 3675
Ann Arbor, M1 48103
Tel (313) 662-6857
Alternative birth resources

International Caesarean Awareness Network

PO Box 152, University
Station, Syracuse, NY 13202
Tel (315) 424-1942
http://www.childbirth.org/secti
on/ICAN.html
Educates women about Caesarean section; working to lower the number of repeat and unnecessary Caesarean sections

International Childbirth Education Association

PO Box 20048
Minneapolis, MN 55420
Tel (612) 854-8660
Fax (612) 854-8772
email: info@icea.org
http://www.icea.org
Trains childbirth educators; provides publications on childbirth and maternity care

Lamaze™ International

1200 19th Street NW,
Suite 300
Washington, DC 20036
Tel (202) 857-1128
Toll-Free 1-800-368-4404
Fax (202) 223-4579
email: lamaze@dc.sba.com
http://www.lamaze-
childbirth.com
Information on Lamaze childbirth technique and assistance locating a group in your community. Check your local YWCA and community centers for prenatal classes

MULTIPLE BIRTHS

Parents of Multiple Births Association of Canada

240 Graff Avenue
PO Box 22005
Stratford, ON N5A 7V6
Tel (519) 272-2203
Fax (519) 272-1926
email: office@pomba.org
http://www.pomba.org
Improve and promote health and well-being of multiple-birth families before, during and after pregnancy

SINGLE PARENTHOOD

One-Parent Families Association of Canada

6979 Yonge Street, Suite 203
Willowdale, ON M2M 3X9
Tel (416) 226-0062

email: oneparent@titan.tcn.net
http://www.tcn.net/~oneparent
Support and activities for single parent families

Parents Without Partners International, Inc.
401 North Michigan Avenue
Chicago, IL 60611-4267
Tel (312) 644-6610
Fax (312) 321-5194
email: pwp@sba.com / http://www.parentwithoutpartners.org

International, non-profit, educational body devoted to the interests and support of single parents and their children

Single Mothers by Choice
PO Box 1642, Gracie Square Station, New York, NY 10028
Tel (212) 988-0993
email: mattes@pipeline.com
http://www.parentsplace.com/readrooom/smc
Information on single

parenthood; fertility methods; support for single mothers

T.E.N.S

Mylon-Tech Health Technologies Inc.

1105 Carling Avenue
Ottawa, ON K1Y 4GS
Tel (613) 728-1667
Toll-Free 1-800-688-1667
Fax (613) 728-9037
email: info@mylontech.ca

http://www.mylontech.ca
Source for T.E.N.S. units

Further Resource Material
Bookstores and libraries are good sources for addresses, and publications on pregnancy, labour, birth and related health, rights and benefits issues. There is information on the Internet; however, there is no means for it to be verified, so discuss your findings with your doctor or midwife.

A GUIDE TO DRUGS IN PREGNANCY

Here is a guide to the drugs you can take in pregnancy and those to avoid. **Consult your doctor before taking any over-the-counter or prescription drugs during pregnancy or while tring to conceive.**

Analgesics (pain relievers)
Acetaminophen is considered safe. Many women at risk of preeclampsia use low-dose aspirin, however, aspirin and other non-steroidal anti-inflammatory drugs, such as ibuprofen, should be avoided in the last two months as they can cause bleeding or problems for the baby.

Acne preparations
Avoid oral medications based on vitamin A, which can cause birth defects. Certain antibiotics used to treat acne should not be taken as they can permanently discolour the baby's teeth.

Migraine medications
Some have ergotamine-based substances and should be avoided as they may contract the womb or cause miscarriage.

Anti-nausea medications (antiemetics)
These should only be prescribed by a doctor who knows you are pregnant. Always see your doctor if you have severe nausea or vomiting.

Antibiotics
These should only be prescribed by a doctor who knows you are pregnant. Most are safe, but avoid minocycline, cotrimoxazole and, particularly near the birth, sulfas.

Asthma medications
These drugs are usually inhaled and are safe in pregnancy. It is important that asthma is controlled during pregnancy.

Allergy and cold medications
Low, limited doses of antihistamines or decongestants that make you sleepy are safe and you can use nasal sprays such as saline and oxylometazoline for a few days.

Anticoagulants
Heparin does not harm the baby, but prolonged use can cause osteoporosis in you. Warfarin may cause birth defects if taken in the first trimester and bleeding in your baby if taken in the last trimester.

Antihypertensives (blood pressure medication)
Some are safe to take in pregnancy. Whether or not you have been diagnosed with hypertension before pregnancy, it is important that your blood pressure be monitored in pregnancy.

Thyroid medication
Drugs for hyperthyroidism (an overactive thyroid) may cross the placenta and affect the baby's thyroid function. Drugs for hypothyroidism (an underactive thyroid) are generally safe. In either case, consult your doctor as it is important that your thyroid function is controlled.

Diuretics
Diuretics for weight loss should not be used during pregnancy. Use of a diuretic should be supervised by your doctor.

Antiseizure medication
Taking these in pregnancy poses a small risk to a baby, but the risk to both of you may be greater if you stop them and have seizures. If you take antiseizure medication, you may need folic acid supplements (ideally, before conception and in the first trimester) because some

medications reduce the amount of folic acid in your body, which is important in preventing spina bifida (see p.12)

Insulin
This is safe for your baby as it does not cross the placenta. However, glucose does, so if you are diabetic you need to maintain good blood sugar control.

Antidepressants
SSRIs (selective serotonin reuptake inhibitors) are thought safe in pregnancy, but they are quite new and there is little supportive evidence. Tricyclics and MAOIs (monoamine oxidase inhibitors) have been in use longer. The use of any antidepressant, particularly MAOIs, in pregnancy must be monitored. Consult your doctor before taking antidepressants.

Lithium
This poses a small risk for birth defects and problems at birth. Do not stop taking this without asking your doctor

Sleeping pills
These should be avoided close to delivery as they may make your baby drowsy.

Narcotics (codeine, morphine, heroin, methadone, meperidine, diamorphine)
If used long term or during pregnancy, these can cause low birthweight. At birth, your baby may be drowsy, have problems breathing, or be addicted.

Steroids
Inhaled steroids, such as those for asthma, are safe. Oral steroids can be used for serious conditions such as arthritis, asthma and inflammatory bowel diesease but tell your doctor you are pregnant.

GLOSSARY

Abruption Premature separation of the placenta from the wall of the womb.

Amniocentesis A procedure in which a small sample of amniotic fluid is removed from around the fetus.

Amniotic fluid The fluid surrounding the fetus (also known as "waters").

Amniotomy (artificial rupture of membranes, ARM) Breaking the membranes using a special plastic hook.

Anemia Lack of hemoglobin in red blood cells, due to iron deficiency or disease.

Antepartum hemorrhage (APH) Vaginal bleeding that happens after 24 weeks of pregnancy and before delivery.

Breech The baby is lying bottom down in the womb.

Cephalic The baby is lying head down in the womb.

Chorion villus sampling (CVS) A method for sampling placental tissue for genetic or chromosome studies.

Cilia The fine hairs that line the fallopian tubes.

Cordocentesis The procedure for taking blood from the fetal umbilical cord via a needle through the mother's abdomen.

Cystitis Infection of the bladder.

Dizygous Nonidentical (fraternal) twins.

Doppler A form of ultrasound used specifically to investigate blood flow in the placenta or in the fetus.

Down syndrome (trisomy 21) A disorder caused by the presence of an extra chromosome 21 in the cells.

Ectopic pregnancy A pregnancy that develops outside of the womb.

Edema Swelling of the fingers, legs, toes, and face.

Embryo The medical term for the baby from conception to about six weeks.

Epidural anesthesia A method of numbing the nerves of the lower spinal cord to ensure a pain-free labor.

Episiotomy A cut of the perineum and vagina performed by a midwife or doctor to make the delivery easier.

External fetal monitor An electronic monitor used to record the fetal heartbeat and the mother's contractions.

Fallopian tubes Two tubular structures (one on each side of the womb) leading from the ovaries to the womb.

Fetus Medical term for the baby from six weeks after conception until birth.

Fibroid A benign (noncancerous) growth of muscle of the womb, usually spherically shaped.

Forceps Metal instruments that fit on either side of the baby's head and are used to help deliver the baby.

Fundus The top of the womb.

Hemoglobin (Hb) The oxygen-carrying constituent of red blood cells.

Hepatitis Viruses (named A, B, C, E, and others) that infect the liver, causing jaundice and generalized illness.

Hypertension High blood pressure.

Induction of labor (IOL) The procedure for initiating labor artificially.

In utero death (IUD) The death of the unborn fetus after 24 weeks.

In vitro fertilization (IVF) A method of assisted conception in which fertilization occurs outside the mother's body and the embryo is replaced in the womb.

Lanugo The fine hair that covers the fetus in the womb.

Lochia Blood loss after the birth.

Membranes Two sets of protective sacs enclosing the baby, called the amnion and the chorion.

Miscarriage The spontaneous loss of a pregnancy before 24 weeks.

Monozygous Identical twins.

Neonatal A baby less than 28 days old.

Nuchal scan A special ultrasound scan that gives an estimate of the risk of Down syndrome.

Oocyte One egg that is released from the ovary at each ovulation.

Placenta A flat, thick disk-shaped organ that supplies the fetus with oxygen and nutrients.

Placenta previa A placenta situated over, or near, the cervix, which makes a vaginal delivery unlikely.

Postpartum After birth.

Postpartum hemorrhage (PPH) Excessive bleeding following delivery.

Preeclampsia A condition that features high blood pressure, edema, and proteinuria. May be mild or serious.

Prenatal Before birth.

Presentation Describes the way the baby is lying in the womb.

Preterm (premature) labor Labor before 37 weeks of pregnancy.

Puerperium Just after and up to six weeks after delivery.

Rhesus (Rh) factor Blood is either Rhesus positive or Rhesus negative.

Rh_o immunoglobulin An injection of antibodies given to women whose blood group is Rhesus negative, if they may have been exposed to fetal blood cells.

Spinal anesthesia An injection of anesthetic into the spine for pain relief in labor (similar to an epidural).

Stillbirth Birth of a baby after 24 weeks of pregnancy, who shows no signs of life.

Sutures Stitches.

Thrombosis A blood clot, commonly occurring in the calf; most dangerous if in the lungs (pulmonary embolus).

Toxoplasmosis A parasite infection that can be caught from cats or other pets.

Transverse The baby is lying sideways in the womb.

Urinary tract infection (UTI) Infection affecting the kidneys and/or bladder.

Uterus Womb.

Vernix Thick, greasy substance covering the fetal skin in the womb.

INDEX

MEDICAL REFERENCES

The papers listed below will give you an opportunity to read for yourself the original papers that help to shape obstetric practice.

Ultrasound scanning: safety and usefulness
Crane J. P., LeFevre M. L., Winborn R. C., et al. A randomized trial of prenatal ultrasonographic screening: impact on the detection, management and outcome of anomalous fetuses. The RADIUS Study Group. *American Journal of Obstetrics and Gynecology* 1994; vol. 172: pp. 382–9
Grisso J. A., Strom B. L., Cosmatos I., et al. Diagnostic ultrasound in pregnancy and low birthweight. *American Journal of Perinatology* 1994; vol. 11: pp. 297–301
Newnham J. P., Evans Michael, C. A., et al. Effects of frequent ultrasound during pregnancy: a randomized controlled trial. *The Lancet* 1993; vol. 342: pp. 878–91

Screening for Down syndrome
Nicolaides K. H., Brizot M. L., Snijders R. J. M. Fetal nuchal translucency thickness: ultrasound screening for fetal trisomy in the first trimester of pregnancy. *British Journal of Obstetrics and Gynaecology* 1994; vol. 101: pp. 782–786
Wald N. J., Cuckle H. S., Densem J. W. et al. Maternal serum screening for Down's Syndrome in early pregnancy. *British Medical Journal* 1988; vol. 297: pp. 883–887

Methods for reducing the risk of postpartum hemorrhage
Irons D. W., Sriskandalaban P., Bullough C. H. A simple alternative to parenteral oxytocics for the third stage of labour. *International Journal of Gynaecology and Obstetrics* 1994; vol. 46: pp. 15–18
McDonald S. J., Prendiville W. J., Blair E. Randomized controlled trial of oxytocin alone versus oxytocin and ergometrine in active management of the third stage of labour. *British Medical Journal* 1993; vol. 307: pp. 1167–71

Yuen P. M., Chan N. S., Yim S. F., et al. A randomized double blind comparison of syntometrine and syntocinon in the management of the third stage of labour. *British Journal of Obstetrics and Gynaecology* 1995; vol. 102: pp. 377–80

Vitamin K and the baby: safety and reasons for use
Grant, J. M. Treating all babies with vitamin K: an "unnatural" policy? (editorial). *British Journal of Obstetrics and Gynaecology* 1996; vol. 103: p. xxii
von Kries R., Gobel U., Hachmeister A., et al. Vitamin K and childhood cancer: a population based case-control study in lower Saxony, Germany. *British Medical Journal* 1996; vol. 313: pp. 199–203

Forceps and vacuum extraction
Hillier C. E., Johanson R. B. Worldwide survey of assisted vaginal delivery. *International Journal of Gynaecology and Obstetrics* 1994; vol. 47: pp. 109–14
Sultan A. H., Kamm M. A., Hudson C. N., Bartram I. Anal sphincter disruption during vaginal delivery. *New England Journal of Medicine* 1993; vol. 329: pp. 1905–1911

Electronic fetal heart rate monitoring in labor
Grant A., O'Brian N., Joy M. T., et al. Cerebral palsy among children born during the Dublin randomized trial of intrapartum fetal monitoring. *The Lancet* 1989; vol. ii: pp. 1233–36
Mahomed K., Nyoni R., Malumbo T,. et al. Randomized controlled trial of intrapartum fetal heart rate monitoring. *British Medical Journal* 1994; vol. 308: pp. 497–500

Vaginal delivery after previous cesarean section
Flamm B. J., Janice R. G., Liu Y., Wolde Tzadik G. Elective repeat Caesarean delivery versus trial of labour: a prospective multicentre study. *Obstetrics and Gynecology* 1994; vol. 83: pp. 927–932

ACKNOWLEDGMENTS

The authors would like to thank:
Christoph Lees would like to thank Deb and Patrick Conner, Hugh and Patricia Sergeant for their helpful comments and input; to Trish Chudleigh; Dr Edward Petch for advice on mental illness in pregnancy; Dr Lesley Roberts for scouring the text and posing for photographs. Finally, thanks to the staff in the obstetric units at Greenwich and King's Hospitals who, although they may not realize it, inspired this book. Grainne McCartan would like to thank her parents Marion and Xavier; also Gretta Duffy, Xavier McCartan, Sen, Brian, Kim, Patsy, Jenny, Juliet, Peter, Sandra, Linda, Briege, Shirley, Alicia, and Jack for all their help and support.

Firefly Books would like to thank the following:
EDITORIAL CONSULTANTS Myla Moretti, B.Sc., Assistant Director of Motherisk™ Program, Toronto; Robin Rowe, Epilepsy Association, Metro Toronto; Association of Ontario Midwives.

Dorling Kindersley would like to thank the following:
DESIGN ASSISTANCE Jennifer Bayliss, Sue Callister, Evan Jones, Claudine Meissner, Kylie Mulquin.
EDITORIAL ASSISTANCE Fergus Collins, Katherine Robinson, Debbie Voller, Pippa Ward.
DTP ASSISTANCE Ian Merrill, Rachel Symons.
ILLUSTRATORS Joanna Cameron, Karen Cochrane, Sandie Hill,

Paul Richardson, Gill Tomblin, Halli Verrinder.
PICTURE CREDITS Collections/Anthea Sieveking 149 br, 168cl, c, cr, 169l, r, 174br, 188br; Sally Greenhill: 37 l, 158 bl; Oxford Scientific Film: /Derek Bromhall 57tr; Science Photo Library: /BSIP VEM 51tr; /Dr. Jeremy Burgess 61tr; /J. Croyle/Custom Medical Stock 88; /Joseph Nettis 215br; /Petit Format/Nestle 8tl, 42, 49tr, 59tr; /Row Sutherland 183br.
Every effort has been made to trace the copyright holders and we apologize in advance for any unintentional omissions. We would be pleased to insert the appropriate acknowledgment in any subsequent edition of this publication.
ADDITIONAL PHOTOGRAPHY Eddie Lawrence.
MODELS Sue Berry, Amber Bezer, Ellie Blancke, Tracey Blancke, Emma Burt, Angie Callan, Sue Callister, Louise Clairmont, Roberto Costa, Felicity Crowe, Duane Duncan, Jo Evans, Yvette Fernandez, Lee Goodger, Joany Haig, Toby Judge, Leesa Kotting, Silvia Lagreca, Andrew Lecoyte, Shahida Majeed, Ian Merrill, Mutsumi Niwa, Kelly Priestly, Eleanor Roberts,Leslie Roberts, Katherine Robinson, Charlie Rutherford, Derek Rutherford, Ellena Rutherford, Faye Rutherford, Jo-anne Skinner, Shannon Skinner, Emily Wood.
MAKE-UP Karen Fundell, Lynn Percival.
HOME ECONOMIST Alison Austin.
PROPS John Bell & Croydon, Kings Health Care NHS Trust.
CLOTHES AND EQUIPMENT supplied with thanks to Mothercare, Blooming Marvellous, Bumpsadaisy, Early Learning Centre.